SCHIZOPHRENIA AND THE FAMILY

SCHIZOPHRENIA AND THE FAMILY

A Practitioner's Guide to Psychoeducation and Management

CAROL M. ANDERSON, PhD
DOUGLAS J. REISS, PhD
GERARD E. HOGARTY, MSW
University of Pittsburgh Western Psychiatric Institute and Clinic

THE GUILFORD PRESS
New York   London

Printed in the United States of America
Second printing, March 1987

LIBRARY OF CONGRESS CATALOGING IN PUBLICATION DATA

Anderson, Carol M., 1939–
    Schizophrenia and the family.

    (The Guilford family therapy series)
    Bibliography: p.
    Includes index.
    1. Schizophrenia.   2. Family psychotherapy.
I. Reiss, Douglas J.   II. Hogarty, Gerard E.
III. Title.   IV. Series.
RC514.A646   1986   616.89′82   85–17218
ISBN 0-89862-065-1

ACKNOWLEDGMENTS

The ideas and techniques described here would not be available without the cooperation and suggestions of the patients and families who participated in this particular project and the other patients and families that we have seen over the last 20 years. Many of the most important coping and management skills were developed by the families themselves, through months or years of trial and error in very difficult times. They have allowed us to learn from and with them in order to be able to contribute their knowledge to others.

The authors also wish to acknowledge the contributions of all of the researchers and clinicians on the Schizophrenia Research Project of which Gerard Hogarty was the Principal Investigator. Their participation in the assessment and treatment of the patients described in this volume has made the development of this family model possible. Special recognition goes to John F. Cahalane, who, as one of the family clinicians, gave his time and energies to the development of many of the interventions that are described. Thanks also go to Dr. Thomas Detre, Director of Western Psychiatric Institute and Clinic, and Dr. David Kupfer, Chairman of the Department of Psychiatry, who provided the support that made this project possible. Additional thanks go to the Psychotherapy Research Branch (now the Schizophrenia Research Branch) of the National Institute of Mental Health (Grant No. MH30750) for providing the funding for this clinical effort and to E. R. Squibb & Sons who provided Prolixin decanoate. Finally, thanks go to Ms. Selma Stone, Ms. Joanne Cobb, and Ms. Bridget Virostek who typed, retyped, and again retyped the manuscript.

v

PREFACE

Schizophrenia[1] is this country's and, in many ways, the world's most serious and abiding, yet enigmatic, mental health problem. It is costly beyond understanding, both in fiscal terms and in the price paid with the tender of human suffering and despair. The "symptoms" of schizophrenia have been described in some of the earliest ledgers of human observation, dating back to thousands of years B.C. Yet schizophrenia has throughout history largely defied an exact description, definition, or classification. Its "treatment" has ranged from burning at the stake to passage on the "ship of fools," from the "dunking stools" of colonial America to early 20th-century innovations such as the daily enema and complete dental extraction. In recent decades we have employed electric shock, insulin coma, chemical restraint, lobotomy, and physical isolation of these patients. And we persist, in some quarters, to psychoanalyze the verbal products of what increasingly appears to be disordered neuroanatomical structures and biochemical processes. We have blamed each other, the patients themselves, their parents and grandparents, public authorities, and society for the cause and for the too often terrible course of these disorders. When hope and money become exhausted, we frequently tear schizophrenic patients from their families, consigning them to the existential terror of human warehouses, single room occupancy hotels, and more recently to the streets and alleys of American cities.

We need a better way. The "psychoeducation" of families and patients, combined with individual and chemotherapeutic approaches of demonstrated efficacy, is a start.

This manual constitutes a detailed guide for implementing our "psychoeducational approach," a method of care that provides attention to the family system without sacrificing the potential contributions of biological, psychological, and vocational systems. The program begins with intensive support and education for families, thus laying the foundation for ongoing work with patients and their families designed

---

1. We use the term "schizophrenia" in the singular, fully aware that multiple disorders might parade under this umbrella. We try, however, to avoid the misuse of the adjective (schizophrenic) as a substantive noun when referring to a human being.

to occur over a period of several years. All interventions aim to develop a good therapeutic alliance which will sustain patients in the community, and minimize relapse *without* undue stress on family members themselves.

The psychoeducational model described in this book is based on the belief that families increasingly are asked to be the patients' primary care providers over the long term, and since family members have something very special to offer, they need and deserve more support and attention from mental health systems. This model attempts to decrease vulnerability, improve cognitive functioning, and improve motivation in patients through the judicious use of pharmacotherapy, while reducing family anxiety through support, structure, and information about the illness. The aim is to improve everyone's quality of life by creating temporary low-intensity home environments and eventually low-intensity work environments, which decrease the likelihood of stress and/or repeated relapses for patients without increasing the burden borne by families.

The psychoeducational program includes a highly specific information sharing session that provides family members with concrete, specific information about the illness and suggested techniques for coping with the problems it causes. After negotiating a contract that includes attainable and realistic goals, ongoing interventions focus on the improvement of motivation and functioning. While certain insights may result from the provision of information or the behavioral changes it produces, insight is neither a goal nor a prerequisite. Rather, this family program attempts to break the cycle of repeated episodes by operationalizing the following principles:

1. Creating a treatment alliance that promotes a supportive working relationship with the patient *and* the family.
2. Providing information about the illness and its management to the patient and family members.
3. Establishing a low-key home/work/social environment that supports the patient's staying in the community.
4. Gradually integrating the patient into familial/social/vocational roles.
5. Creating a sense of continuity of care and an "institutional transference" for both the patient and family.

Chapter 1 reviews the theory and research on which this program is based and gives the basic philosophy and assumptions underlying the interventions. This chapter therefore tends to be somewhat "heavy," but the details of experimental design and statistical analyses have been minimized as much as possible for the sake of brevity and understanding. Chapter 2 describes the connecting phase of treatment, those early interventions that establish working relationships between clinician, patient, and family members and set up the rules for working together. Chapter 3 describes the survival skills workshop, the component of treatment that provides general information about schizophrenia and how to cope with it. Chapter 4 describes the early outpatient phase of treatment, when patient survival in the community is the primary goal. Chapter 5 focuses on how to help patients become better able to work and socialize outside the home. Chapter 6 discusses the issues in the final stages of treatment when patients and their families move to maintenance sessions, other treatments, or termination. Chapter 7 introduces issues of training and the application of the model in other mental health systems.[2] The examples used in all chapters are derived from actual cases. Names and other identifying information have been changed and certain dialogues have been modified or shortened for the sake of clarity.

A few final words of caution are in order. First, an attempt has been made to be sufficiently specific to allow others to duplicate this model of treatment. However, clinicians must always respect the individual needs of patients and families, as well as their own clinical skills and abilities as they attempt to apply these principles and techniques. Modifications will always be necessary.

Second, while this approach offers help to families who must cope with a severely disturbed member, the authors wish to emphasize that they do not believe that all families should be encouraged or even asked to provide daily care for patients. Some patients are simply too disturbed and disruptive to be managed consistently in this way. Furthermore, some families have other obligations and stresses that could interfere with their ability to provide a patient with the kind of time, energy, and support that is necessary to be maintained at home. Thus, the relative success of models such as these should not be used as evidence that they are the answer for all patients or that more comprehensive care programs are not necessary. Inpatient emergency care, long-term hospitals, day care centers, halfway houses, and rehabilitation programs all play a vital role in the treatment of schizophrenic patients. The techniques presented in this book are intended to help families and patients obtain the option of living more positively and comfortably with each other should both be able to so choose.

2. Gerard Hogarty assumed primary responsibility for those sections imparting information about schizophrenia (Chapter 1 and the first half of Chapter 3), while Carol Anderson and Douglas Reiss assumed primary responsibility for the family treatment sections. Inquiries to the authors will be more easily facilitated with this division of labor in mind. The effort represented an increasingly necessary (and rewarding) collaboration between professionals with theoretical/research interests and those with clinical experience and skills.

CONTENTS

SCHIZOPHRENIA AND THE FAMILY

CHAPTER ONE

BACKGROUND AND RATIONALE

If only somebody had offered us this kind of help before, life would have been so much better.—*Wife of a patient who had been ill for 21 years*

INTRODUCTION

In public mental health systems, the ultimate repository for the least endowed and least monied patients, the obligation to improve the long-term "quality of life" of many schizophrenic patients has tended to fall upon the least trained, least experienced, and least paid "professionals" or "case managers." Only upon the onset of acute psychosis requiring hospitalization are "therapists" called in, with little administrative acknowledgment that the best defense against a new psychotic episode is a continuing, interepisodic, prophylactic offense. In third-party reimbursement systems, principally Medical Assistance support for the most economically disadvantaged, preventive aftercare is largely ignored (psychoeducation, for example, is a nonreimbursable service), while limited resources are depleted in providing treatments for what are too often unnecessary and preventable acute psychotic episodes. Mental health professionals are not helped to develop rational, humane, and effective outpatient interventions or the means to implement them. The system, at times, seems more blatantly "crazy" than the disorders it presumes to treat.

Why?

We contend that the lack of understanding regarding the nature and treatment of schizophrenic disorders does not represent conscious vindictiveness or deliberate neglect. Rather, the knowledge base supporting the relationship between treatment techniques and patients' needs has only been thinly developed, particularly in the case of rational treatment strategies that are shaped and guided by psychological, biological, and environmental factors. Until recently, these factors had been poorly understood and rarely studied interactively. Some years ago, for example, Philip May (1975), in an excellent review of the treatment literature on schizophrenia, lamented that "with the exception of drug effect studies, the abundance of opinion and prejudice

1

[was] equalled only by the dearth of scienfitic evidence." It was, however, from the ashes of these worn hypotheses, negative findings, name calling, defective experimental designs—and what could only be described as atheoretical, if not wholly altruistic, treatment approaches—that there arose a redefined model of schizophrenic disorders, steeped in a theory that contained the seeds of a more logical, sensitive, and effective therapeutic response. No longer is it enough to approach the treatment of severe mental disorders with strategies developed from expediency and intuition. Treatment has to come from knowledge, and that knowledge, in turn, from the results of careful, legitimate, demonstrable studies in the clinical and basic sciences. Legislators, the public, and patients and their families *demand* it. Our collective guilt allows no alternative.

HISTORICAL ROOTS

The rationale for our model of treatment had its origins in more than 20 years of clinical and research experience, leading to the formation of our current clinical research team in 1976 and the explication of a grant proposal during the early months of 1977 [Grant No. MH30750 from the National Institute of Mental Health (NIMH)]. Clinically, we became increasingly aware that the traditional approaches to dealing with families of schizophrenic patients were at best ineffective and at worst injurious. The clinicians among us had tried a variety of treatment interventions, some based on the latest theory in vogue, others based on an intuitive sense of what these patients and families "needed." None of us felt that we were positive and effective "agents of change." Experience taught us that unstructured treatment approaches such as those that were confrontational or that encouraged the expression of highly charged feelings between family members were problematic. Intense family therapy sessions too often stimulated an increase in patient symptoms and in family anxiety. As we became increasingly aware of the vital role of family needs and stresses in the assessment and treatment of patients (Anderson, 1977; Anderson & Meisel, 1976), we also began to wonder if most "real" family therapy was in fact antitherapeutic. We began to experiment with other, more educational, formats for use in the posthospital phase of treatment (Anderson, Meisel, & Houpt, 1975).

Meanwhile, the research component of our group was moving toward an evolution of a new "theory of change." Some of the movement was influenced by the research of others, especially the initial reports about the importance of the "expressed emotion" of relatives on patients' tenure in the community (Brown, Birley, & Wing, 1972). At the same time, the results of our own research on the treatment of schizophrenia were making us consider what we might be doing right, what we were more likely doing wrong, and whether results of our past trials and the recent contributions of our psychosocial and psychobiological colleagues could place us on a more reasonable course. Only the time constraint imposed by a large, experimentally controlled trial (n = 103) had precluded an earlier detailed description of our own method and process. We felt that evidence regarding the efficacy of our psychoeducational strategy for the family as contrasted to an individual psychotherapeutic approach and a drug-treated control group was a first and necessary condition for publication of our rationale for a different treatment approach to schizophrenia.

In the late fall of 1976, we had before us the findings of a randomized, controlled trial that sought to "prove" that schizophrenic relapse was in large part due to the failure of patients to take their maintenance antipsychotic medication (Hogarty et al, 1979). This study had been conducted in Baltimore through 1976 and supervised between 1974 and 1976 by one of our team (G.E.H.) from Pittsburgh. Some patients had been treated with fluphenazine (Prolixin) decanoate, a long-acting, injectable, antipsychotic drug. These 55 patients also simultaneously received daily inert, *placebo* tablets that resembled fluphenazine hydrochloride in appearance. Another 50 patients had just the opposite treatment. They received active fluphenazine (Prolixin) hydrochloride tablets and received a placebo injection of sesame oil. In each of these conditions, patients were further randomized to social therapy or no social therapy. Schizophrenic relapse, if caused by drug noncompliance, should have been greater in the oral fluphenazine hydrochloride group.

First year relapse rates were sobering. The expected (as based on past research findings) 40% relapse rate was observed on the daily oral dose of fluphenazine hydrochloride, but 35% of patients on the long-acting, injectable fluphenazine decanoate experienced a psychotic relapse as well. Over 2 years of treatment, there was no statistically significant difference in observed relapse rates between oral and depot fluphenazine-treated patients, although patients on depot fluphenazine who also received a *social therapy* did have a decrease in relapse over time. In the latter part of 1976, however, preliminary results from a multihospital, NIMH study of oral and depot fluphenazine (later published in Schooler et al., 1980) were made available to us: It contained essentially the *same* conclusions. Thus, two large, well-controlled studies failed to confirm what had been up to then (and in some quarters still is) a steadfast belief held by most clinicians: "Schizophrenic patients relapse and reenter the hospital simply because they stop taking medication." Our results, the NIMH results, and, as we discovered, a

British study that used a long-acting oral and a long-acting injectable antipsychotic medication (Falloon, Watt, & Shepherd, 1978) now demanded an explanation and a response. Why did these patients relapse while receiving medication?

We privately began to realize, and then publicly began to share the idea that it was no longer wise or useful (under the guise of science) to indiscriminately throw drug and/or ill-defined psychosocial treatments at poorly understood patients, or to sit around for years anticipating research results and waiting for the dust of research findings to settle. Nor was it possible to hide behind our own passive, nondirective (and often arrogant) stance when dealing with families who, from the sidelines, begged and cajoled us in their desperate attempt to secure information about schizophrenia and its practical management.

Internationally, the community of "clinical" schizophrenia researchers also seemed restless. Studies of the family had been abandoned for the most part. Except for occasional sojourns into psychopharmacology and its side effects, the field seemed demoralized, if not a bit worn out by "me-too drugs" and "me-too psychosocial treatments." Dr. John Wing at London's Maudsley Institute was, to our knowledge, one of the first to begin a synthesis of modern psychosocial and biological data that affected the understanding and treatment of schizophrenic disorders (Wing, 1978). But we had our own experience—and data—from the previous decade as well. The task before us was to attempt an integration of findings from the behavioral and neurosciences; an integration from which the principles of clinical practice might *logically* and *immediately* flow.

We do not in the least suggest that there are "answers" to the problems of schizophrenia. We offer no cure. As a matter of fact, we have only a few comments on the possible causes (etiology) of schizophrenia. We do feel, however, that selected evidence available today, indirect and incomplete though it may be, does support a theoretical model that directs clinicians, patients, and families in positively influencing the *course* (pathophysiology) of schizophrenic disorders. This distinction between "etiology" and "pathogenesis" is real, important, and in the mainstream of contemporary health care. Most of life's chronic illnesses are of unknown causes, but do nonetheless respond sometimes to therapeutic intervention. We realize that "theory," particularly theory with a biological basis, is not the pad from which popular "how to" manuals are launched. But theory is the necessary base on which the blocks of an effective treatment program must be built.

Our own experience and review of available supporting evidence led us to conclude that schizophrenia, in spite of what we may have been taught, is not a "myth" secondary to social labeling, nor is it a rational response to an irrational environment. Neither is schizophrenia simply a failure in problem-solving ability or the sequelae of traumatic experiences, particularly early parenting experiences; nor is it another "problem in living" in need of authoritative control. These formulations, even when individual circumstances might provide an intuitive validation, are incomplete, if not inaccurate, and more often seem to be the result of other primary processes.

We believe that *schizophrenia is an environmentally sensitive and too often persistent or recurrent thought disorder with a rather convincing substrate of cerebral dysfunctioning* (cognitive, perceptual, anatomical, or biochemical) *that has been acquired* (via trauma, infection, etc.) *and/or inherited through one's genes.* In this sense, we are clearly in the camp of the "stress–diathesis" and "vulnerability" proponents but we also steer a course independent of psychological, biological, or environmental determinism. While this definition might seem a truism to some, it borders on heresy for others. "Medical model," "biological reductionism," and "linear thinking" are often the epithets thrown when we suggest that a process of experientially influenced cerebral dysfunctioning might ultimately determine the course of schizophrenia. Yet, it is a process most responsive to principles of education and subsequent modification of the patient's external *and* internal environment. After all, the organ of impairment in schizophrenia is the *brain.*

"THEORIES" OF SCHIZOPHRENIA

In many regards, it is probably incorrect to state that there are multiple theories of schizophrenia. Rather, there are numerous "hunches," few of which can be supported by the empirical data needed to elevate such speculation to the realm of hypothesis, let alone theory. A careful appraisal of contrasting beliefs about schizophrenia reveals that the differences separating "theorists" seem, at times, more semantic than real and can be traced to: (1) points of emphasis; and (2) a varying concern as to whether the theory represents etiology or pathophysiology.

Our concern is with the psycho-social-biological parameters that seemingly underlie the pathophysiology of schizophrenic disorders. We want to examine those variables that are likely to influence the subsequent course and treatment response of *already affected* individuals, rather than variables that may have caused the disorder in the first place. Nevertheless, within these parameters diverse theoretical approaches can be loosely defined according to the component of the psycho-social-biological trinity that is stressed.

Students of Kraepelin have tended to emphasize the biological component, that is, an acquired or inherited "organic" disposition to schizophrenia that frequently portended a chronic and/or deteriorating course. (Kraepelin, however, did recognize spontaneous remissions.) While Bleuler challenged the inevitable and terminal "dementia," he too believed that a *restitutio ad integrum* was not characteristic of schizophrenic disorders. In recent years, biological theorists have justified their theories with convincing evidence of the effectiveness of somatic therapies and the obvious role of genetics and biochemical and anatomical factors in the transmission and manifestation of schizophrenic disorders. Perhaps the biological basis of schizophrenia can best be viewed in such representative contributions as those offered in recent years by Gottesman and Shields (1982) who are proponents of the stress–diathesis school of thought. In their etiologic formulation, as much as 70% of the cause of schizophrenia is biological (i.e., genetic), and 30% environmental. We do not adopt a strong position against such etiologic speculation. However, while recognizing that few biological theorists entirely discount the role of psychosocial factors, we argue that the available evidence suggests a relatively greater role for psychosocial variables in the *pathophysiology* of schizophrenic disorders, that is, with respect to those factors that influence subsequent course and outcome.[1]

Similarly, most psychoanalytically oriented theorists would readily admit the role of genetics and exogenous cerebral insults in the development of schizophrenia. Only among the extremists of the group does one find claims that schizophrenia is entirely a learned behavior, that is, an unconscious, developmentally acquired, maladaptive repertoire of behaviors.

Sociologically, many theorists over the past 40 years have recognized a primary disease process in schizophrenia (e.g., Waxler, 1974), but tend to focus on the secondary or residual effects of having been ill. Behaviors such as amotivation, social withdrawal, blunted affect, and poverty of speech are viewed as the sequelae of society's tendency to warehouse patients in "deskilling" and "dehumanizing" institutions, or as the culture's response to primary deviance. Again, only extremists in the group claim that schizophrenia is simply the "normal" behavior of a minority of the population, pejoratively "labeled" as deviant by the culturally determined value judgments of the majority. Surprisingly, at a time of more empirical data regarding schizophrenia, unsupported, if not peculiar speculation on causality

---

1. It is the relative emphasis on classification systems and "disease" concepts that has, unfortunately, brought the unfair charges of "reductionism" and "linear thinking" against more biologically oriented theorists.

and treatment seems to be emanating from family theorists as well (e.g., Stierlin, Wynne, & Wirsching, 1983).

Fortunately, a good deal of balance can be found today and is articulated in, for example, the writings of Zubin and Spring (1977), under the rubric "vulnerability theory," and in those of Richard Day (Day, in press; Day, Zubin, & Steinhauer, in press). Vulnerability theory gives broad recognition to the relative contribution of the neurosciences as well as the fields of environmental and personal psychology. Our differences, if any, with these formulations are the speculative, second-order inferences that arise from the theory (Zubin, Magaziner, & Steinhauer, 1983). "Negative symptoms" of schizophrenia, for instance, are viewed as consequences of impoverished environments, though recent evidence suggests the contribution of organic factors (see Chapter 3). Episodes of schizophrenia are seen as intermittent and time-related (even if separated by hours or days) and unequivocally persistent primary symptoms as rare or nonexistant. One also gets the feeling that the interrelationships among intrinsic and extrinsic variables in vulnerability theory are linear or curvilinear. In fact, much of what we know about schizophrenia might ultimately be captured in such "new wave" formulations as "catastrophe" theory (MacCulloch & Waddington, 1979), a model derived from the field of mathematics. This theory suggests that "discontinuity phenomena" characterize the state of the organism at any given time such that minuscule changes in one system (e.g., biochemical) might have quantum or "catastrophic" consequences in another system (e.g., behavior). If this is true, the experimental and mathematical methods available to clinical researchers today would be largely inadequate for hypothesis testing.

With this background, we examined the psycho-social-biological literature with caution and chose to focus upon empirical contributions to the pathophysiology of schizophrenic disorders that suggested reasonable and relevant clinical applications.

THE THERAPEUTIC ENVIRONMENT

Drug Therapy

Guaranteed drug therapy, as we learned, did not always prevent a schizophrenic relapse. A review of the world's better conducted drug studies (Hogarty, 1984) revealed that in the first year following hospital discharge, 41% of 814 drug-treated patients relapsed and 68% of 189 placebo-treated patients also relapsed. These relapse rates, of course, varied widely according to the type of patient under study (a point that we elaborate at some length in our educational workshop for family members). The rates are rather constant among types of antipsychotic medications as well as among methods of administration, either oral or long-acting injectable. At the end of 2 years of controlled study, about 48% of drug-treated patients and 80% of placebo-treated patients suffer a psychotic relapse.

However, if one were to start a drug–placebo study with patients who were already *out* of the hospital for a year or more, or had achieved a good remission of psychotic symptoms prior to study, then the rate of relapse for those on medication would decline dramatically in the following year (Hogarty, 1984). Of 500 patients observed in several countries, 15% experienced relapse in the subsequent year, but once again, nearly two thirds of the patients (65% of 448 patients) experienced their relapse following drug withdrawal. It appears, then, that a majority of schizophrenic patients will relapse *whenever* medication is stopped.

Johnson and associates (Johnson, Pasterski, Ludlow, Street, & Taylor, 1983), for example, withdrew medication from groups of schizophrenic patients who had been successfully maintained on drugs for 1, 2, or 3 years. In the following year, across these three groups, those on medication who relapsed averaged 16%, while among those discontinued from medication, relapse averaged 65%. The corresponding relapse rates after 18 months of study were 23% for the drug maintenance and 80% for the discontinued groups. These relapse rates following drug discontinuation were nearly identical to our own findings (Hogarty, Ulrich, Mussare, & Aristigueta, 1976). After 2 to 3 years of study, 104 patients on medication were still doing well in the community. Staff selected 43 patients who not only had maintained a stable course, but who were judged by treating psychiatrists to be at low risk for relapse and perhaps not in need of continuing medication at all. Following an open, gradual discontinuation of medication, 65% of these patients relapsed in the next year, most within 7 months of discontinuation. Thus, the need for continuing medication can be justified for at least 4 years following the resolution of a psychotic episode. While relapse on drug does indeed decline with the passing of time (Hogarty & Ulrich, 1977), the number of patients affected by psychotic relapse still remains a considerable public health concern.

Further, it is important to note that the risk of relapse following drug discontinuation is very much influenced, it seems, by the type of patient involved and the stage of the patient's illness. Two prominent characteristics that researchers have identified are the number of prior psychotic episodes and the patient's sex. One carefully controlled study has involved *first* episode patients randomly assigned to drug or placebo following hospital discharge (Kane, Rifkin, Quitkin, Noyak,

& Ramos-Lorenzo, 1982). In this trial, 40% of placebo recipients experienced a psychotic relapse at the end of 1 year, but none of the drug maintained patients relapsed at all. On the other hand, our review of controlled studies (Hogarty, 1984) has convinced us that 80% to 100% of chronic, multiepisode patients will relapse when removed from medication and a greater proportion will relapse on drugs as the number of prior episodes increases.

An ongoing study is illustrative (Grant No. MH30750). Among 157 schizophrenic patients who remained on drug for the first year following hospital discharge, 35% experienced a relapse. However, only 7% of first episode patients relapsed, while 38% of those with one to four prior episodes experienced a relapse and 52% of those with five or more episodes relapsed. For those who refused medication in this trial (i.e., those who refused injections of the long-acting fluphenazine decanoate), the relapse rate was 58% of first episode patients, 66% of those with one to four prior episodes, and 83% of those with five or more episodes. Patients with multiple hospitalizations thus represent a "high risk" group, one for whom the prophylactic effects of medication are incomplete because of a severe pathophysiology of the disorder and/or the preponderance of enduring or periodic stress in their lives.

Since the advent of psychopharmacology, many studies have shown that male schizophrenic patients relapse at a greater rate than female schizophrenic patients (e.g., Brown, Birley, & Wing, 1972; Hogarty, Goldberg, & Schooler, 1974; Vaughn & Leff, 1976; Vaughn, Snyder, Jones, Freeman, & Falloon, 1984). However, all studies that demonstrated this difference involved the use of an *oral* antipsychotic medication. On the other hand, two of our own trials (Hogarty *et al.*, 1979; MH30750) that guaranteed the receipt of medication via a depot neuroleptic, had relapse rates that remained quite high (averaging 35%), but the rates of relapse were *not* different between men and women. Thus, while it appears that there is a greater risk of relapse for male patients, the risk is likely due to their propensity to noncompliance with an oral medication regimen.

Therefore, from our reviews, we were able to conclude that drug therapy was the most effective form of treatment known to psychiatry, but it was by no means a panacea. About 10% to 20% of patients over a 30 month period could probably avoid a psychotic episode without maintenance chemotherapy, but there was no means for effectively identifying these patients. About 30% of schizophrenic patients who would otherwise relapse if drug therapy was discontinued remained well *on* medication. But 40% to 50% of patients relapse within 2 years *in spite* of medication, with chronic patients having even higher rates. It should be noted that only in uncontrolled, retrospective studies are claims made for the possibility of identifying those fortunate patients who do not need medication. This is a most important point to emphasize. All studies, to our knowledge, that claim to identify patients who do not require antipsychotic medication have been conducted *after the fact* (e.g., Leff & Wing, 1971; Young & Meltzer, 1980; Carpenter, McGlashan, & Strauss, 1977). It is crucial to remember that in every long-term study, there is a small group of patients who survive without medication. The only way to answer definitively the question of who does not need medication is to select a group of these low-risk patients, (allegedly first episode, good premorbid, rapid onset schizophreniform disorders) and randomly to assign them to either drug or placebo. Our assumption is that the risk of relapse with this group would be less on both drug and placebo, but that the difference (regarding relapse) between these treatment conditions would continue to be dramatic.

There is something of this same philosophy that underlies current efforts to "stop and start" medication. Even though the risk of relapse on drug declines over time, many professionals today believe that discontinuing medication when the patient achieves a remission of symptoms, and reinstating medication when signs of relapse appear, is the proper strategy and best defense against long-term, unwanted side effects such as tardive dyskinesia (Herz & Melville, 1980). (To be sure, some believe that stopping and starting medication might be one of the precursors of tardive dyskinesia [Jeste, Potkin, Sinka, Feder, & Wyatt, 1979].) We have attempted this strategy in selected patients and believe that the *social costs* of a decompensation are significant and too often overlooked, particularly if the patient is working or has recently renegotiated a tenuous position in the family. Also, the strategy of intermittent medication usage requires the patient, the family, and the professionals involved to be acutely aware of early prodromal signs, and to monitor them. This places added pressure and stress on all. Johnson *et al.* (1983) have further demonstrated that over an 18-month period, the dosage increases needed to restabilize discontinued patients often exceed that which patients might have accumulated had they remained on the prewithdrawal dose. In another ongoing study, we have learned that we can maintain 80% of stabilized schizophrenic patients on very low doses of medication averaging 4 to 5 mg of fluphenazine decanoate injected once every 2 weeks (Hogarty, 1984). At the moment, we are inclined to accept the value of a continuously administered low dose of antipsychotic medication as the preferred dosage strategy. However, we realize that this is an interim decision that must await further research. A collaborative study of differing dosage strategies has recently been initiated by Schooler and Keith of NIMH's Schizophrenia Research Branch.

(This important investigation will also place under study various conditions of family education and management as well.)

Finally, our review of the literature regarding medication and relapse led to the "theory building" observation that if the patient can survive for the 1st year on medication, then the risk of relapse in the next year will decrease. For this reason, we have come to believe that a psychosocial program should emphasize "holding on" during these early critical months and avoid overly ambitious or premature attempts at a rapid resumption of role performance.

Psychosocial Therapy

With the information on the strengths and limitations of maintenance chemotherapy in mind, we next examined the results of an earlier controlled study of drug and social therapy in the aftercare of schizophrenic patients conducted by Hogarty between 1968 and 1973 in Baltimore (Hogarty, Goldberg, Schooler, & Ulrich, 1974). Three hundred seventy-four schizophrenic patients discharged from three state hospitals and admitted to three participating outpatient clinics had been randomly assigned to a social therapy or to no social therapy at clinical admission. At 2 months, they were again randomly assigned to identical-looking tablets of the antipsychotic drug chlorpromazine (Thorazine) or its placebo. Patients were treated under these controlled conditions for 2 years or until they relapsed. As mentioned earlier, 48% of these patients relapsed on drug by 2 years, but 80% of those assigned to a *social therapy* and a placebo had relapsed, as had 80% of those assigned to placebo *alone!* Thus, it was very clear that a psychosocial form of treatment *by itself* offered no advantage to the schizophrenic patient in forestalling a relapse. In combination with drug, however, there did appear to be gains in forestalling relapse (37%) for patients receiving both drug *and* social therapy in this study, and in the later study where depot fluphenazine and social therapy were employed (Hogarty *et al.*, 1979).

Why had some patients done well and others fared so poorly on drug and/or a psychosocial treatment? Detailed analysis revealed that it was not possible, for the most part, to predict who would do well or poorly on drug or placebo. However, patients who did well or poorly with social therapy could, it turned out, be well defined (Goldberg, Schooler, Hogarty, & Roper, 1977). At hospital discharge, patients who seemed more withdrawn, disorganized, and anxious, and who had little "insight," relapsed much more quickly when assigned to a "high expectation" social therapy than when they had simply been left alone. This observation has subsequently been supported by Linn, Klett, and Caffey (1980) regarding the increased relapse among schizophrenic patients discharged to high-activity foster homes; and also characterized patients who tended to relapse more often in "dynamic" Day Treatment Centers as well (Linn, Caffey, Klett, Hogarty, & Lamb, 1979). Later in the "negative finding" study of injectible and oral fluphenazine (Hogarty *et al.*, 1979), further data about why patients relapsed on medication were obtained. If the patient had returned to a household characterized by conflict and tension, the risk of relapse was greatly increased. This result was similar to another finding from the chlorpromazine and social therapy study. The greatest relapse difference between drug and placebo was found for patients in families with the least "distress." Relapse rates on placebo and drug were higher and more similar as family distress increased (Goldberg *et al.*, 1977).

The inferences from our own study were further developed when we looked at the personal and social adjustment of *nonrelapsed* patients (Hogarty, Goldberg, & Schooler, 1974). Here the provision of a social therapy had a clear "interactive" effect; that is, the psychosocial form of treatment increased the performance and adjustment of patients when combined with medication. But when psychosocial therapy was offered in the absence of medication (i.e., placebo), the personal and social adjustment of schizophrenic patients actually got worse. Rummaging through 10,000 "process" recordings of these therapeutic encounters led to the conclusion that the treatment differences of patients who did well or poorly on social therapy could not be identified. The outcomes more likely had to be explained on the basis of the disorder itself, principally as the illness was mediated by medication.

Since this study had been the first long-term, controlled study of a drug and nondrug treatment in the *aftercare* of schizophrenic patients, we wondered whether earlier *inpatient* studies of drug-and-psychotherapy might provide confirmation of these inferences concerning the absence of a psychotherapy effect per se and the negative effect among patients not treated with drug therapy. A few, well-controlled inpatient studies, primarily the classic trial conducted by Philip May (1968) as well as 11 partially controlled studies, were available (see Hogarty, 1981). These studies generally concluded that drug therapy was superior to psychotherapy and that the combination of drug and psychotherapy (on an inpatient basis) offered very few, if any, advantages over drug treatment alone. Julian Leff (1980) had suggested that the process of changing environments from home to hospital could represent such a "powerful therapeutic source" that little could be achieved by the application of inpatient psychosocial programs. There were, however, a few exceptions to the negative findings concerning psychotherapy worthy of note. Gordon Paul demonstrated that among long-term treated, chronic, and apparently drug-refractory inpatients, medication could be withdrawn in a special hospital environment without precipitating psychosis (Paul, Tobias, & Holly, 1972). Karen and Vanden Bos (1972) felt that experienced psychotherapists achieved gains in adjustment and in avoiding relapse without drugs, although design problems, critics argued, precluded valid inferences from this study. A further study of insight-oriented psychotherapy offered by trained and experienced analysts, however, provides little support for this form of treatment (Gunderson et al., 1984). Mosher and Menn (1978) compared a special psychosocial residency program without chemotherapy (Soteria) to the inpatient drug treatment of a community mental health center and found no differences in symptom reduction or subsequent relapse rates. The experimental subjects were more often employed and living apart from their families at followup. The patients were not randomized in this study, however, and the length of time needed to resolve psychosis was considerably longer in the experimental program.

Thus, it appeared that the contributions of psychotherapy were not overwhelming regarding the inpatient studies of schizophrenic patients. However, there was an observation often made in a number of uncontrolled studies that bore a striking similarity to the important inference made from our aftercare trial. It seemed that over the past 20 years there had been a series of inpatient studies directed toward the social rehabilitation of chronic schizophrenic patients (see Van Putten & May, 1976; Wing & Brown, 1970), from which one could conclude that certain patients, when exposed to intensive rehabilitation ("total push"), or an enriched milieu responded with the *emergence* of long-dormant psychotic symptoms; a phenomenon that seemed to represent a side effect of the psychosocial inpatient treatment of schizophrenic patients, much like the side effect observed in our outpatient study.

THE NATURAL ENVIRONMENT

If aspects of the therapeutic milieu may be sufficient to elicit psychotic symptoms in certain schizophrenic patients, what could be said about macro influences on the environment (such as culture), on the one hand, and micro influences (i.e., family life) on the other? The literature regarding environmental "press" in schizophrenia is formidable. Psychological and social pressures that range from stressful "life events," to induction into military service, to membership in socially disadvantaged classes in North America have all been associated with higher rates of schizophrenia (see Anderson, Hogarty, & Reiss, 1980). Data from British investigators in the 1960s and 1970s suggested that life events in the history of schizophrenic patients are clustered in the weeks immediately preceeding a psychotic episode. If severe or numerous enough, they seem sufficient to overcome the protective influence of chemotherapy and result in a psychotic episode (Leff, Hirsch, Gaind, Rhode, & Stevens, 1973). Contemporary theory suggests that life events are more likely "triggers" of an episode than formative of the illness, and are clearly modified or influenced by other important social and environmental variables such as one's social network, support system, prior experience with the event, or means of coping (Rabkin, 1980). Nonetheless, for selected patients, environmental stressors that might otherwise be negotiated by most people in the general population appear to exacerbate the symptoms of severe mental illness in people already affected, even when maintained on medication. For those who are off medication, life events exact an even greater toll in the form of relapse. By definition, these patients have to possess some particular vulnerability to social stimuli (including perhaps, the stimulation provided by a psychosocial treatment). Otherwise, if it were "stress" alone that causes schizophrenic relapse, we could literally be awash in a world of psychotic individuals.

Elsewhere, there is evidence that culture itself exerts a potent influence over the form and course of schizophrenic illness. For many decades it was believed that schizophrenia was "universal," a belief that argued against the role of culture as a possible causative agent of severe mental illness in its broadest sense. However, Torrey (1973) had raised questions about this assumption, arguing that most cases of severe illness observed in so-called "primitive cultures" either appeared at hospitals established by Europeans or in highly westernized villages and towns. Other "cases" of schizophrenia were to be found in rural areas where more "reactive" types of psychosis were prominent, and for which a reasonable link to infectious disease could be established. If anything, it appeared that rates of psychoses varied more within developing countries than between countries, with rates increasing as contact with western (industrializing) influences increased.

Some intriguing evidence for culture as formative of severe psychotic conditions can be found in the work of H.B.M. Murphy (1978). Incidence rates among Catholics of Southern Ireland, for example, appeared two and one half times greater than for Irish elsewhere and three to four times greater than non-Irish controls. Murphy concluded that the role of complex tasks, perhaps the complexity of communication and ridicule "inherent in the land of double-think and double-speak" was the cultural pathogen sufficient to exploit some deficit in certain individuals who were prone to schizophrenia. But independent of whether culture "caused" schizophrenia was the important observation drawn from the follow-up study of the World Health Organization's

International Pilot Study of Schizophrenia, as well as similar studies in other Third World countries (Warner, 1983). These studies suggested that the course and outcome of patients meeting rather uniform diagnostic criteria for schizophrenia, were significantly better in such developing countries as India, Nigeria, Sri Lanka, and Mauritius than in developed countries such as the United States, England, Denmark, and the Soviet Union.

More convincing evidence for the effect of the *natural environment* on the course and outcome of schizophrenia could be found in studies of the micro environment, particularly studies of the family. There is no evidence supporting the family's role in the *cause* of schizophrenia. Historically, there has been a great deal of interest in the family environment of schizophrenic patients, primarily from the standpoint of attempting to establish a causal role. Early psychoanalytic writers focused on various parental behaviors which they viewed as causative, with Fromm-Reichman (1948) contributing a phrase that has come to haunt the mothers of these patients, the "Schizophrenogenic Mother." Early family researchers expanded this etiologic focus to examine family interactional patterns that they believed could influence a patient's sense of self and ability to perceive and interact with the world in a coherent manner. The researchers conducting these studies claimed that problems in families such as skewed parent–child relationships, structural irregularities, marital discord, and communication disorders contributed to the development of schizophrenia (Bateson, Jackson, Haley, & Weakland, 1956; Bowen, 1960, 1961; Lidz, Cornelison, Fleck, & Terry, 1957: Lidz & Cornelison, 1965; Singer & Wynne, 1963, 1965; Wynne & Singer, 1958). Several investigators have concentrated on the study of patterns of family communication in an attempt to identify one or more such patterns that might play a crucial role in the development of this illness. They have suggested, for instance, that for schizophrenic patients interactions among family members lack clarity and acknowledgment and are often vague, amorphous, tangential, or unrelated to the topic at hand (Goldstein & Rodnick, 1975; Jacob, 1975; Jones, 1977; Singer & Wynne, 1963, 1965; Wynne & Singer, 1958). To clinicians who believed in the idea that families could cause schizophrenia, these observations were so compelling that they immediately undertook to modify these family interactional patterns as a method of treatment. Unfortunately, early programs of family intervention concentrated on relatively unstructured attempts to help family members to express their thoughts and feelings more clearly and directly to one another. These therapeutic efforts were not particularly rewarding for either clinicians or the families they attempted to treat. Certainly, as we have mentioned, it was the experience of the clinicians in our own group that the family interventions which they had attempted in the early 1960s were ineffective, and, at times, actually seemed to have made things worse.

Meanwhile, in considering the results of previous clinical research, we began to conclude that while it was unlikely that problematic family interactions were causing schizophrenia, they were nevertheless relevant. Certain data suggested that families (and, so it appeared, therapists and others involved in the lives of schizophrenic patients) could manifest patterns of interaction that exploited a preexisting vulnerability in patients. Minimally, they might constitute precipitating stresses for vulnerable individuals or signal serious family distress caused by living with an impaired individual for an extended period of time.

Overall, the results of family studies have contributed important data to our understanding of families with schizophrenic members, and even of families in general. But as follow-up studies either failed to confirm, to expand upon findings, or to have direct clinical applicability for the design of intervention strategies, interest in family research with this population decreased (see Hirsch & Leff, 1975, for an extensive review of both the original and subsequent studies).

In the 1950s, however, British investigators began a series of studies that focused on the course rather than the etiology of schizophrenia. These studies led to the observation that the type of living situation to which patients returned following hospital discharge, particularly a return to conjugal or parental households, was associated with an increased risk of relapse compared to patients returning to other living conditions (Brown, 1959). Brown and his colleagues (Brown, Monck, Carstairs, & Wing, 1962; Brown et al., 1972) pursued the notion that the emotional level of a home with close familial ties contained something of a specific stress for schizophrenic patients that might lead to relapse.[2] In the two independent studies by Brown (Brown et al., 1962, 1972), a third replication conducted by Vaughn and Leff (1976), and in a study conducted recently in California by Vaughn and her colleagues (1984), it was observed that families manifesting high "expressed emotion" (EE), principally reflected in criticism, hostility, and levels of emotional overinvolvement, tended to have relapse rates of 50% or more in the first 9 months following a hospital discharge, compared to rates of 13% to 15% relapse among patients

2. Other British studies had found that an unstimulating environment in the form of interpersonally sterile hospital wards was associated with "negative" symptoms of schizophrenia, such as poverty of speech, blunted affect, and amotivation (Wing & Brown, 1970). We feel, however, in light of recent evidence on the relationship between cerebral atrophy and defect state, that these symptoms might be more fruitfully traced to an organic basis.

returning to low EE households. Within the high EE households, continuing face-to-face contact with relatives appeared to increase relapse, even when patients received medication. Relapse rates, however, were greatest in high EE households where patients were not protected by maintenance chemotherapy and remained in face-to-face contact with the high EE relative more than 35 hours each week.[3]

At this point in our thinking, we came to a critical juncture: Was the study of EE simply the most recent exercise in a long series of attempts to blame close family members for the recurrent illness of their schizophrenic member? *Or, was there a common denominator in the findings from the studies of culture, life events, the family, drug- and psychotherapies?* We believed that there was.

This common denominator suggested to us that the "triggers" could be traced to any one of a number of characteristics of the therapeutic or natural environment that required the schizophrenic patient to make an adaptive response to complex, vague, excessive, or emotionally charged expectations capable of precipitating a cognitive or affective dysregulation. The theory would be most compelling if there existed literature from the neurosciences capable of demonstrating that the "internal" environment of the schizophrenic patient was altered or sufficiently impaired in such a way that the processing of information, internally and externally derived, represented a most difficult task. The literature was there, greatly enhanced by the theory of, and developments in, the neurosciences of the previous decade.

THE UNDERLYING DEFICITS

At the core of most theories concerning the deficits that underlie schizophrenic symptoms, is an acknowledgment that typical schizophrenic patients simply fail to adequately process stimuli or bits of information from their internal and external environments. When we first attempted a review of this literature, we had available such eclectic statements as those by Broen and Storms (1966), Lang and Buss (1965), Payne, Mattussek, and George (1959), Shakow (1962), Silverman (1972),

---

3. Our own ongoing studies (MH30750) indicate that the influence of EE on schizophrenic relapse seems related more narrowly to *unmarried males* living in *parental households*, and that other sources of stress, particularly conflicted interpersonal relationships, might better explain the relapse of "ever married" female patients, particularly those with schizo-affective disorders. Further, males *and* females, still actively psychotic, who are discharged from the hospital and return to a high EE household, experience further increases in persisting symptoms, that is, a Type II relapse. The ability of this family approach to "buy time" for these symptomatic patients has been demonstrated and will be described below.

Tecce and Cole (1976), and Venables (1964, 1978). In recent years the excellent, integrating reviews of Gjerde (1983) and more recently Nuechterlein and Dawson (1984) and Dawson and Nuechterlein (1984) have been offered, and serve the needs of the educator–clinician very well.

In these theories, the problems variously appear as extraordinary difficulties for schizophrenic patients in selecting relevant stimuli, inhibiting irrelevant stimuli, or as an inability to sustain or flexibly shift focused alertness. Schizophrenic patients have been observed to have problems in recognizing stimuli and identifying them, as well as in integrating, storing, recalling, and using them appropriately. This process, which has been broadly defined as "attention," in turn appears to be adversely affected by the extremes of autonomic "arousal" that "energizes behavior unselectively," thus affecting the intensity of a person's response to a stimulus (Tecce & Cole, 1976).

In spite of conflicting results from this vast literature, one very important observation has consistently been made: Schizophrenic patients are *slow* to process stimuli, even under predictable conditions. If anything, the field of information processing has tended to move away from the "Trade School" approach to information processing (pigeonholes, bundles, filters, and channels) and has, in recent years, focused on a concept called "capacity theory." According to this theory, different tasks require different processing capacities (see Nuechterlein & Dawson, 1984). Information processing demands appear less at the initial perceptual level, but increase at the "response end," an observation further supported by evidence that schizophrenic patients have less difficulty in "encoding" messages, but fail at short-term and recognition memory tasks (Calev, Venables, & Monk, 1983). As the information in need of processing *increases*, or as the task is made more *difficult*, (e.g., by tasks that "degrade" or weaken the stimuli), performance on laboratory tests, at least, tends to become impaired. A greater intrusion of "irrelevant stimuli" is observed when high levels of competing information are introduced (as in dichotic listening tasks where the patient is asked to "ignore" a message in one ear, and attend to the message in the other ear). This literature has some support for its functional significance from the study of verbal behavior among schizophrenic patients. While the syntactical use of language by schizophrenic patients is not necessarily impaired, the "loosely connected" responses, for example, have been seen as failures to "self-edit," particularly as a failure to self-edit very personal material (Cohen & Camhi, 1967). Others have described failures to "disattend" during communication as the control function of attention becomes arrested, thus leaving the patient unable to "follow" or "develop" an idea (Singer, 1978). As such, the "information processing" tasks put before the vulnerable schizophrenic patients seem formidable indeed.

We should note (this is of specific relevance for our purposes) that the criticism contained in the expressed emotion of family members as well as the verbal and nonverbal stimuli generated from high-expectation therapeutic encounters is likely to contain the highest levels of information in need of processing. In the least, these stimuli require the highest processing demands at the response end. Nuechterlein and Dawson (1984) have speculated that the reduced capacity among schizophrenic patients that impedes important cognitive functions could implicate either an impaired "executive" or "control" function (even in the face of an otherwise normal capacity) or a "reduction in normal capacity." Or, the capacity available to a patient may be devoted to "irrelevant" information, an idea for which a large, supporting literature exists. Most intriguing in the explanations by these authors is that a conscious process might be required to complete cognitive tasks that are usually done automatically. Information processing seems to occur in critical midbrain structures and their projections that represent higher order centers of control over human behavior (Fish, 1961; Stevens, 1973). The behavioral sequelae that follow upon impairment of these structures are compatible with the principal signs of schizophrenia (Corbett, 1976).

A closely related literature on "arousal" describes electrodermal responses in the form of skin conductance levels (SCLs) and skin conductance responses (SCRs) to stimuli as indicators of sympathetic nervous system arousal. (Again, it is Dawson & Nuechterlein, 1984, who have recently provided us with a succinct, yet conceptually clear review of this difficult literature.) Overall, many populations of schizophrenic patients have been observed to have abnormally high "baseline" levels of arousal, that is, tonic SCLs. Significantly, several recent studies (Sturgeon, Turpin, Kuipers, Berkowitz, & Leff, 1984) indicate that patients residing in households with high levels of EE tend to have correspondingly high skin conductance levels. However, it is generally agreed that only half of schizophrenic patients subsequently demonstrate high levels of orienting skin conductance responses (ORs) when faced with novel or noxious stimuli, while the other half can be classified as "nonresponders," a phenomenon which one doesn't encounter very often among normal people. This latter group of nonresponders has been characterized as being more withdrawn and cognitively disorganized than responders. Responders, alternatively, tend to be more active and excited and often fail to "habituate" (i.e., return to baseline) following a repetitive experience with the same stimulus. It is, in many ways, as though each repetition of the same stimulus is a novel experience for the patient! This characteristic also appears to predict poor response to treatment. When integrated into the information processing literature, Dawson and Nuechterlein (1984) have described how "responding" but "slow habituating" patients have been thought to "allocate processing capacity indiscriminately," while nonresponders "fail to allocate sufficient processing capacity" (Dawson & Nuechterlein, 1984, p. 214). For us, it is enough to appreciate the extraordinary difficulty in the form of arousal that the schizophrenic patient faces when attempting either to respond cognitively or to maintain affective regulation in the midst of an emotionally charged or high-expectation environment.

Closely associated with this literature is an extensive series of studies recently reviewed by Nassrallah (1982) that focuses upon hemispheric laterality, that is, the "differential activation of left and right cerebral hemispheres for motor, perceptual, cognitive, and emotive functions" (Nassrallah, 1982, p. 273). Studies of skin conductance, lateral eye movements, dychotic listening tasks, EEGs, evoked potentials, cerebral blood flow, and cerebral atrophy (CAT and PET scan studies) seem, in general, to indicate that there is a "lateralized dysfunction in the left cerebral hemisphere of schizophrenic patients" (Nassrallah, 1982, p. 284). The areas of cerebral impairment appear to be those most central to information processing and most central to the presumed inability of many schizophrenic patients to respond cognitively. The difficulties are found most often in left temporal lobe, temporal-frontal, and temporal-limbic cortical connections. Problems in the interhemispheric transfer of information have also been observed among schizophrenic patients. Further, increasing evidence suggests that many of the information processing or arousal dysfunctions observed in these patients tend to occur among their first degree family members, particularly their children (Nuechterlein & Dawson, 1984).

Antipsychotic medication plays an important role in this whole process. Among its many wanted (and unwanted) effects, medication clearly regulates if not normalizes the extremes of arousal and enables the patient to "deploy" attention appropriately (Spohn, Lacoursiere, Thompson, & Coyne, 1977). The loci of this remarkable therapeutic effect represent the very midbrain (mesolimbic) structures that appear crucial to the processing of information, the control of arousal, and the regulation of one's thinking and feeling life (Meltzer, 1979).

The causes of these impairments remain largely unknown. As we explain to families, some of the impairments possibly find their cause in heredity, or from the sequelae of infectious disease, birth trauma, and other perinatal events. Some impairments remain invisible, as it were, even with "high tech" pictures of the functioning brain. Increasingly, however, studies of the brains of certain living schizophrenic patients have revealed signs of actual cell loss, as with cerebral atrophy (Weinberger, Wagner, & Wyatt, 1983); functional impairment, as in the case of reduced blood flow to critical frontal lobes (Farkas et al., 1984; Buchsbaum et al., 1984); and insufficient pumping of cerebral spinal fluid to frontal lobes, that is, ventricular reflux (Sedvall, Oxenstierna, Bergstrand, Bjerkenstedt, & Wik, 1984). A recent study of cerebral blood flow, for example, indicates that when confronted with the higher capacity, abstracting tasks of the Wisconsin Color Card Sort, the frontal lobe blood flow of some schizophrenic patients actually appears to be reduced (Weinberger, 1984). Further, a sophisticated series of autopsy studies have yielded these discoveries: an actual "thinness" of parahippocampal tissue; the reduction of the crucial neuropeptides, somatostatin and cholecystokinen (Crow, 1984); increased concentration of left amygdala dopamine (Reynolds, 1983); as well as the presence of certain cells (gliosis) that indicates an earlier infection or lack of oxygen (Stevens, 1982). This fibrillary gliosis, for example, has been found specifically in brain areas (mesencephalic tegmentum and substantia innominata) rich with nerve fibers that extend from these important centers of "feeling" regulation to the cerebral cortex, which governs our rational life (Stevens, 1982). Moreover, about a quarter of schizophrenic patients, on CAT scan, show cell loss in the limbic cortex that surrounds the cerebral ventricles, giving rise to the finding of enlarged ventricles in many schizophrenic patients (Weinberger et al., 1983). From twin studies, the source of the enlargement seems not to be genetic, but due to exogenous insults of the brain (Reveley, Reveley, Clifford, & Murray, 1982). While the functional significance of these findings remains a matter of debate, poor treatment response, the dominance of "negative" symptoms of schizophrenia, and a gradual loss of intellectual capacity (i.e., what appear to be old "Kraepelinean" schizophrenias) increasingly characterize this subgroup of schizophrenic patients (Weinberger et al., 1983). Thus, we believe there is a biological basis to many, if not all, of the schizophrenias. Schizophrenia is in the brain, yet its manifestation is brought to view by environmental stimuli, external and internal, broadly and narrowly defined.

THE THEORY

It seemed to us that if either the demands of the environment or the underlying cerebral deficit were sufficiently severe, then these factors operating alone or more likely *together* might represent the sufficient causes for a schizophrenic relapse, even when antipsychotic medication was assured. Alternatively, antipsychotic drug regulation of attention and arousal (via its influence on neurotransmitters), or the provision of a more benign, stimulus-controlled, external environment, or a combination of these two approaches, might account for a reduction of schizophrenic exacerbations and thus increase the chances for a patient's recovery. If the preceding were true, there was an immediate and necessary obligation to put these ideas into practice in ways that could help patients and families. As part of that effort, it made consummate sense to attempt to give an explanation to both families and patients as to what these disorders were all about, at least to the extent that current data would permit. With this beginning, we hoped it might become more clear just what important roles both patient and families could effectively assume in dealing with the illness over time, what they could avoid in the way of stress or inappropriate expectations, and what might be achieved given enough time. Graduated tasks, their rehearsal, the rational use of medication, and carefully negotiated moves toward resocialization, prevocational and vocational rehabilitation all seemed to make sense in light of our developing model.

While no one had attempted the type of psychoeducational program we had in mind, we were encouraged by the positive results of the first controlled study that included an attempt to provide patients and families with some understanding of the illness and ways to cope with it. Goldstein, Rodnick, Evans, May, and Steinberg (1978) at UCLA designed a 6-week program of family therapy in which patients were randomly assigned within a two-by-two design; high- or low-dose drug therapy and family therapy, or no therapy. The Goldstein model of family intervention was brief, concrete, and problem-focused. The goals of the program were to identify the events that were stressful to the patient and then to prevent the occurrence of these events or to mitigate their destructive impact. Family sessions began by exploring the psychotic experience, with the therapist helping the patient and the family to discuss the illness and its symptoms. Out of these discussions, the therapist helped the family and patient to identify and agree on two to three specific stresses that were of particularly current concern. Conflicts with significant others, or stresses that were viewed as having the potential of precipitating a psychosis were emphasized. Although symptoms themselves were often labeled as stressors by family members, attempts were made to focus on the interpersonal consequences of symptoms rather than symptoms per se.

Following the identification of stressors, the therapist's task was to help families develop strategies to avoid these stresses or methods of coping with them when they occurred. With the therapist's guidance, the need for the family and the patient to accommodate to one another was emphasized. Once coping strategies were developed, the therapist helped the patient and the family to implement them. When necessary, coping skills were developed using direct teaching, coaching, and practice. When problems arose in the use of these new coping strategies, obstacles to the implementation process were analyzed and the strategies were modified. Finally, therapists helped families and patients to anticipate and plan how they would handle future stress.

The results of this short-term program were extremely positive. After 6 weeks of treatment, the low medication/no family therapy group had a relapse rate of 24% while the high medication/family therapy group had no relapses at all. After 6 months, relapse rates increased to 48% for the former group, but remained at 0% for the latter. In other words, this intervention program achieved its primary goal of helping patients maintain themselves in the community during the high risk period immediately following hospitalization through the provision of only six sessions of family therapy. Although the differences between the groups were less dramatic at long-term follow-up points (Goldstein & Kopeikin, 1981), the initial impact of this program (Goldstein et al., 1978) was dramatic enough to inspire increased optimism regarding attempts to develop further the idea of a family intervention program for schizophrenic patients.

A grant application designed to support our work was thus submitted to the NIMH in March of 1977 and its subsequent approval ultimately gave birth to the psychoeducational family approach in the winter of 1979. This volume describes the family component of the aftercare research project that compares the relative effectiveness of medication management and two types of psychosocial intervention (social skills training and family therapy) for patients whose families are rated as high in EE. The highly structured model of family intervention described here was designed to be used in conjunction with a program of maintenance chemotherapy and to simultaneously decrease environmental stimulation and the patient's hypothesized vulnerability to it. In this program, a variety of supportive and educational techniques are used to lessen the emotional tensions of the family while maintaining sufficient pressure on patients to avoid the pitfalls of negative symptoms.

EVIDENCE OF EFFECTIVENESS

In the years since these attempts at theory building were initiated, the results of our own trial as well as the results from two family studies that used a similar conceptual basis have been obtained (Leff, Kuipers, Berkowitz, Eberlein-Vries, & Sturgeon, 1982; Falloon et al., 1982; Falloon, Boyd, & McGill, 1984). There are several unique characteristics of our own study: We accepted *all consecutive admissions* who met Research Diagnostic Criteria for schizophrenia or schizo-affective disorders, and who lived with at least one family member who was rated high in expressed emotion; we *randomly* assigned all of these patients to one of four treatment cells; and we began treatment during the acute psychotic episode rather than waiting for stabilization. The individual treatment (social skills training) was developed for this population based on the same vulnerability model making the individual–family comparison a particularly salient one. We conducted separate analyses that distinguished patients and families assigned to the various treatments and those who actually met criteria for engagement. This is unusual in that most studies select appropriate cases for the modality, and do not report differences in their results, considering them "no takes" or dropouts. Finally, to insure medication compliance and remove this factor as a possible intervening variable, all of our patients, whenever possible, were maintained on a minimal, effective dose of fluphenazine decanoate.

Results of our outcome study using this model during the first year of posthospital treatment have been encouraging in terms of the usefulness of family interventions. Among treatment takers ($n = 90$), 19% of those receiving family therapy alone experienced a psychotic relapse in the year following hospital discharge. Of those receiving the individual behavioral therapy, 20% relapsed, but *no* patient in the treatment cell that received *both* family therapy and social skills training experienced a relapse. These relapse rates constitute significant effects for both treatments when contrasted to a 41% relapse rate for those receiving only chemotherapy and support. Further, the combination of treatments yields an (additive) effect not possible with either treatment alone. When patients who were entirely faithful in adhering to their maintenance chemotherapy were included, a clear and significant effect for family therapy was also observed. Analyses regarding the adjustment of these patients are not complete as of this writing, but in general, there is no evidence that family therapy or social skills training are simply maintaining poorly adjusted patients in the community just to make the relapse rates look good.

Studies conducted at the University of Southern California by Falloon et al. (1982) and in London by Leff et al. (1982) reveal that 6% to 9% of family therapy treated patients experienced a relapse by 9 months, but that 44% to 50% of controls treated with drug and individual therapy had relapsed in the same period. These figures for the experimental group are consistent with our own 9 month results, although our 1 year results are somewhat higher. Nevertheless, all of these studies provide an increasingly broad validation of the effectiveness of family approaches, at least in the forestalling of a psychotic relapse. This, in turn, increases the potential for helping the patients to be reintegrated into their communities.

We wish, however, not to be intemperate in our claims. The results, at least from our own study, have demonstrated that these approaches forestall relapse but in no way provide "prevention" per se. To date, relapse rates continue to rise as patients near the end of their 2nd year of treatment. An uncensored estimate of relapse into the 2nd year of treatment reveals that relapse continues to rise in all treatment conditions, although an effect of family treatment is still present. Further, we feel that investigators familiar with the EE method and associated family therapists (ourselves included) have succumbed to a profound error in judgment in limiting these modern interventions to high EE patients and their families. High EE, it seems, has become the exclusive definition of high risk in these studies. Admitting patients to studies who come from high EE households tends to place under observation, for the most part, a group of unmarried males living in parental homes. In our own studies, this group represents only a subsample of the "at risk" schizophrenic population. Other samples, including married and unmarried females, are also at high risk for relapse and we believe they might also profit from these or similar interventions.

We surmise from our results, thus far achieved, that the primary effect of family treatment is one of delaying relapse and hospital readmissions. The family approach appears to buy time for patients, permitting them to recover more fully by decreasing family distress and helping them to understand the illness that reduces their expectations, and otherwise promotes the development of new coping strategies. Patients in both the family therapy and social skills training are *not* simply being maintained in the community in an impaired condition. Both treatments appear to produce improved adjustment. A limitation of the social skills training approach, however, seems to be its lessened ability to engage or maintain patients who are actively psychotic at the time of discharge. However, in facilities with long-term hospitalizations, or that otherwise discharged patients in a more clinically stable condition, both family therapy and social skills training could probably constitute effective interventions in significantly lowering schizophrenic relapse. The combined treatment approach provides an additional and important prophylactic advantage.

Thus, while we have no "panacea," no "cure," there is strong evidence that a method of intervention based on theoretical notions of schizophrenic pathophysiology has been able to reduce the traditionally high relapse rate of patients maintained on drugs alone. It is a new beginning, no more and no less.

CHAPTER TWO

CONNECTING WITH FAMILIES

I think professionals should show more empathy to the families and know what the problem looks like from our side, not the professional side. If all the hospitals we've had contact with even did that, things would be a lot better for all of us.—*Mother of a patient*

When a person develops schizophrenia, it has an impact on everyone in his or her family. Family members see someone they care about develop strange ideas and perceptions, heightened anxiety and agitation, unusual rituals or belief systems, and sometimes extremely disruptive, even violent behavior. The despair and anxiety family members feel at such times often is complicated by fears that they may have contributed to the patient's problems; fears that may be reinforced and exacerbated by the very professionals who are supposed to offer help and support.

Most families with schizophrenic patients initially seek help from professionals because the patient has ceased to function appropriately. When this occurs, it is not surprising that family members themselves also feel anxious and vulnerable. Whether it be the family's first contact with psychiatry or their 20th, a psychotic episode constitutes a crisis during which family members need immediate help and relief. If it is the patient's first episode of the illness, family members are usually frightened and confused by the inexplicable behaviors the patient has begun to display. In fact, many families describe the period during which the early episodes occur as the most difficult in the course of the illness. They have not yet given up the hopes and dreams they have had for the patient, nor have they mourned the loss of his normality (Hatfield, 1978). If it is the patient's fifth or sixth episode, family members can be overwhelmed by a sense of hopelessness and loss.

In either case, because patients often do not seek help on their own, families are likely to have gone through a prolonged period of stress before they are able to convince their loved one to get professional help. All too often, contact with professionals only occurs when patients are ill enough to require emergency assessments, middle of the night admissions, or even forced hospitalizations through legal commitment (Vine, 1982b). Unfortunately, the need to use coercion to get patients to accept treatment can make things worse by stimulating conflict, accusations, and angry feelings between families and patients. All of these problems are complicated by the process of getting patients into hospitals, which can be, in itself, a frustrating one under current legal statutes and mental health policies. As one relative of a chronic schizo-phrenic patient stated:

> The just and human spirit which today prevents one relative from placing another in an uncaring hospital where many people wasted 30 years ago also provides little comfort for a mother who sees her daughter slowly starving to death, a man who sees his brother aimlessly wandering and taking refuge on a bus bench, or a child who watches a parent isolate himself to the point of nonexistence. (Vine, 1982a)

Even if a legal commitment is not the issue, the way mental health systems handle patients and families during emergency admissions often contributes to family pain rather than diminishing it. Both patient *and family* arrive in need of protection, support, structure, and a sense of control, but most systems are geared to offer such things only to the patient. When patients are evaluated by most mental health systems, families are seen briefly, if at all. These brief contacts are generally used only to gather information about the patient. Not only do questions focus entirely on the patient, but they also tend to be negative; what was wrong, abnormal, or atypical about the patient's development, the family's interaction, or its social, genetic, or biologic history. The psychiatric system's preoccupation with deficits, coupled with a lack of attention to assets, often leads already upset families to believe that professionals seek to establish family responsibility for the patient's problems. With this impression, it is not surprising that family members give their information and their "patient" to the hospital system and quickly leave, wondering to themselves what happened, how, and why. One mother, referring to a past intake interview by a competent and even empathic social worker, stated, "She was very nice, but I could tell by the questions she asked that she was trying to find out what we had done wrong." While her mother shared as much infor-mation as she could and defended herself well in the session, she went home and spent a tearful, sleepless night worrying about the things she may have done to cause her son to develop schizophrenia. It was not until months later that she began to get angry.

Given the attitudes of many professionals, it is not surprising that family members are not always very eager to get involved with mental health treatment systems. Unless the professionals that families first encounter are genuinely attuned to family issues and respectful of family needs at such a difficult time, most families are likely to be defensive, resistant, and may even withdraw from contact with professionals. This is most likely to be true for those families of patients who have been ill for many years. Even though care today is more humane than in the past, patients and families have learned the hard way that there is no cure. After family members have adjusted to this harsh reality, they may be less upset, but they may also have less energy, less hope, and less motivation to get involved. After multiple hospitalizations and multiple treatments, they have found no treatment to be effective over the long haul. In fact, they have probably encountered some treatments that made the patient worse. Almost certainly they have encountered professionals who have mistreated them somewhere along the way by ignoring them, and/or by implicitly or explicitly accusing them of being destructive.

To add to the problem, many professionals who work with this illness make a causal connection between the patient's illness and family behaviors. Based on the observation that patients often are more agitated during and after family visits, many of the staff of inpatient facilities have learned to see families as destructive and responsible for causing the patient's illness. In their desire to protect and help patients, they tend to view families as threats to patient progress. They ignore the fact that family interaction is likely to be intense in even the healthiest and most supportive of families. When patients are as vulnerable to stimulation as these patients undoubtedly are, they are likely to react with agitation to any intense situation, including contact with their family members. While it does not logically follow that families cause schizophrenia, the relatively positive response of patients to the less intense and more structured atmosphere of an inpatient unit, as opposed to the emotional complexity of their families, is used as evidence that families are the villians in these tragic plays. Considering that this is the perspective from which many mental health professionals view families, it is not surprising that they tend to develop attitudes and behaviors that are not helpful to families, and even less surprising that many families come to distrust and avoid contact with mental health professionals.

The withdrawal of families from hospital systems is particularly problematic because, following hospitalization, they are likely to become the primary caretakers of patients. Over 65% of patients discharged from psychiatric hospitals return to their families (Minkoff, 1978). Whether this is the most reasonable plan for either patients or their families is a topic of debate. Nevertheless, in most situations the choice is not between returning patients to their families or to truly independent living. Rather, it is a choice between returning them to their families or to grossly inadequate residential programs. In some communities, patients have no alternative at all, except perhaps that of living on the streets. If patients return home, the family's participation in treatment is crucial, since with their support, it may be possible to maintain many patients in their communities, eventually helping them to return to a more normal lifestyle. Without the family's support, any treatment plan is less likely to succeed. For instance, if professionals must depend only on the patient's motivation, they are unlikely even to see these patients once they leave the hospital. Up to 50% of these patients fail to connect with aftercare services, or discontinue treatments after just a few visits (Taube, 1974).

Without ongoing treatment, patients receive neither the protection of medication nor the ongoing support and guidance they need, leaving them more vulnerable to stimulation and to relapse. The repeated hospitalizations that result when outpatient treatment is inconsistent, unavailable, or unused are stressful to both patient and family, and eventually can result in a loss of the skills necessary for even minimal functioning in the community. While families can be the patient's and the professional's most important allies in the treatment of the patients, family members themselves also can benefit from receiving help in managing this difficult and painful illness while continuing to function and live productive lives.

GOALS

The family clinician's initial contacts with both the patient and members of the family are crucial in that these contacts help to decide whether or not treatment will occur, and help to establish the ongoing treatment relationship. Since the needs of family members are so often neglected, it is important to pay explicit attention to beginning the process of "connecting" with the family immediately, and to continue this effort over several sessions. Optimally, the family should be seen while the patient is being initially evaluated, not just to gain information about the patient, but also to assess their stresses and resources, and to provide them with support. This connecting phase has five primary goals that lay the foundation for the entire process of treatment:

1. A relationship should be established between clinician and family in which there is a genuine working alliance, a partnership that aims to help the patient. All treatment requires the establishing of a working relationship between patient and clinician. For treatment to be successful, patients must respect their clinician and believe that he or she can help them. Clinicians must feel they understand their patients and must believe their treatment has something to offer in resolving their problems. In any sort of family treatment, the establishing of this working relationship is more complicated than in other forms of therapeutic intervention since therapists must establish a special relationship with each family member simultaneously. Clinicians who work with families must be able to understand the needs of each family member and find ways to make each feel that participating in treatment will be beneficial. A basic requirement for establishing a therapeutic alliance in family therapy is "joining" with the family system before attempting change-producing interventions (Minuchin, 1974). By taking the time to become a part of the family system, clinicians diminish a family's natural tendencies to exclude them, to resist their interventions, or to discontinue treatment prematurely.

In working with the families of schizophrenic patients, general techniques of joining (social conversation with each member, displaying an interest and concern for everyone's viewpoint, etc.), should be augmented by specifically addressing the problems and themes specific to patients and families dealing with this illness. First, a special attempt must be made to help family members see the logic of their participation in family sessions without intimating that they play any sort of causal role in the patient's illness. Second, attention to the views of family members about the course and impact of the illness, as well as the family's current life situation, helps to enlist families as allies of clinicians and begins to define their roles as partners in the attainment of therapeutic goals.

2. *Clinicians should understand family issues and problems which might contribute to the stress level of the patient or family members.* Although the psychiatric illness of a member has an overwhelming impact on a family, it is usually not the only issue family members are attempting to manage at any given time. For this reason, stresses that might be influencing each family member, and thus the family as a whole, must be assessed. Ongoing demands on individual family members, chronic family conflicts, and any major change, be they positive or negative, could constitute stress. Issues such as unemployment or promotion, marriage or divorce, physical illness or death, trouble with the law, or school problems all have an impact on both family and patient, and on everyone's ability to tolerate the stress of psychiatric illness and the demands of participating in treatment. Family members who are currently struggling with their own issues may have little energy left for coping with the illness or treatment of another family member. Thus, at least some attention to the problems and needs of each family member is essential before making requests of them in the best interests of the patient.

This goal is complicated by the fact that family members often tend to minimize their own problems during initial interactions with those professionals primarily committed to helping the patient. They may feel it is inappropriate or disloyal to focus on themselves when a relative is in such an acute crisis. They are sometimes hesitant to share information that they feel could be interpreted as evidence of their inadequacy. Whatever the reasons, an accurate assessment of family stresses takes some time, and may only be possible after family members have had a chance to assess the clinician's sincerity, interest, and expertise.

3. *Clinicians should gain an understanding of the family's resources and their past and current attempts to cope with the illness.* Families naturally attempt to do what they think is best for a member who becomes ill. During the long course of a chronic mental illness, most families will have at one time or another tried to ignore or adapt to the patient's symptoms, to coax the patient to function as before and to control aberrant behavior, or to convince the patient that his or her unusual ideas are unfounded. Some of the coping mechanisms families have developed are effective, hard-won skills developed by trial and error over years of experience, while others have not worked and may even have resulted in increased stress for the patient and for the rest of the family. In either case, it is helpful to understand what family members have done to cope in the past so as to be better able to help the patient and family to cope in the future.

Gaining an understanding of the coping mechanisms that have been used must, in part, involve a discussion of what the patient was like before he or she became ill, and how much the family has been able to deal with the changes that have occurred as a result of the illness. Some families will have had a chance to mourn the loss of the patient's normality and their dreams of what might have been, while others may still be struggling with the grief inherent in this process. The extent to which they have dealt with these issues will have an impact on their ability to cope and to accept information and advice.

Attention must also be paid to the resources available to the family, such as the availability and extent of each family member's support network. The stigma of a psychiatric illness, the pain of the experience, or simply a lack of awareness of the availability of relevant resources, may have prevented some families from using possible support systems. The level of contact and comfort received from friends, extended family, and self-help groups is another important consideration in determining whether the family can (or should) allow the patient to return home, or whether a more structured long-term living arrangement must be found.

4. *Family strengths should be emphasized and maximized.* Both professionals and families themselves sometimes underestimate family strengths. Simply to have survived over time while living with an

acutely psychotic person requires patience, tolerance, and significant coping skills. Because these abilities will continue to be needed in order for the family to cope effectively over the long course of treatment and rehabilitation, it is the task of the clinician to ascertain and emphasize the family's strengths, and their ability to use them. If the family is particularly frustrated at the time of initial interviews, they may feel helpless, as though they have no resources, and that nothing they have done has been helpful to the patient. At such times they may not even be aware of the tremendous strength and caring they have brought to bear on this chronic problem, strength that may well be available again after a respite from the acute crisis. For these reasons, it is necessary to take considerable initiative and time in conducting a careful assessment of strengths, not just weaknesses, emphasizing for the family the good things that have happened, the negative things that have been avoided, and the strength inherent in just "hanging in there" over the years.

5. *Rules and expectations of treatment should be established through the creation of a contract with mutual, attainable, and specific goals.* People are most comfortable when they have a sense of structure and predictability. With families of the mentally ill, many of whom are in acute crisis, the need for structure is usually essential. Giving the family and patient specific information about the treatment process, establishing clear and attainable goals to be achieved through mutual effort, along with communicating a realistic time line for goal accomplishment, can decrease anxiety and provide a focus that allows for a remobilization of hope. Amorphous, ambiguous, or overly grandiose treatment goals simply increase the family's sense of confusion and can lead to a negation of the professional's ability to help.

IMPLEMENTATION OF THE PRINCIPLES OF CONNECTING

Being Immediately Available

The crisis that brings patients and families to hospitals or mental health settings offers an opportunity to show families that a treatment experience can be a helpful one, differing from some of the negative experiences they may have had in the past. Although these families often have good reason not to trust professionals, in a crisis they at least may be open to giving it a try, even if they do so out of desperation, not desire.

The initial contacts with the family, therefore, should be made immediately, before the crisis has passed or diminished, since this is when families are most likely to be open and in greatest need. These first contacts, out of necessity, must serve multiple purposes. First, they must be used to begin to establish a good working climate, one in which the family is given support and treated with respect. Second, they must be used to gather information about the patient, including information about past history and the present episode. Third, they must focus on assessing the family, with attention paid to the respective individual needs and aspirations of each family member, as well as to the coping style of the family as a whole. These contacts must attend to the family's response to the crisis, their immediate needs for support and information about the patient and his or her illness, and their general needs unrelated to the current crisis. (See Table 2–1 for an outline of the issues to be covered in the family assessment.)

Focusing First on the Present Crisis

The first family contacts must focus on the present crisis and the family's reasons for getting help for the patient at that particular time. After gaining some understanding of this issue, the clinician should focus, at least briefly, on the feelings and needs of other family members. Some families, because of the length of the crisis, or the existence of other concurrent stresses, may be particularly vulnerable and require additional support during this period. If the clinician does not know the needs of family members, he or she will be unable to help them effectively. Establishing a working relationship with the family during the crisis involves listening to their feelings about what they have been through, discovering other present or potential stresses in their lives, explaining the procedures and policies of the treatment system, and making them feel comfortable in a strange and confusing environment.

Avoiding Treating the Family as the Patient

During the initial contacts, clinicians must demonstrate to families that they respect their priorities and concerns, and recognize all they have done to help. They must also communicate their belief that the family has taken a positive and necessary step in seeking professional help for the patient. It is important to avoid treating the family as "the patient." Such tactics deemphasize family strengths, impose unilateral therapist-initiated contracts, and deny the fact that family members have something to offer to the treatment process. Instead, family members should be helped to feel that they will be entering into a cooperative relationship with the treatment team *to help the patient*.

In the following example, a family arrived at a psychiatric emergency room with their son and the police, having just had to file for

TABLE 2-1
Initial family assessment

	Task	Methods
Part I Crisis assessment	1. Determine extent of the patient's dysfunction. 2. Determine current level of family distress. 3. Determine extent of professional support needed by the patient (hospitalization, medication, frequency of sessions).	Ask about patient's symptoms and impact on family functioning. Ask about how family members are coping (other current stresses and resources). Ask family about perceived needs and desires from the treatment facility at this time.
Part II Assessment of family reaction to illness and treatment	1. Determine level of long-term impact of illness on family life. 2. Determine response of family members to past treatment(s).	Review course of the illness. Review in detail past treatment experiences, especially negative ones, and the family's perception of their effectiveness.
Part III General family assessment	1. Determine general family factors that might contribute to current stresses or constitute special strengths in coping with the illness: a. history b. structure c. communication patterns d. life cycle stage e. family–community relationships 2. Determine current stress tolerance of family and its members.	Take family genogram. Explore patterns of relationships regarding activities and alliances, generational boundaries. Observe style of communication, including conflict resolution processes, feedback mechanisms (clarity of messages, listening skills, etc.). Ask about each family member's extrafamilial contacts and relationships. Ask about recent events, changes, both positive and negative.

a legal commitment after a long, painful process of deterioration of their son's behavior. They were upset by his anger at them, and guilty about forcing him to come to the hospital. They were sure, however, that they had to take drastic action for everyone's sake. While the patient was being seen, the family representative met with the family.

CLINICIAN: While Dr. S is seeing your son, I'd like to get your views on what just happened.

FATHER: Well, it got so bad, we had to call the police.

MOTHER: I don't even know if I can tell you. It's all been so confusing. He's been acting strange for weeks, but these last few days. . . .

FATHER: (*Interrupting*) He's been up all night for weeks—laughing and talking to himself. First, he just told us God was talking to him. Then, he started talking about how people were out to get him. When he asked about where I kept my gun, I really got scared. I knew there was no way this was going to settle down.

MOTHER: I've tried to get him to call his old therapist, but he wouldn't. He needs help.

FATHER: So, I told him, "You have to come with us to the hospital," and he swung at me and locked himself in his room.

MOTHER: When he's himself, he's very gentle, but when he gets like this, we get scared.

CLINICIAN: I'm sure you do. So this has been getting worse for weeks?

MOTHER: At least. We've put up with a lot, you know. We don't like to do this to him.

CLINICIAN: I guess you wouldn't have gotten the police involved unless things were really bad.

FATHER: He was talking about "getting even" with the CIA.

MOTHER: We don't exactly know what he means, but we get scared. Now, he blames us for everything, he says the CIA is controlling our minds. I'm afraid he might hurt us. Himself, too.

CLINICIAN: Clearly, you've been through a lot in the last few weeks and particularly tonight. It must be tough when he blames you.

MOTHER: It's terrible, and you know, no one ever understands. He's had problems for 6 years and no one ever has really helped him.

FATHER: (*Angrily*) And now you can't get him into a hospital unless he's out of control. I got him to come down 2 weeks ago before things were so bad, but when he wouldn't sign himself in, they just let him go. They could *see* he was crazy.

MOTHER: It's the law, Joe. They can't make him stay unless he's dangerous.

FATHER: What kind of a law is that? Do they think we *want* to see him in a hospital just for the fun of it?

CLINICIAN: It must be really frustrating to see someone you love getting worse and not being able to do anything about it, not being able to get anyone to help.

FATHER: It sure is. I've about had it. And, I'm still not sure we did the right thing.

MOTHER: I know—he'll blame us for making him come here, and it will be *more* trouble.

CLINICIAN: Really, it sounds as though you did the only thing you could under the circumstances. You coped as well as anyone for as long as you could.

MOTHER: I guess so, but it breaks my heart to see him go through it again.

As the session went on, the clinician continued to review the immediate crisis, allowing the patient's parents to express their feelings about the patient, the helping system, and eventually to become less upset about the events leading up to and surrounding the commitment. During this process, he took care not to tell them that everything would be fine, a fact every family knows to be untrue. Offering false reassurances when family members know the seriousness of the illness from personal experience is never helpful. Families know what problems the patient has experienced, and they know their own sorrow. Too rapid reassurance can only serve to alienate them, making them feel the clinician either does not understand the situation or is trying to dismiss them with platitudes.

Attending to Family Supports and Stresses

As assessment contacts progress, an attempt must be made to discover in more detail the current stresses experienced by each family member. In so doing, attention must be paid to potential stresses and resources of each member concerning their workplace, extended family, and social network. In addition to the importance of collecting this data for use in making treatment decisions, the process of demonstrating concern about the issues of family members other than the patient can be used to communicate caring and to form a treatment relationship.

In the following example, the clinician inquires about supports following a discussion of the impact of the illness and other stresses.

CLINICIAN: Is there anyone who you can talk to about all of this?

MOTHER: It's a family matter. I can't discuss it.

CLINICIAN: How come?

MOTHER: I don't know.

CLINICIAN: Isn't it your brother who comes over?

MOTHER: My brother, yes, but he's like one of us.

CLINICIAN: So, he's a resource?

FATHER: Yeah, but her sister, whenever you talk to her about this, she says, "I have enough problems of my own," and—

MOTHER: Well, she doesn't exactly say that, she says she doesn't want to hear it because it upsets her. And things may be better at her home, but she's still upset. And I can understand her point.

CLINICIAN: So, she kind of steers clear?

MOTHER: So then once I didn't tell her about Art taking the overdose, and she heard through somebody else, and she got mad at me. You can't win for losing.

CLINICIAN: Is there anyone else? (*To father*) Maybe someone you could talk to?

FATHER: No. (*Tearfully*)

CLINICIAN: You're the silent one of the family?

FATHER: Yeah, I don't . . . I don't even talk to my brother about it because. . . .

MOTHER: He has his problems. He's laid off now. He worked down at the steel mills. They closed. He and his son are both laid off. They've closed it up, so. . . .

CLINICIAN: But you never have really talked to anyone? It's been a long time.

FATHER: Yeah. I see him in church once in awhile, but . . . , no I don't even bring it up with them.

MOTHER: It's something that you just don't like to talk about to outsiders. You know.

Clearly, while this family has relatives and friends, these supports are not useful to them in specifically discussing the problems related to the patient's illness. Understanding the vulnerability of families to this particular type of isolation can alert clinicians to the need to provide experiences in which family members can interact with others who genuinely understand these issues. In this case, the clinician will eventually suggest participation in a multiple family or self-help group involving other families coping with similar problems.

However, an assessment of the social support networks of family members should not be limited to an assessment of whom they can talk to. Those extended family members and friends who do not understand the illness still may be available to provide for other needs of the immediate family, such as providing chances to be distracted by social activities, practical help with household chores, or getting a respite from having to constantly think about the illness. These are valuable functions which clinicians may want to emphasize over time.

Preparing for the Treatment Contract

Toward the end of the session(s) in the connecting phase, clinicians should tell families specifically what is to happen to the patient and what the hospital system will ask of them. They should stress the importance of and need for the family's ongoing involvement in the patient's treatment, and the staff's need for their input in order to help the patient. Clinicians should be prepared to be explicit about these issues, and prepared to answer questions posed by families.

It is rare that the initial contact will involve the entire family. Frequently, it is only the primary caretaker(s), that is, spouse or parents, who accompany a patient to the hospital. Thus, one task of the first session is to discuss the involvement of other family members in future sessions. This is important for a number of reasons. First, it emphasizes the clinician's awareness that the illness has an impact on everyone and that everyone's needs and perceptions will be taken into account in the process of treatment; and second, it reinforces the message that everyone's help will be needed to help the patient. In the end, clinicians should make sure family members have the phone numbers of all team members, information on how they may be reached in an emergency, and the next appointment time. Most of all, they should leave the family with the feeling that, this time, a caring expert has joined them in their efforts to cope with this debilitating illness.

In the following example, the family clinician, having described the treatment program and its requirements, attempts to negotiate the next appointment time with a patient's somewhat disbelieving parents.

FATHER: I must say, it all sounds good . . . but we've been this route. You asked about what's happened before. Well, let me tell you: We were in family therapy and had to sit each week while our son yelled at us! When we asked the therapist a question, all he'd say was, "What do you think?" If we knew, we wouldn't be asking him.

MOTHER: It was terrible. We used to leave the sessions feeling miserable. We'd go home, asking each other over and over what we did wrong. And nothing changed . . . just a lot of pain.

FATHER: That's why I'm not sure we want to get involved.

CLINICIAN: I can certainly understand your feelings and I don't blame you for being skeptical. As I've said, we're asking for a totally different kind of involvement. To put it bluntly, we *need* your help. You know your son better than anyone, and we know about schizophrenia. Working together, I think we can come up with some ideas that may help to make things better for him, *and* for the family.

FATHER: (*Still skeptical*) As I said, it *sounds* good. . . .

CLINICIAN: I know it's hard to believe things could be helpful when it hasn't worked in the past. But, I really think it's important that we work together. If it doesn't feel right to you or if at any time you have a complaint or are unhappy about what I say or do, please let me know and we'll discuss it.

MOTHER: *(Looking at husband)* Well . . . of course we care enough to keep trying. . . .

FATHER: What choice do we have? He'll be home soon. If this has *any* chance of making it less of a nightmare. . . .

CLINICIAN: I know how hard it is to keep trying and I really appreciate your giving it a go. Now, what would be a good time for you to come for an appointment?

In this session, the clinician stressed the differences between the new treatment approach and past ones by focusing on the collaborative nature of the treatment relationship. Past therapies were neither attacked nor defended. The clinician expressed an understanding of how difficult it must have been to have had these negative experiences and did not try to convince these parents to believe that the new therapy would be better, only that it would be worth a try. Their doubts about its efficacy were accepted as appropriate and healthy, and communication channels were established to enable family members to provide feedback about treatment on an ongoing basis.

Solidifying the Treatment Relationship

In all sessions, but particularly the early ones, it is helpful to give family members a chance to settle into the session before launching into a discussion of highly charged issues. This technique reinforces the sense that clinicians care about the family members themselves, in addition to their commitment to helping the patient. Some discussion of neutral topics also tends to increase the family's comfort and feelings of being accepted, and facilitates the transition to the work of the session (Minuchin, 1974; Minuchin & Fishman, 1981). For this reason, clinicians are advised to begin each session with a few minutes of appropriate social conversation (i.e., greetings, small talk).

The following dialogue occurred at the beginning of the third session with the family of a young schizophrenic patient who was still on the inpatient unit and unable to attend sessions.

CLINICIAN: Hi, how are you folks today?

MOTHER: Fine, how's Andy [the patient]?

CLINICIAN: He's doing fair. We'll talk about that in detail in a few minutes. Before that *(Turning to father)* . . . you look beat.

FATHER: I'm always tired.

JOEY: [brother] That's for sure.

CLINICIAN: I think if I had to work at the furnaces, I'd be more than tired. . . .

FATHER: *(Laughing)* It sure ain't easy being in the mills. . . . I must sweat gallons. . . .

MOTHER: (*Laughing*) And he puts it back on with his beer.
CLINICIAN: (*Smiling*) Every job has to have benefits.
FATHER: Right on!

While the content of the interaction in this example is not addressed in a serious manner, emphasizing the social nature of the conversation gives everyone a chance to settle in. At some point, the clinician may address the mother's reference to her husband's drinking, but, for the moment, this is ignored. The clinician chooses to demonstrate both a genuine concern for the father's health after a hard day in the steel mills, and a sense of humor that can make the work of the session seem a little less formal. These social interactions also can make the therapy less intense, less patient-focused, and more cooperative over the long haul. When the patient joins the sessions, these dialogues can serve as models of appropriate social conversations, a skill that patients with schizophrenia often have lost over time.

After a few minutes of social interaction, attention must turn to the work of the session. In these continuing connecting sessions, the major tasks are the review of the course of the illness and its treatment, the disconnection of the ideas of family etiology and family treatment, the establishment of the clinician as the family's representative to the hospital system, and the creation of a treatment contract.

Reviewing the Course of Illness and Treatment

Once the immediate crisis has passed and a patient is either admitted to an inpatient unit or entered into outpatient treatment, time can be taken to review the course of the patient's illness in greater detail, including previous level of functioning, past responses to treatment, and the family's response to both. A detailed review not only gives the family a chance to tell their story, but also allows the clinician to gain a more thorough understanding of what the family has been through, and what resources are available to them. This is important for several reasons. Unless family members feel that their experiences with the patient have been understood and appreciated, they will be less receptive to suggestions about treatment options or different coping strategies. The family's reactions to past treatment attempts must be given particular attention, since their past experiences will influence their current expectations, assumptions, and tendencies toward cooperation or resistance.

In the following session, which occurred the day after Jim's admission to an inpatient unit, the clinician begins to explore the patient's history with his wife.

WIFE: I can't believe it. It's never going to end. This time I thought it would be different.

CLINICIAN: Was it different for awhile?

WIFE: Oh, yes. This time, Jim promised he would take his medicine, and he did for awhile. Things were going really well. . . .

CLINICIAN: Oh?

WIFE: Every time—he stops his meds and then, Bam! It's driving me crazy. I think *I* need to be in here [the hospital].

CLINICIAN: I doubt it. In fact, I'm amazed with your strength. Coping with this problem for 8 years has taken a lot. I don't know if I could have done it.

WIFE: I've put up with a lot.

CLINICIAN: (*Emphatic voice*) Can you tell me a little about it?

WIFE: (*Deep sigh*) Well, you know he first became ill just after we moved to Pittsburgh. . . .

The patient's wife goes on to describe the years of frustration with her husband's illness and the treatments that didn't work or didn't engage him sufficiently even to get started. She describes her attempts to get the best possible help for him and her attempts to deal with his strange behavior. The clinician listens and asks questions respectfully and empathically, appropriately reinforcing her attempts to handle difficult situations. The manner in which this review of the illness is done can help family members begin to feel better about psychiatry, themselves, and particularly about their ability to cope with the illness in a way that enables them to be a positive resource for the patient.

In this review, attention must be paid to potential stresses brought on by the patient's most recent episode and hospitalization. A discussion of these issues provides the family with a chance to decompress the impact of these events and to see the clinician as understanding their difficulties. For this reason, common emotional responses experienced by family members should be explored. For instance, one of the more frequent emotional reactions is that of guilt. Most families, particularly parents, ask, "What did we do wrong?" or "What could we have done that we didn't do?" Some families also feel stigmatized, since behaviors related to this mental illness can be socially embarrassing. When patients accuse neighbors or employers of attempting to poison them, cease to care about personal hygiene, or rudely ignore other people's needs, both they and their families may be rejected by the community in which they live. It is also not surprising that many family members come to feel justifiably angry about the strange rules, unreasonable rituals, and just plain inconvenience imposed by patients over the years. In fact, it is often surprising that they have managed so well for so long. Here, the clinician reviews the family's attempts to help the patient.

CLINICIAN: You say that Joe has been ill for a long time, and that when he's sick, he's pretty hard to live with. Can you tell me more about that?

MOTHER: I guess the worst thing has been the worry that he'll do something. Not that he's ever been violent or hurt anybody, but he has no judgment. I mean he smokes constantly and drops his ashes everywhere. I'm afraid he'll burn the house down.

FATHER: And then his ideas that people are out to get him. . . .

CLINICIAN: How have you tried to handle these things in the past?

MOTHER: Mostly we've talked to him. I tell him people aren't really out to get him. I try to convince him that his ideas aren't true.

FATHER: And we just try to ignore a lot of it because nothing seems to work. Like the rituals, you know. We just sort of let them be. We can take it, we have sort of built our lives around them.

MOTHER: Yes, like we never leave him alone because of the smoking. We take turns going out when we have to. At least if one of us is there, if a fire starts. . . .

CLINICIAN: So you really haven't gotten away from all this in . . . how many years?

FATHER: I'd say five where it's been this bad . . . not constant, you know, but most of the time.

MOTHER: And when he's in the hospital, we can rest a little. He seems to go in at least twice a year.

CLINICIAN: Sounds rough on everyone.

FATHER: More on my wife than on me. I can at least go to work. And my daughter just went away to college.

MOTHER: He's *my* son. It's hard, but I would never forgive myself if something happened.

The discussion continues with an exploration of the family's fears of what would have happened if they left the patient alone, and the lengths to which they have gone to protect him over the years. The clinician discovers that their coping mechanisms have included, at one time or another; attempting to coax their son to behave according to society's rules; using logic to convince him that his paranoid ideas were not true; ignoring his bizarre behaviors; attempting to make sense out of his tangential confused communications; and taking on extra chores themselves in order to compensate for what Joe was no longer able or willing to do. In this situation, as in many, the patient has been maintained in the home only because his entire family has learned to curtail their social and vocational activities and to ignore many of their own needs. Like many families, they turn to the mental health system for help only after these techniques have failed to work.

After reviewing other treatment experiences, every attempt is made to stress that the present treatment approach will be different from past treatment efforts. Without criticizing other professionals, it is possible to stress that more is constantly being learned about this illness and how to treat it. Reassurance can be given that the family clinician will attempt to protect the family's interests, and that the treatment team will be made up of competent professionals who expect to be able to facilitate change. In the following example, two very upset parents discuss their feelings after visiting their son who had recently been admitted to the inpatient psychiatric unit.

FATHER: Do you know the last thing he said to me? He said, "I hate you." I can't believe it. After all I've done. And then . . . that damned nurse told me I'd have to leave because I was upsetting him. I should have told her what for. . . .

MOTHER: What do you expect? It's just like the times at the other hospital. Like we're the enemy. Well, let me tell you; We're not. And you guys don't know what the hell your doing. If you did, we wouldn't have to keep coming back.

CLINICIAN: I don't blame you for being hurt and angry. This has been a really upsetting time and then to have the staff imply you were making things worse . . . I'm surprised you're not even more angry.

FATHER: (Sighs) I guess we're used to it by now.

CLINICIAN: That probably doesn't make it any easier.

MOTHER: No, it still hurts. And the hard thing is I can't see any end to it. We've been through this over and over. . . .

CLINICIAN: It's been a rough road for everybody, and you're right, we don't have any magic answers. But, I do think this time can be different—no magic—but better. The program we've been discussing has had a lot of success. Many patients are able to stay out of the hospital, some even out of crises.

FATHER: Hm . . . hm, but were those patients as bad off as Tom?

CLINICIAN: Some were worse, some were better. I don't want to con you. There is no cure. I guess you know that, after all you've been through. But, with your help and patience, I think we can work together to help Tom.

Throughout the review of the history of the illness and past treatment, the feelings of family members about the patient and the illness begin to emerge. Those families who are not angry are often overwhelmed by sadness, feeling that their loved one will never be the same again. They are painfully aware that the patient's capabilities have diminished and the hopes and dreams they have had for his or her future may be lost forever. In the following example, two parents struggle with their feelings about their son's illness, and the clinician begins to try to diminish feelings of guilt and responsibility.

MOTHER: I don't understand it. We brought Neil up just like his sisters and they're fine. But then, I keep saying maybe we should have been stricter.

FATHER: I don't know either. Looking back I guess we should have seen the problem coming long before we did. If we had gotten help then, maybe this never would have happened.

CLINICIAN: It must be really easy to do "What if's." That's probably the worst game we all do to ourselves—myself included. I don't know if things would be different today if you did those things, although, to be honest, I doubt it.

MOTHER: Really? . . . I just don't know.

Later in the session, after a good deal of discussion of the parents' feelings, talk moves to their feelings about what they have lost and the issue of defining reasonable expectations for the future.

FATHER: I can remember when Neil was in junior high, he had as many friends as anyone else. (*Laughs*) There was never a time when there wasn't a kid over to the house. And he did well in school. Not brilliant, you know, but well. I had such hopes. We talked about him taking over the business—and now, this.

MOTHER: (*Crying*) I guess we all had such high hopes for him. Now, what can we hope for?

CLINICIAN: I can imagine how hard it is to feel you might have to give up your hopes and dreams. And you are probably right. Neil may never be able to take over your business.

MOTHER: (*Cries*)

FATHER: (*Deep sigh*) I know he can't do it. I've tried not to think about it, but I know he'll never be right.

CLINICIAN: I do think you can hope that he will be able to do things in the future though, like get a job, make friends again. . . .

MOTHER: Do you really think that?

CLINICIAN: There's a chance.

MOTHER: (*Pause*) That's even more than I could dare hope for right now. I've been thinking of it as hopeless. That gives me something to hang on to . . . if I can believe you.

In this example, the therapist encourages the family to express their feelings of sadness and to begin to mourn the loss of their hopes and dreams. It is only *after* this process that he begins to suggest there might be some hope for a better future. Again, reassurance that is too rapid sounds and *is* insincere, and is quickly dismissed by families of schizophrenic patients.

Often the process of mourning the loss of a family member's mental health, and of developing realistic expectations, is helped by exploring what he or she was like before becoming ill. In this session, the entire family spends time remembering what Sheldon was like before he became ill and socially isolated.

BROTHER: He was sort of a class clown, I think.

MOTHER: Yes, he was much more socially oriented.

FATHER: When he was growing up, he could have a bunch of friends around and it always seemed like they would come and wait for Shelly to finish what he was doing, for him to join them. He wasn't exactly a leader, but someone who was the center of attention. I thought some things he did were really funny, humorous.

MOTHER: (*Proudly*) He was witty and interesting, and *very* outgoing.

FATHER: I remember one time there were about four or five boys in the backyard and they were playing touch football. It got a little too rough and two of them took exception to it and they were squaring off to fight each other, and Shelly was making all these side comments. It was just impossible for the two who wanted to fight to be serious. Sounded like the dialogue from *MASH* . . . like, you know, "Don't let him kiss you," or something like that. . . .

SISTER: He broke the whole thing up.

FATHER: He just turned that thing around in about 2–3 minutes, and there was no way they could be serious because he was just breaking them up.

CLINICIAN: Sounds like he had a lot of positives.

FATHER: Yeah, he did. It just seemed as though he was capable of so much and then it kind of just all went, and I don't know where it went. I don't know if I'm to blame . . . I just don't know where it went.

CLINICIAN: It's really sad that that liveliness doesn't seem to be there, but I don't think it helps to blame anybody.

FATHER: (*Pause*) I just don't know.

CLINICIAN: Do you feel guilty?

MOTHER: (*Tearful*) "No, except that. . . ."

CLINICIAN: I got the feeling last time . . . a couple of things you said. . . .

MOTHER: Well, I worry. Maybe if we would have been stricter and more like policemen and laid down rigid hours, and maybe if we would have been more firm, but we weren't with the other kids and it never entered our minds, we trusted him just as we did the other kids.

CLINICIAN: You must spend a lot of time wondering what you could have done.

FATHER: I do, but you can go nuts doing that.

CLINICIAN: Sure can.

This family had been so busy coping with the crises of overt psychotic symptoms and the frustration of negative symptoms for several years that they had rarely discussed what their son was once like, and the sad feelings they had about the loss of that person. Mourning the loss of health can serve to release tension in and of itself, to uncover and at least partially resolve fears of having unwittingly contributed to the patient's problems in some way, and to lay the groundwork for more realistic plans and expectations for the future.

Disconnecting Etiology and Treatment

Frequently, when professionals suggest family sessions, family intervention, or family therapy, that recommendation can be interpreted by families as a suggestion that they probably have caused the patient's illness and therefore need to be treated themselves.

It is important to dispel these notions (in staff *and* in families) before the type of family work recommended in this book can be done effectively. Families will otherwise tend to appropriately resist the attempts of the staff to involve them in the patient's treatment. In the following example of what *not* to do, a clinician has attributed causality to the family. This has led not only to a focus on helping the family to adjust to Margie's dysfunctions and complaints, but to the promotion of a separation from her parents for which no one was prepared.

MARGIE: If they would treat me as an adult instead of a 2-year-old, everything would be fine, and I could get on with my life.

FATHER: We would like to treat you like an adult, but we can't trust you. If only. . . .

CLINICIAN: It sounds like Margie feels you've never given her a chance to grow up.

MARGIE: Exactly. They don't want me to grow up.

FATHER: No, that's not true. We'd be happy if you could. (*To the clinician*) Her brothers and sister have grown up. We treated them all the same.

CLINICIAN: Did you?

MOTHER: Well, we tried to. But Margie started having problems and we got worried. She needed more of our time.

MARGIE: I don't need your time.

CLINICIAN: So, you were really more involved with Margie?

MOTHER: Yes, but . . . she needed us.

CLINICIAN: Hm. . . .

The session continued to focus on the parents overinvolvement with Margie. Among other things, the clinician implied that the parental "enmeshment" was causing Margie's problems and impeding her developmental growth. Two sessions later, at the clinician's suggestion, the parents agreed to pay for an apartment for Margie. Seven weeks after that, Margie was back in the hospital. While in many cases, eventual emancipation may remain the final goal of family, patient, and clinician, it is a goal to be worked on directly only after a patient has been able to *prove* his or her ability to function independently.

In handling familial involvement with the patient, it is again important to emphasize the strengths of family members and to reinforce and normalize their attempts to cope. When a mother says, "Our son is ill and our hearts are breaking; when our son suffers, we suffer," it is better to stress the normality of her concern and the inevitable emotional contagion that occurs when a family member is severely ill than to emphasize the potentially negative effect of enmeshment. The family's overinvolvement may simply be a result of coping with a seriously dysfunctional child. Only when anxiety is allayed and effective functioning has been restored is it reasonable to work towards increased differentiation, or decreased enmeshment, if it in fact still exists.

The following interchange took place between a clinician and the parents of a patient during the first family session following an emergency commitment. In this session, the clinician begins to redefine what is appropriate to expect in terms of emancipation of a seriously disturbed young woman.

FATHER: I want you to know, I don't want to be here, and I don't know why I'm here. Where's Sandy? *We've* been seen before and it never helped. In fact, it only made things worse!

CLINICIAN: I think it's important to answer your questions of why you're being seen.

FATHER: Yeah, how's that going to help Sandy?

CLINICIAN: This has been a very painful experience for everyone. It's also been going on for a long time. We believe you've done your best to help, and we want to help you in your efforts.

MOTHER: What do you mean?

CLINICIAN: Well, it's obvious that Sandy needs you now, and will continue to need you when she gets out. Maybe working together we can come up with ideas that will make her next time at home better for everyone and help her to feel and do better.

FATHER: Wait a second. Are you saying she's coming home? Every other shrink we've ever seen has thought it was bad for her to come home, that she's got to live on her own.

CLINICIAN: You and I both know she's not going to be ready for that for quite awhile. I guess we all hope that someday down the line, she will be, but that's *way* down the road.

FATHER: I agree! But these doctors, they seem to think you can push your kids out of the nest even when you *know* they can't fly. It made me feel like they thought our home was a bad place. . . . It sounds like you have children, too. Do you?

In this example, the clinician acknowledged the family's concern and recognized their potential resistance to family treatment based on past experiences. What the clinician said is true: Sandy was not ready for independent living. In so saying, he confirmed the family's perception of reality but left the door open for emancipation to be considered as a future goal.

The father ended this session still checking out the clinician and his qualifications. These challenges to the clinician's competence are reasonable and common, but they often anger professionals who further stimulate family doubt and resistance by responding defensively. Checking out a clinician's qualifications makes good sense for those who have had negative experiences with professionals in the past. After attempting to follow innumerable suggestions, plans, and medication regimes that have failed to help the patient, it seems healthy for patient and family to look at helping professionals with a skeptical eye. As the wife of one patient in our project said, "I've heard all the promises before." Thus, the challenge must be understood, accepted, and responded to with appropriate reassurance. In the case discussed above, the interaction continued in this way:

CLINICIAN: Yes, I have two children, a son, 9, and a daughter, 2.

FATHER: Hm . . . then maybe you understand. But I guess it's different when they're young.

CLINICIAN: (*Laughing*) Yeah, I don't know if I'm looking forward to adolescence.

FATHER: (*Smiling*) It can be tough, but you gotta be firm. My sons did pretty good.

CLINICIAN: So I heard, two bankers and a lawyer.

MOTHER: So, we must have done something right.
CLINICIAN: I'm sure you've done a lot right, even with Sandy.
FATHER: (*Smiling*) Were you born here?
CLINICIAN: No, I grew up in New York; but I've lived here 10 years.
FATHER: Been doing this all that time?
CLINICIAN: Yes.
FATHER: Don't you get bored?
CLINICIAN: Not as long as I think I can help, and I think I can.
FATHER: (*Smiling*) I hope so, but I have to let you know, we're not going to be easy.
CLINICIAN: I got that feeling.

In this case, the clinician enhances the connecting process by joining around the common identity of parenthood. He gives the strong and accurate message that Sandy's parents were and are competent in childrearing. By answering the father's questions directly, he implies that it is reasonable and appropriate to check out his credentials before agreeing to go along with the treatment program. Finally, the clinician offers a statement of hope for the future, while at the same time acknowledging the father's message that therapy will not be an easy process.

Establishing the Clinician as the Family Representative

Clinicians must establish themselves as family representatives or ombudsmen in relationship to the psychiatric system. The staff of most hospital and mental health systems find it easy to establish relationships with patients since their pain and disorganization are obvious. Particularly on inpatient units, staff come to know patients and to identify with their problems. Since staff members have not had to spend 24 hours a day with a decompensated patient in an uncontrolled environment, they are less likely to be sympathetic about, or to fully understand the family's plight and are thus more likely to be critical about the family's attempts to cope.

In their role, as liaison between families and the mental health system clinicians attend to the needs of other family members, provide the glue between inpatient and outpatient care, provide information to families, and help raise the consciousness of other members of the treatment team about the family's concerns.

Being an ombudsman requires a consistent effort to see things from the perspective of the patient's family. Procedures, policies, and decisions about patients must be explained to family members so that they come to feel they are genuinely being included in treatment.

Hospital systems themselves can be a source of concern and confusion. As the husband of one patient said, "The worst thing is not understanding what is going on. Is she going to get better? What are they doing to help her?" Frequently, the reports of patients only serve to cloud the family's understanding of the situation. When a hospitalized wife complains to her husband that the staff are all against her, he doesn't know if these ideas are a part of her illness or if the staff is being punitive. When she complains about group therapy, he may not know what group therapy is, much less whether there is a good reason for the confrontations between staff and other patients that his wife describes. Giving family members information about and reasons for the treatment plan and the hospital routine helps them to understand the system and elicits their support for treatment. Family members can feel that they are still important to the patient and that their own involvement and cooperation in treatment is meaningful.

In the following example, the clinician talks with the husband of a patient early in the course of the patient's hospitalization. She gives him specific information to help him understand what is happening to his wife.

CLINICIAN: I wanted to let you know that Joan is beginning to settle in on the unit and seems a little less agitated.

HUSBAND: She usually settles down as soon as she's in the hospital.

CLINICIAN: Oh, that's important to know.

HUSBAND: I visited yesterday and saw that she was calmer, but now she's just lying in her room.

CLINICIAN: That's because it was Sunday. Let me tell you about the ward routine. During the week, she'll be going to group therapy. (*Continues to describe the various therapies of the unit.*) And over the next 2 weeks in particular, they'll be evaluating her and trying to find out the right dose of medication—enough to get the symptoms under control, but not so much that she's oversedated. They'll keep adjusting it until things seem okay.

HUSBAND: Well, she sure seems out of it now . . . She's like a zombie. You know, she could hardly keep her eyes open when I visited. It doesn't seem to me that they're changing her drugs like you say. She's been on the same dose 2 days.

CLINICIAN: Well, 2 days is a short time with these drugs. It takes a while to get things to the right level. They also tend to have a sedating effect at first and some of that wears off. (*Gives more detail on the nature of the drug regime.*) But your feedback about how she seems is important and I'll share it with the inpatient staff. It will be taken into consideration in making any changes in her medication.

HUSBAND: Well, that's an all time first . . . I'll believe it when I see it.

CLINICIAN: You let me know if you don't see it. Okay?

In this example, the channels of communication are beginning to be established. The clinician gives specific information to help the husband understand the patient's lethargy and the behavior of the treatment staff. The clinician also gives the message that the staff and the family will be partners in the treatment process. Once again, the husband's statement of doubt is seen as reasonable, not as resistant. The clinician also establishes an agreement that the family's opinions, suggestions, and reactions will be shared with the treatment team. This is essential for two reasons: First, families really do know patients best. They may not be sure of what to do, but they are usually most aware of the patient's strengths and weaknesses and what has worked best in the past. For instance, a patient on an inpatient unit recently was refusing to take his medication. Threats and inducements by the staff were ineffective and were stimulating an increase in anger in both staff and patient. A major power struggle was brewing. The clinician reported this to the family, and the patient's father told him that the patient had done this during past hospitalizations in a different facility.

FATHER: He's done it three or four times. Once he told me he liked the staff getting upset. It showed they cared.

CLINICIAN: What happened that time?

FATHER: Well, what worked was me telling him to stop crapping around and take his medicine . . . and the nurses stopped pushing him.

The clinician took this suggestion to the treatment team and after some discussion, it was decided to try just what the father suggested: to ask the father to tell his son to "stop crapping around" and to stop pushing as a team. The problem cleared up almost immediately.

The second reason for incorporating family input into the decision-making process is to attempt to defuse or avoid potential problems that could occur in the future. If families adamantly disagree with treatment decisions, they will make it known sooner or later. If families are not included in the early plans, and if the goals are not mutual, it could impact negatively on treatment compliance and even destroy the therapeutic relationship altogether. For example, John's parents were very much against a placement in a halfway house. The inpatient staff, sure that it was in John's best interests, went ahead with the discharge planning, insisting that the reluctant family give the plan a try. After 3 days at the halfway house, John called his family and asked them to come to take him home. He said that he hated the halfway house, and his family didn't insist that he stay. He became noncompliant with medication 2 days later. After 5 weeks, he was back in the hospital. This time, the family was angry at the staff, and the staff was angry with the family. The family felt the staff had made a bad recommendation and the staff felt the family had sabotaged their plans by allowing John to come home. The staff had not really listened to the family's ideas in formulating the treatment plan, had overridden their concerns about a halfway house, and had not really prepared either John or his family for such a radical change in living arrangements. The staff thought they knew best and thus refused to use the family's experience in the formulation of a discharge plan.

Connecting with Patients

While connecting with the family is essential, it is important to establish a relationship concomitantly with the patient. These contacts should also begin as soon as possible, even when the patient is severely ill. Brief individual contacts with the patient, especially if he or she is on an inpatient unit, allow the clinician to establish familiarity and a beginning relationship even before including the patient in family sessions.

Although the notion of conducting separate connecting sessions with patients alone is inconsistent with the practices of most family therapists, it is useful for a number of reasons. First, it is difficult to establish a relationship with acutely disturbed patients in a family context. If they are not overtly psychotic during this time, they are likely to be angry and distressed. Many patients enter psychiatric treatment either involuntarily or under duress. During the course of their inpatient stay, they are likely to be ambivalent or even unwilling participants in their own treatment. Many of these patients do not believe that they are ill, and therefore, do not believe they require treatment. It is not surprising that, initially, they are uninterested in or unable to tolerate family sessions. Thus, enhancing the patients' willingness to cooperate with future treatment is best accomplished through brief individual contacts with the clinician. These talks help to develop a working relationship which offers some reason for returning for outpatient treatment.

Second, it is important for clinicians to establish themselves as sources of support for both family members *and* patients. While the ease with which staff can become overly aligned with patients has been discussed, the opposite also can happen. Since clinicians must (for reasons already cited) meet with family members a number of times without the patient, it is important that there be a number of contacts with the patient to insure a more balanced perspective. These individual contacts will help clinicians begin to gain some understanding of patients' perceptions of their families, their own problems, and their own needs. If clinicians are then able to convey their acceptance and understanding to patients, they can help patients to appreciate the potential usefulness of treatment in resolving the issues of greatest concern.

The initial contacts with patients by family clinicians should be kept very brief until the acute psychotic symptoms have been at least partially controlled. This is not to say patients must be able to make sense consistently, but it is best if they are aware enough of the events around them to remember the contact. If during a contact, patients begin to lose focus, clinicians should politely terminate the interaction and come back at another time. In the following example, the clinician makes one of several brief contacts with a patient who moves in and out of contact with reality.

CLINICIAN: Hi, Ellen. Do you remember me?

ELLEN: No. . . .

CLINICIAN: I'm Jack Carter, the clinician who sees your family. We talked yesterday.

ELLEN: (*Distractedly*) Oh, yes. Thanks for coming.

CLINICIAN: I saw your husband and children yesterday after we talked.

ELLEN: How are they? Are my kids okay?

CLINICIAN: They're fine and they asked me to say hello and tell you that they miss you. Is there anything you'd like me to tell them?

ELLEN: Could we conjugate the verb "to be" in Latin?

CLINICIAN: I'm afraid that doesn't make sense to me. Would you rather not talk about your family now?

ELLEN: I guess not. "To be" tells it all. Don't you think Latin is powerful?

CLINICIAN: It's okay. We don't have to talk right now. I just wanted to let you know I'm seeing them.

ELLEN: That's good. The staff here is very tense. I can tell by the way the shadows are falling on the wall that it's a plot.

CLINICIAN: I can see that it's hard for you to keep on a topic right now. How about if I come back later and we'll try again?

ELLEN: Okay.

The specific content of discussions at this point in time is less important than actually making contact and beginning to establish expectations about the kinds of communications and interactions that will be acceptable in treatment.

Through several very brief meetings, occurring for as long as the patient is able to stay in contact, the beginnings of a relationship can be facilitated. It is important to note, however, that prolonged discussions with an acutely psychotic patient are rarely productive. In particular, discussion of family issues when patients are this disorganized may stimulate anger and intense reactions and interfere with, rather than enhance, the formation of a therapeutic relationship. The following example came from the fourth meeting between the family clinician and Patrick. Patrick had been in the hospital for 10 days and although he was more stable then he had been on admission, he was still quite symptomatic.

> CLINICIAN: Hi, Pat. How are you doing today?
> PATRICK: Hi, Mrs. Norman. I'm pretty good. How about yourself?
> CLINICIAN: Not bad, a little tired, but otherwise fine. What have you been up to?
> PATRICK: Same stuff. Groups. I like talking to my nurse. She understands. Did you see my family?
> CLINICIAN: Last night. They're concerned about you.
> PATRICK: Yeah? (*Very skeptically*)
> CLINICIAN: Very much. You sound like you don't believe that?
> PATRICK: Well, I don't know. . . .
> CLINICIAN: How do you think they feel about you?
> PATRICK: I can't.
> CLINICIAN: Why not? It might be good to talk.
> PATRICK: Don't I know you from somewhere? Maybe MacDonalds?
> CLINICIAN: Don't you want to talk now?
> PATRICK: There's something wrong with my legs. (*Getting up*) See the way they bend. (*Laughs and starts to pace*) I don't like it here.

After this brief interchange, the clinician had to call another staff person to help Patrick settle down. What had started out as a pleasant exchange rapidly deteriorated because interaction moved too quickly into a discussion of highly intense family relationships. It is important that the clinician be sensitive to potentially "charged" issues, and to limit discussion of these topics as soon as emotions begin to rise.

During the initial contacts with patients, family clinicians are generally viewed as just one of a number of professionals assigned to the case. This is an important perception to encourage since a long-term goal is for both patient and family to accept and to relate to the entire treatment team. Nevertheless, it is also important for the patient to recognize that the family clinician has been meeting with the patient's family and keeping them informed about the patient's progress and the hospital program. Patients should be made aware of the purpose of these meetings, and any questions they pose should be answered clearly and directly.

Even during these initial contacts, the focus should be on how treatment can potentially help the patient. As in the family meetings, however, care must be taken not to reinforce unrealistic goals. It is easy to begin a relationship by agreeing with patients about their grandiose plans or unachievable goals. But, in the long run, this practice will lead to severe difficulties and conflicts. It is best to be realistic about what clinicians can and cannot do to help, even if this may prolong and complicate the joining process.

The following example came from the first meeting between Roger and the family clinician. Roger was court committed and had been in the hospital for 7 days. The meeting took place on the inpatient unit.

CLINICIAN: Hello, Roger. I'm Dr. Simon. I was wondering if I could chat with you for a few minutes.

ROGER: (*Long pause*) Who are you?

CLINICIAN: My name is Dr. Simon. I'm part of the treatment team. I've been meeting with your wife and children since you've been in the hospital.

ROGER: You've what? She put me here. I don't want to see her— or you.

CLINICIAN: I can understand your anger. Let me explain why I've been seeing them.

ROGER: (*Silent glare*)

CLINICIAN: They have been very concerned and upset about what happened and how you are feeling.

ROGER: They're upset? What about me?

CLINICIAN: I hear that you're upset also. That's why I wanted to talk with you, too. Your wife and children care a lot about what's been going on and how you're doing.

ROGER: They do? Well they had a funny way of showing it.

CLINICIAN: They do care and certainly would like to see you to tell you themselves.

ROGER: Well . . . I'll think about it.

CLINICIAN: Fine. I'd also like to chat with you occasionally. That way we can get to know each other, and also I can better let your family know how you're doing.

ROGER: I guess it's okay. I talk to enough people already. One more won't hurt.

During the initial contact the clinician focused on the exclusive goals of introducing and identifying herself and defusing the patient's anger. She acknowledged the patient's upset but avoided pursuing it any further. Two contacts later, the clinician explained her role in more detail.

CLINICIAN: I've told you a couple of times that I've been meeting with your family and would like to continue to meet with all of you.

ROGER: You mean me and them together?

CLINICIAN: Right. I'd like to explain why I think it's important.

ROGER: I can think of one reason. I'm still angry.

CLINICIAN: That's true, I guess, although it sounds like you're a little less angry. Anyway, I think there may be some ways to make it possible for you and your wife to have fewer problems after you're discharged from the hospital.

ROGER: Like how?

CLINICIAN: Well, that's what I'd like to discuss with you now and also with you and the family together when they come in. You mentioned one thing last time we talked about having trouble keeping jobs, and how that stirs things up with your wife.

ROGER: Yeah, I've got a family to support.

CLINICIAN: I know—and I know you want to support them. I think helping you get a job after you're feeling better and more energetic is one thing we can do.

ROGER: Really? That would *really* help.

CLINICIAN: Really. I also think I may be able to help you and your family to deal better with your illness and help prevent another hospitalization.

ROGER: Hm. . . . Well, a job would be great. You say we'll be meeting with you even after the hospital?

CLINICIAN: Yes. I don't want to kid you. I don't think you'll be ready for a job overnight. But, I'd like to work with you and the family toward that and other goals you all may have, as well as dealing with your illness better.

ROGER: Well, maybe it doesn't sound as bad as I thought. I'll think about it.

CLINICIAN: Fine. We can talk more about it the next time we meet.

During this connecting session, the clinician begins to offer some reasons for the patient to engage in treatment. She stresses the relevance of involving Roger's family and introduces the issue of learning new ways to cope with the illness (obviously a significant issue) without focusing on it to the point of creating conflict. She accepts Roger's hesitancy, and does not force an immediate decision. Finally, she

attempts to connect treatment with the goal that seems most relє
to the patient, that of getting a job.

Establishing a Treatment Contract

The need for the patient and the family to participate in ongoing treatment is made explicit and operationalized by the creation of a treatment contract. The contract specifies a step-by-step move from crisis intervention to the limited goal of patient survival in the outside world, to the long-term goal of encouraging genuine reintegration into social and work functioning. Such a contract involves a mutual agreement about the goals, content, length, and methods of therapy. The family's main complaints and concerns are translated by the clinician into clear, specific, and attainable goals. If a complaint is unreasonable or a goal is unattainable, the clinician negotiates with the family toward "the possible." If there are crucial goals the family has not mentioned spontaneously, the clinician can suggest they be placed on the treatment agenda, but should never do so unilaterally.

If treatment begins while a patient is hospitalized, specific efforts must be made to have the contract differentiate between the goals of hospitalization and the goals of outpatient treatment. Based on the realities of time constraints, the major goals of short-term inpatient care with this population can only be to provide the patient with a beginning sense of control, to provide the family with a brief respite from having to cope with the illness, and to get some initial agreement as to the terms of aftercare. Therefore, during this time, no emphasis should be placed on behaviors, insights, or feelings that do not directly aid the patient's return to the community. In this way, the goals of inpatient treatment can be kept specific and focused on concrete issues and practical management techniques. Making this message explicit with families will keep expectations low and help to dispel any remaining myths that hospitalization can solve all the patient's problems. As the patient and family move into outpatient treatment, the basic goals change. The first goal is to keep the patient out of the hospital by decreasing stress for both patient and family. The second goal is to return the patient to effective functioning in the community.

The initial contract formation process usually has two phases: the inpatient component and the ongoing outpatient treatment component. These two components are interrelated. The former deals with the establishment of short-term goals necessary for the patient to leave the hospital, as well as focusing on the family's preparations for the patient's reentry into the home. The family is helped to understand that because hospitalization tends to be brief, it is highly likely that the patient will return home still symptomatic. Families are helped, as part of the contract, to decide on the most basic rules for behavior that they will expect the patient to abide by at home. The clinician negotiates these rules with the family (first with family members alone and then with the patient present), and together they develop realistic guidelines based on a knowledge of the illness, the patient, and the needs of other family members.

Whether the patient begins treatment as an inpatient or not, the first major emphasis of the contract should be on the phase of treatment that occurs immediately after the acute psychotic episode. Careful attention to symptoms and stresses at this early time can be extremely useful in avoiding recurrent crises. Chronic illnesses require continuity of care over time, rather than crisis oriented care. In preparing the patient and family for such long-term treatment, the slow nature of change and the need for mutual goals of treatment must be emphasized. The family must agree to attend sessions and to work on the goals that have been established. The clinician must agree to be available to both patient and family, to represent them in their dealings with the treatment system, and to provide advice and practical help as needed.

Although many issues will not be addressed directly for months or even years to come, long-term goals for the patient and family should be formulated. (Making these goals explicit helps to make the short-term goals seem more relevant, and helps to maintain hope for more significant change over time.) Long-term goals may include such things as beginning or returning to work or school, more social interaction, and, finally, more independent living. In most cases, however, the emphasis is placed on first negotiating the intermediate steps or tasks needed for the achievement of long-term goals. In the following example, taken from the first family session with the patient present, just such a negotiation took place.

TONY: I don't know how these sessions will help me. I just need a job and a place to live that's safe.

FATHER: Oh, no, here we go again. What do you mean "safe"?

TONY: (*Long pause*) I can't talk about it.

MOTHER: I can't believe it, you still have those worries. (*To clinician*) That's part of the problem, these worries.

TONY: (*Looks down uncomfortably*)

CLINICIAN: Okay, there are two separate issues here. One, Tony's goals for the future and, two, the presence of some symptoms. I'd like to talk about them one at a time. First, let's discuss the fact that you still have some worries.

In this session, the clinician first addresses the fact that Tony is still symptomatic, feeling that unless this fact was adequately handled, neither Tony nor his family would be able to focus on contracting for future goals. After he felt Tony's parents had some understanding about why Tony still had some symptoms, the clinician focused the discussion on goal negotiation.

CLINICIAN: Tony, if you feel as though you can control your worries for a while, I'd still like to discuss some goals. (*To the family*) Tony mentioned two: work and living on his own. Tony, you asked how these sessions can help. Well, I think we can help you to achieve those goals—and they're really good ones.
TONY: Really?
CLINICIAN: Really.
TONY: The doctor told me "no way."
CLINICIAN: Well, I guess I'm looking further into the future. I think we need to first talk about some of the steps needed to get there. First, let me hear how your family feels about these goals.
MOTHER: It's our dream.
FATHER: I agree. We're afraid to even think about it. You know he hasn't worked since he got out of high school 5 years ago.
CLINICIAN: Well, I still think they are achievable goals—in the long run. We've had a lot of success in getting people back to work but it's taken some time. (*To Tony*) I know you're eager, but our best success has happened when we've taken a slow, step-by-step approach. Let's talk about some short-term goals that will help to get you ready to go to work.

In this example, the clinician suggests that Tony's goals may be achievable, offering hope to the entire family. However, in beginning the process of goal negotiation, he states that the time schedule will be an extended one. He reinforces his own credibility by stressing his experience with other patients, mentioning the success other patients have achieved in following a relatively slow-paced schedule. He proceeds to connect the long-term mutually agreed upon goals to short-term goals that otherwise would not seem important.

CLINICIAN: I wonder if we can't focus on the next couple of months right now. Tony will be leaving the hospital soon. I think he'll be feeling better than when he first came here but he's still going to need some recuperation time.
TONY: I told you what I need.
MOTHER: The doctor already answered you about that, you can't—
CLINICIAN: That's true, but Tony, you did mention needing a place to live that's safe. I'd like for our first goals to be focused on how to make your home a comfortable and safe place for everyone.

TONY: (*Pause*) Well, it won't be . . . there is no place I can go to be my myself—not even my room.

MOTHER: We were scared to let him out of our sight.

CLINICIAN: I can understand that. Luckily, things seem calmer now, and everybody needs privacy now and then. I'd think both Tony and you two could use time outs once in awhile.

FATHER: I know *I* could, but only if I didn't have to worry about Tony.

CLINICIAN: Well, then our first goal should be to build in comfortable ways for everyone to have privacy.

As the session continues, the clinician makes this goal more concrete and begins to work on developing other achievable short-term goals. Thus, through negotiation, the family evolves a contract consisting of a hierarchical series of small goals leading toward the achievement of Tony's stated long-term goals of work and independent living.

Not only the patient's problems, but also the needs of family members should be considered in making decisions about the terms of the contract. The current emotional, social, and financial stresses of family members is relevant to the patient's continuing care and also for its own sake. During the crisis of an acute psychosis, many of these stressors are overlooked or put aside since everyone's energy must be directed toward helping the patient. The following example came from the second session of contract negotiations with Charles and his family.

CLINICIAN: I think we've come up with a number of excellent goals and some good ways to go about achieving them. . . .

FATHER: I agree.

CLINICIAN: But, you know in reviewing our discussion last week, I realized I had overlooked something important and wanted to bring it up this time.

MOTHER: What's that? I thought we covered almost everything.

CLINICIAN: Well, regarding Charlie, yes. But a couple of weeks ago, you mentioned that Carl [the patient's brother] was having some school problems recently, and I wanted to check that out. Is that true, Carl?

CARL: Yeah, well . . . sort of.

FATHER: His grades dropped a lot the last marking period.

CLINICIAN: Right. You brought that up before, and I thought perhaps we could discuss it now briefly, if that's okay with you, Carl.

CARL: I guess so . . . I don't know. Nobody seemed to care much and there was so much going on, I guess I didn't care either.

MOTHER: Of course, we care. It's just that . . . well, we had our hands full.

CARL: I know.

FATHER: You've got to understand. Charlie needed us. I thought you *did* understand.

CARL: (*Looking down*) I do.

CLINICIAN: We've talked about how it was a rough time for everyone, including you, Carl, and we've also been talking about goals. With your permission, I'd like to suggest that we put getting your grades back up on the list also.

CARL: This is silly. You don't have to worry about me.

MOTHER: We do worry and we do care. I guess we haven't shown it much lately.

CLINICIAN: Maybe we can come up with some ideas as to how the family can help you in achieving this goal.

CARL: (*Visably brighter*) Well, okay.

Although not part of the initial contract negotiations, the clinician brought up another issue that had come up during the assessment. He felt it was important enough to be addressed at that point because Carl clearly felt neglected, and it was better to attend to the problem before it escalated and created even more stress for the family. Nevertheless, he solicited the family's permission before placing an issue not immediately related to the presenting problem on the agenda.

Occasionally, clinicians become aware of other family difficulties (i.e., marital conflict that, while important, would be unlikely to interfere with the achievement of the initial goals of the contract). At those times, it is often better to postpone dealing with the issue until other stresses have been at least partially resolved. Sometimes focusing on these other family issues actually increases stress and decreases the amount of energy the family has to cope with the immediate crisis. In the following example, the clinician gently postpones dealing with the marital issues of two parents whose son, George, was only recently hospitalized.

MOTHER: You asked about other problems, well . . . to be honest we haven't gotten along in years. We don't agree on anything.

CLINICIAN: Is that so?

FATHER: Well, she's been so involved with George she never had time for me. I moved into the guest room 4 years ago, I think. . . .

MOTHER: You just don't see him the way that I do. He needs us. You go to work, you don't see the things he does.

FATHER: He wouldn't do half the stuff if you'd set some limits.

MOTHER: He doesn't understand, but it isn't only George . . . it's been that way. . . .

CLINICIAN: So what I'm hearing is that there are problems in your relationship and problems in coming to some agreement about how to handle George?

FATHER: Yes.

MOTHER: (*Nods*)

CLINICIAN: Well, those are certainly both important issues. What I would like to suggest is we work first on coming to some agreement about how to manage George. You don't even have to like each other a lot to do that, since you both care about George. After things are more settled with him, if you want to work on the marriage, we can talk about it.

FATHER: That makes sense, I guess. Maybe if we could agree on him, we wouldn't have so many problems with each other.

Before anyone agrees to a contract, they must be convinced that it will benefit them. The first step in negotiating the contract, therefore, is to deal with the sense of hopelessness that is often encountered in people who have lived with this illness for any length of time. As shown, sharing the positive experiences of other families tends to help give a sense that change is possible. Defining the family as a powerful agent of positive change also can be helpful. Over the years, many families lose sight of their potential to be a positive influence on the course of the patient's illness. For this reason, the concern that most families feel is defined as caring that can be put into effective action by learning about the illness and following some of the prescriptions of the program. In the following example, a clinician begins to deal with one family's sense of hopelessness.

FATHER: You know we've been talking about this contract for the whole session. It sounds all well and good but look at her [the patient, Laura]. I don't think we'll ever get anywhere. She doesn't want to get better.

LAURA: (*Looks angrily at father*)

CLINICIAN: How does everyone else feel?

MOTHER: I hate to say so but, I don't have much hope either.

MELISSA: [sister] It's been the same way for 4 years.

CLINICIAN: I certainly can understand everyone's feelings. It has been a long time, and I guess I'd be a little doubtful, too. But, I've got to say that in listening to the family talk earlier, I'm impressed with how well everyone has done in dealing with a tough situation.

FATHER: I think we've done a great job, too, but nothing we've done, nothing anyone else has done for that matter, has ever really helped Laura.

CLINICIAN: Well, I don't know about that. You've helped her to avoid going into the hospital a number of times, and you've been able to get on with your own lives at the same time. I'd say that's a sign of just how strong the family is. . . .

MOTHER: It is a good family. We're really proud of our children.

CLINICIAN: You should be. And I know this strength and caring can be used to help Laura. I also believe that Laura wants the help. With the strength of this program and your help, I believe we can achieve the goals that we've discussed.

LAURA: I *do* want to get better.

MOTHER: It's good to hear you say that.

FATHER: Like I said, the contract idea sounds good. We're not really ready to give up. We just get discouraged.

In this example, the clinician refuses to accept the family's sense of impotence. He avoids dealing directly with the issue of Laura's motivation but rather focuses on the family's abilities to cope and the fact that they care enough to have remained involved through years of frustrating attempts to help their daughter. In addition, he links the strength of the program with the strength of the family as a powerful dyad to help effect change. While he has not convinced the family that change will occur, he has begun to combat their sense of discouragement.

Although it is important to stress the possibility of change, care must be taken not to imply that it will be a simple task. Families who have been coping with schizophrenia for a long time are acutely aware of the enormity of the problems involved, and will rightfully challenge any clinician who minimizes them. Those families who are dealing with the illness for the first time have another struggle. They must come to recognize that recuperation is a slow process that will require an enormous amount of time and energy, from the patient and from them.

In either case, to concretely reinforce the messages of the program, it is best to push for a renewable contract of at least a year. A contract of this length (in contrast to the short-term contract used in most family approaches) is important for a number of reasons. It stresses the severity of the problem and the length of time needed for recuperation. It reinforces the importance of maintaining relatively low expectations for the immediate future, which eases pressure on the patient, the family, and the clinician. Finally, it says to the family that the clinician is also making a commitment to them to be available for advice and support during the many difficult months that will follow.

In the following example, the clinician is attempting to renegotiate a treatment contract with Ron and his family a few months after Ron's first psychotic episode. As with many patients and families experiencing a first episode, once the acute crisis has passed, the need for treatment begins to be questioned. Everyone has the hope that the patient will never become ill again, and therefore, the belief that the patient may not need treatment on an ongoing basis.

FATHER: Don't get me wrong, we appreciate your help. We've sure learned a lot. When Ron got sick, it was frightening and confusing. But, he's better now.

MOTHER: What Joe's saying is, we're not really sure as to why we're talking about goals. Ron's doing better. We'd all just like to forget about the past. We don't think we need to keep coming here.

CLINICIAN: I can certainly understand your feelings. It would be nice to be able to put this behind you and get on with it.

FATHER: Right.

CLINICIAN: Well, as we've discussed, there is a chance that this will never happen again, and I really hope for that.

RON: It won't.

CLINICIAN: Good . . . but it was frightening and it is a serious illness. As we've mentioned, the first year is the time of highest risk. I'd like to help to make sure things continue to go well during this time and that the whole family can get back on track.

FATHER: Well, I'm still not sure we need it, but I guess we can talk about it some more. Maybe it wouldn't hurt to come for a while, just to make sure. How about it, Ron?

RON: I guess.

The clinician attempts to present an accurate picture without becoming too pessimistic, all the while respecting the family's desire to put the illness behind them. In this manner, she negotiates a contract that focuses on helping the patient and family through a high-risk time that everyone seems willing to accept, albeit reluctantly.

Preparing the Patient and Family for a Team Approach

A group of professionals, available to both the patient and the family, is central to an effective program for patients with a chronic illness. One clinician may be responsible for the patient's medication while another is responsible for the family, and perhaps even a third responsible for issues of vocational and social rehabilitation. Usually, each clinician also has a supervisor, so the number of professionals who know about a given case is quite large. It is helpful if all of these individuals can work together to maximize the possible benefits of treatment.

In the treatment of schizophrenia, effective therapy for patients and families begins with effective support for staff. Patients with schizophrenia usually make slow progress. Working with these cases takes a great deal of time, energy, and patience. Months of therapeutic work can go down the drain with an attempt to push the patient back to work before he is ready. Hard-won stability of functioning for a patient can be threatened by something as simple as a brief vacation of a clinician. For these reasons, staff treating patients with chronic disorders and their families are unusually susceptible to clinician fatigue, hopelessness about the possibility of change, and increased vulnerability to the acceptance of resistance.

A team approach provides some protection from these problems (Beels, 1975). Team members can support one another and supply a dose of reality when one member becomes overinvolved or develops too high or too low expectations. Those members of a team who are less involved with day to day treatment can observe and identify subtle signs of change or progress unseen by the more directly involved clinicians, thus increasing objectivity and morale. Team members can cover for one another's absences, providing ongoing availability to patients and families. Furthermore, rather than encouraging an intensive relationship between the patient/family and one professional (which in itself can be stressful to such patients), patients and their families can be encouraged to use the entire treatment team as a resource. An "institutional transference" can be stressed, one in which all members of the team *together* are regarded as "the clinician."

The presence of a united team of professionals communicates to families a general availability and a joint philosophy of care. Families should be helped to use the entire team in the best interests of the patient. The following interaction between the clinician and the parents of a patient new to the psychoeducational program begins to establish the availability of team members and how they can be used.

MOTHER: What should we do if a problem comes up?

CLINICIAN: I was just going to bring that up. A member of the team is available 24 hours a day if a crisis arises or if you have any questions. I'm going to give you a list with our telephone numbers and also the telephone numbers of the emergency room and the switchboard. The switchboard can get in touch with a team member at any time.

FATHER: Are you serious? You're always available? You must get exhausted.

CLINICIAN: Well, you can always call me. But one of the benefits for me and for your family is that there's always someone covering for me in my absence.

MOTHER: Wow! This is something new.

Like many, these parents are reacting with surprise and pleasure to the accessibility of the staff. Many family members and patients have occasion to test out the validity of this promise early in treatment, as questions and crises arise. Once assured that a staff member truly is available when needed, most become more comfortable with trying new techniques of managing things at home.

Common Problems in the Implementation of Connecting Strategies

When Families Won't Come at All

Some families have become so alienated from treatment systems or so hopeless about the possibility of change that they absolutely refuse to come in for sessions, or if they do, they seem unable to mobilize any energy to consider psychiatric help again. They tend not to hear supportive messages either because they have become defensive about the patient, the patient's illness, and their own perception of their role in it, or because they cannot afford to have their hopes once more raised and disappointed.

There are a number of options open to clinicians trying to convince such families about the potential usefulness of the psychoeducational family program. First, the clinician's attitude and the information shared during the initial phone contact is important. The message to be conveyed is that the family's involvement is not only important, but essential in treating the patient appropriately. Clinicians should be neither defensive nor angry about the family's negative or skeptical responses which are reasonable under the circumstances. Thus, time should be taken to explain how family members can help and what clinicians have to offer this time. If these explanations fail to work, the family should be encouraged to come in for just one trial session. Most families will agree to try anything once. However, if even this fails, the clinician can ask if it is possible to visit the family in their home. The perseverance, sincerity, and consistency of the clinician's message about the importance of the family's involvement is crucial in beginning the process of joining. If reluctant family members agree to come, the clinician should be as accommodating as possible about the time of a trial session, without necessarily implying that this will always be the case. This flexibility gives the important message that the clinician is aware of the family's reluctance and is attempting to meet their needs.

The following example was taken from an initial phone contact with the mother of the patient. The family had not accompanied the patient to the hospital although he was living at home at the time of the hospitalization.

CLINICIAN: Hello, Mrs. P. This is Peggy J. I'm the family representative from the hospital. I've just been told that Rich is a patient here, and I wanted to talk to you.

MRS. P : Yes?

CLINICIAN: I was hoping that I could meet with you and the rest of the family to discuss Rich and what we both might be able to do to help him to get back on his feet.

MRS. P : Well, this is a very bad time for us. My husband is working a lot of overtime.

CLINICIAN: Hm . . . that's tough. Well, I can understand that. Perhaps there's a time that's more convenient for you than others?

MRS. P : I don't see why you need to see us anyway. We've been in therapy before. All that happened in those sessions was that Rich yelled at us. We don't need that.

CLINICIAN: I don't blame you for feeling that way. No one needs that. I'm sorry that you've had a bad therapy experience. This time will not be like that, I promise. I'd like to work with you in helping Rich. You folks know a lot more about him than we'll ever know, and we're going to need your help to best help Rich.

MRS. P : Well, as I said, this is a busy time . . . and our car is in the shop. My husband is exhausted when he isn't working . . . it's just bad. . . .

CLINICIAN: I understand, and yet I feel it's essential to get your help. I was wondering . . . perhaps I could come to your home at a time convenient to you to discuss this with you.

MRS. P : (*Pause*) You'd come here? Well, maybe . . . I'd have to talk to my husband, but maybe some evening.

CLINICIAN: That would be fine. How about if I call back tomorrow morning to set up a time?

MRS. P : Fine.

In this example the clinician acknowledged Mrs. P's perceptions of past treatment, and then focused on her needs for the parents' expert help in dealing with Rich. She reinforced this message by being as accommodating as possible to the family, attempting to diffuse any resistance with her understanding, flexibility and perseverance.

When Family Problems Interfere with Initiating Treatment

There are times when the chaotic state of some families interferes with the formation of an appropriate treatment contract. This is often likely when the patient is one of the parents. Even if the family in such cases is willing to be involved in treatment, the focus of treatment sessions can become diffuse when one of the individuals responsible for providing leadership in the family is disturbed. The focus of treatment can also wander when families are dealing with multiple crises that deplete the energy needed to deal with the illness and its treatment.

In both situations, it is necessary for clinicians to take a more directive role. They must help establish an external structure that enables families to form a treatment contract that states clear priorities and offers guidance in taking the initial steps to achieve them.

In the following example, the patient, is the 52-year-old widowed mother of eight children ranging from 10–21 years of age. The excerpt comes from the seventh session with the family, but only the second session in which the patient was present since the acute phase of her illness was very slow to resolve.

CLINICIAN: Well, everyone made it again. I'm impressed. Who organized the caravan?

JOAN: [18 years old] I did. But what a hassle! Up until 5 minutes before we left almost nobody was home.

CLINICIAN: Well, I appreciate your efforts. . . .

TOM: [14 years old] (Sarcastically) Yeah, sometimes she thinks she's Mom.

JOE: [16 years old] (Resentfully) Yeah.

JOAN: That's not true, but somebody had to get everyone together.

CLINICIAN: I agree on both counts. No one can take the place of your mother. She's the boss. But at this time, until your mother gets back on her feet, we need someone who can help out.

MARY: [19 years old] We all help out, but we have our own problems to deal with, too.

CLINICIAN: I understand, and they're important. I also believe that everyone helps out. I don't want to overburden anyone. In fact, I'd like to make it easier for everyone. One way is for all of you to know what's expected in this helping out. Your mother is going to take more charge soon, but, until then needs some help and also needs to know what to expect.

MOTHER: I'd appreciate it.

CLINICIAN: Okay, I know things can get disorganized at home, but I'd like to come up today with a list of exactly what each person will do to make things easier—no more or less.

In this example, the clinician attempts to bypass the issues between siblings which tend to stimulate conflict and dissension. He gives the message that the mother is a parent who may actively resume that role in the future, but stresses the fact that everyone must pick up some of the responsibility until that happens. Finally, he acknowledges that the children are helping out, while emphasizing the need to come up with a more systematic way of helping to avoid chaos.

Families that are dealing with multiple crises have less energy to direct toward the goal of helping a specific patient to recuperate. In these situations, clinicians must determine how much help other family members may need. Since the crises that arise in the treatment of multiproblem families are often not related to the illness and are not part of the original treatment contract, decisions to focus on these areas must be negotiated with relevant family members (see p. 61). The ultimate goal does not have to be complete resolution of any given crisis, but rather to help the family gain a greater sense of control.

The following example came from an emergency session, scheduled following a phone call from Mrs. L who was highly distraught because her 17-year-old daughter, Lisa, had run away from home. Their son, Stuart, the patient, had been home from the hospital for 4 weeks.

MOTHER: I don't know what to do. We're frantic.

FATHER: I've been driving all over looking for her, and Elizabeth [his wife] has been calling everyone we can think of. We're ready to call the police.

CLINICIAN: I don't know Lisa that well. What do you think were her reasons for leaving?

STUART: (*Obviously symptomatic*) She knows about the plot!

FATHER: He's been a lot worse, too. And that sure doesn't help.

CLINICIAN: I'm sure everyone is upset and worried. I sure would be. It sounds like you have taken all the right steps. . . .

MOTHER: Do you think we should call the police?

CLINICIAN: Well I'm still not sure exactly what Lisa's reasons were for leaving, but—

FATHER: She's been having a rough time lately. Some school problems and then her boyfriend broke up with her. I think Stu's coming home was the last straw, but I don't think he caused it.

STUART: I warned her.

CLINICIAN: Okay. As I said, I think you've taken the right steps and I think it's fine to continue to call around. I hope that Lisa will come home on her own accord, but perhaps you should notify the police since they can cover a lot more territory than you can.

MOTHER: That's true.

CLINICIAN: I also would like to suggest three other things that may help to tone things down a little during this time. First, it's obvious that Stu is very upset and concerned also. (*To Stuart*) I'd like to have you talk to Mary [his nurse clinician] just to check on your medication.

MOTHER: We'd appreciate that.

STUART: Well, all right.

CLINICIAN: Second, if it's all right with you I'd like to call you each day until Lisa comes home. That way, I know what's going on, but also I can offer some support. Also, I'd like to speak with Stuart briefly at those times, just to see how he's doing. Third, when Lisa returns, I'd like to see her since she's obviously pretty upset right now. Perhaps I can arrange for someone to talk to her.

FATHER: That's just fine.

CLINICIAN: I realize my suggestions don't solve the problems.

MOTHER: They help. It just helps to know someone has some ideas of what to do.

Although the clinician could not offer any concrete solutions to this significant crisis, she recognized the family's need for support and greater control. She offered suggestions designed to do both. By suggesting that Stuart check with his nurse clinician, she attempted to tone down the familial stress and give the parents one less thing to worry about. By offering someone special just for Lisa, she demonstrated respect and concern for Lisa's issues, not just those of the patient.

SUMMARY

The major task of the connecting phase of treatment is the development of a working relationship between the clinician and all members of the family, including the patient. This working relationship is achieved by using sessions to review the course of the illness and its treatment, and to discuss the impact of both on the lives of family members. It is further facilitated by making a specific effort to give family members the message that the clinician does not believe that families cause this illness, while emphasizing that families do have the ability to influence its course positively.

During the connecting phase, the clinician plays the role of family representative to the rest of the treatment system, prepares the family for ongoing family sessions, and establishes a treatment contract with patient and family that contains specific, attainable, and mutual goals. The contract specifically differentiates between the sessions immediately following the acute episode which must concentrate on the patient's survival in the outside world, and later sessions which must deal with long-term issues such as a gradual return to work and social functioning. In all sessions during the connecting phase attention must be given to providing a reasonable sense of hope for the future, without encouraging unrealistic expectations. Finally, clinicians should be prepared for reluctance on the part of some families to become involved in treatment, and more specifically to be prepared for challenges of their own competence and ability to help. If these challenges are accepted as reasonable ones under the circumstances, and if clinicians can avoid becoming defensive, the process of connecting with patients and families can be greatly enhanced.

CHAPTER THREE

THE SURVIVAL SKILLS WORKSHOP

What bothers me most is not knowing. I don't know what they're doing for her. I don't know what has to be done. Not knowing is what's getting to me.—Father of a patient, shortly after the 15th hospital admission in 7 years

Our understanding of schizophrenia and its underlying biochemical and neurological processes has expanded over the last 2 decades. While professionals still cannot fully explain the causes and effects of schizophrenia we believe it is time to begin sharing what is known with patients and families who are understandably confused about schizophrenia's pathogenesis, course, and treatment. Information is a valuable asset to a family trying to cope with this devastating disorder. This chapter will provide a rationale for giving families of patients the best available information about the illness, describe one format for doing so, and list some of the possible content that can be shared.

RATIONALE

This model of psychoeducational family intervention is based on the assumption that providing information to families with a severely ill member is extremely important and valuable. Under current mental health policies, patients with schizophrenia are maintained in their communities whenever possible. Families have become the primary caretakers of these patients, and thus they are more involved than ever in determining the patient's fate. Caring for a severely disturbed patient is a difficult task. Information helps family members to develop a sense of mastery about a sometimes chaotic and seemingly uncontrollable process. A sense of mastery is associated with a decrease in fear, anxiety, and confusion that, in turn, can free up energies that could better be used for coping with the illness and its ramifications.

Considering the complex nature of schizophrenia, the normal instinctive responses of both patients and families to the crises of illness and hospitalization may not always be the most helpful ones.

When someone in a family becomes ill, whatever the illness, most families attempt to help that person by being supportive, involved, tolerant, and by doing all they can. For patients with schizophrenia, these normal responses, which would be helpful in coping with most illnesses, can make things worse. Intense interpersonal involvement and permissive, unstructured environments tend to increase stress and reinforce inappropriate behaviors. Distressed, disorganized, and amotivated patients are more likely to respond positively to limit setting, control, and moderate interpersonal distance. Information about these unusual needs of patients with schizophrenia can help many family members create a more controlled, predictable, low-key environment that will aid patients in their own attempts to cope.

Knowledge about the illness and its course can help family members develop realistic expectations and plans for the future. Rather than clinging to unrealistic hopes that the illness will go away, or becoming overwhelmed with hopelessness, family members can begin to understand and accept limitations imposed by the illness. Thus, information can allow the establishment of appropriate and achievable short-term and long-term goals for patients, and even for other family members and the family as a whole. Hopefully, this will decrease the likelihood that pressure will be placed on patients early in the course of the illness, when they are least able to tolerate it. It also can help family members to understand when to begin to expect and demand more from patients to prevent them from stagnating at levels below their functional abilities.

The provision of information changes the relationship between professionals and family members. Traditionally, the mental health community has been reluctant to share information related to diagnosis, course, and outcome of psychiatric illnesses with patients and their families. The reasons for this lack of communication are multiple but most probably relate to our own discomfort and prejudice. Because we know neither what causes nor cures these illnesses, we tend to maintain covert beliefs that psychiatric disorders are not illnesses, but rather moral weaknesses, pathological responses to pathological environments, or self-indulgent malingering. We also tend to feel that these illnesses are hopeless and that accurate information could only serve to make things worse by making everyone more pessimistic, while inaccurate information would give false hope.

Whatever the reasons for not sharing information with patients and family members in the past, this position has become increasingly untenable. For years, out of guilt, confusion, and the desire not to alienate professionals, patients and families have stood by and accepted the treatments that were offered, often without explanation. Rarely was their input asked for or heard. More recently, however, the "informed consent" movement, along with patient advocacy and self-help groups, have enabled patients and families, individually and collectively, to stand up and demand information and to be included in decisions that impact on their lives (Deasy & Quinn, 1955; Hatfield, 1979; Kint, 1977; Lamb & Oliphant, 1978). Nevertheless, many mental health professionals still fail to tell either patients or their families much about the illness, its treatment, or the treatment system itself. Family members are sometimes given sympathy but they are rarely given information that might help them to develop effective methods of coping with very disturbing behaviors. This usually leaves them ill equipped to manage severely disturbed patients who frequently are discharged from inpatient units only partially recovered. Ironically, when problems then arise in maintaining such patients in their homes, professionals often blame families, and a cycle of mistrust and misunderstanding between families and professionals begins. Professionals argue that information can be upsetting or discouraging to families. However, most families claim that not knowing about the illness is worse than any information they have ever received, no matter how grim the data about course and prognosis may be. No professional has *all* the answers. No one is yet able to say that if you do X, patients will not relapse, and if you do Y, they will. Nevertheless, it is possible to begin to share what *is* known with families.

The change in the atmosphere of therapeutic relationships that occurs with the provision of information has a number of ramifications. For instance, dealing with an increasingly sophisticated public no longer allows professionals the luxury of "assumed omnipotence." Providers of psychiatric care and medical care must be explicit about what they are doing, by what method, and with what potential risks and benefits. It is expected that procedures will be explained in a way that allows patients and their families to make choices and to give truly informed consent, thus establishing the possibility of greater openness and increased mutual respect. While these changes may be uncomfortable for professionals initially, in time it may help them by decreasing unwarranted professional arrogance about unproven treatments while stimulating a commitment to an ongoing pursuit of knowledge.

Information can be provided in a number of ways, including the written word or conversations over the course of treatment. It can be given in a series of multiple family group sessions (Plummer, Thornton, Seeman, & Littmann, 1981; Zelitch, 1980) or in the day-long workshop format described here and elsewhere (Anderson *et al.*, 1980; Anderson, Hogarty, & Reiss, 1981; McFarlane, 1983). The last two methods are advantageous since a format can be used that allows several families to come together to learn. A group format is not only less threatening to those family members who otherwise may be reluctant to ask questions, but may also be of help in beginning to overcome isolation by providing a special kind of support for family members who are not connected with a network that understands the problems with which they are coping. In a group, family members can compare experiences and find comfort in the knowledge that they are not alone in their struggle. The group format can also help to create a less formal relationship between families and professionals.

The physical setting of the workshop must also be considered. Some professionals choose to impart information by visiting individual families in their own homes (Falloon et al., 1982; Leff et al., 1982; McGill, Falloon, Boyd, & Wood-Siverio, 1983), while others conduct workshops within institutions (Anderson et al., 1980; McLean, Greer, Scott, & Beck, 1982; Thornton, Plummer, Seeman, & Littmann, 1981). We believe that there are special advantages to conducting these programs within the sponsoring institution. Home care for most schizophrenic patients is unlikely to become a common treatment practice in the near future. Practically speaking, it is more expensive in terms of staff time and resources. It is more likely that third-party payers will reimburse treatment sessions in an authorized facility than in the patient's home. Sound community maintenance of schizophrenic patients tends to involve many professionals cooperating to provide a total "systems" approach. Treatment programs that involve maintenance chemotherapy, individual supportive therapy for the patient, implementation and coordination of resocialization and vocational programs, as well as family education and treatment are best provided by a team of professionals. The cost in terms of time, money, and the logistical problems of bringing patients and families to the team for one or more of these services is far less than bringing an entire team to each home. More importantly, the development of an "institutional transference" is often beneficial. The institution can come to symbolize qualities that aid the therapeutic process: The institution is a legitimate and informed authority; it is the repository of treatment resources; and it represents a permanent and durable entity which exists beyond the individual personalities of the service providers. Thus, if a particular clinician leaves the program, other ties are already in place and will serve a maintenance function until a new primary treatment relationship is formed.

It should be noted here that the patient's family members and any significant others are asked to attend the workshop in this program. Patients are excluded for two specific reasons. First, in our particular program, families are asked to attend a workshop close to the beginning of treatment. In fact, the workshop usually occurs relatively early in the course of a specific psychotic episode, at a time when it would be difficult for patients to tolerate the stimulation of a day-long session. Even patients who stabilize relatively quickly tend to have neither the energy nor the attention span to tolerate a 7-hour meeting so early in the course of treatment. Second, we have found that family members at this early phase seem more comfortable in discussing their concerns without patients present. This does not mean that the patients are denied any information or that they are not intimately involved in the experience. Families are encouraged to discuss their workshop experience with the patient if they wish to, or if the patient expresses interest. In addition, clinicians eventually share all of the same information with patients during later sessions. However, this sharing is done over time at a pace and level determined by the patient's ability to tolerate and understand the information. While they were not a part of the design of this particular project, it would certainly be possible to provide patients with similar, perhaps abbreviated, workshops somewhat later in the course of treatment. In fact, in our particular project, a good number of family members attending workshops also had a mental illness. They not only seemed able to use the information to understand the patient, but often these individuals claimed they achieved a better understanding of their own struggles.

While the specific content of any educational program must be based on the particular belief system and philosophy of the professionals providing the information, there are a number of topics so universally raised by family members that they should be covered in one way or another. These topics are listed in Table 3-1, which is the outline for our day-long "Survival Skills Workshop." In the remainder of this chapter, the content of our particular educational workshop is described in greater detail. This description is meant only to serve as a possible model for others and can easily be modified as new information becomes available, or to fit the particular philosophy and beliefs of a particular group of professionals or treatment system. Whatever information is ultimately disseminated, it is important that those providing it distinguish between facts and belief systems, and emphasize that there is no conclusive evidence for any particular theory of causation or method of treatment at this point in time.

The underlying philosophy of our workshop is roughly based on the acceptance of a model that suggests that schizophrenia is a serious illness, involving a biological vulnerability of unknown origin that makes patients particularly susceptible to stress from their environments. The use of the terms "schizophrenia" and "illness" is controversial because it has been suggested that labeling causes, or at least

TABLE 3-1
Outline of the psychoeducational workshop day

9:00–9:15	Coffee and informal interaction
9:15–9:30	Formal introductions and explanation of the format for the day
9:30–10:30	Schizophrenia: What is it?
	History and epidemiology
	The personal experience
	The public experience
	Psychobiology
10:30–10:45	Coffee break and informal discussion
10:45–12:00	Treatment of schizophrenia
	The use of antipsychotic medication
	How it works
	Why it is needed
	Impact on outcome
	Side effects
	Psychosocial treatments
	Effects on course
	Other treatments and management
12:00–1:00	Lunch and informal discussion
1:00–3:30	The family and schizophrenia
	The needs of the patient
	The needs of the family
	Family reactions to the illness
	Common problems that patients and families face
	What the family can do to help
	Revise expectations
	Create barriers to overstimulation
	Set limits
	Selectively ignore certain behaviors
	Keep communication simple
	Support medication regime
	Normalize the family routine
	Recognize signals for help
	Use professionals
3:30–4:00	Questions regarding specific problems
	Wrap up
	Informal interaction

perpetuates, mental illness or fixates patient-type behaviors (Doherty, 1975; Erikson, 1962). We feel, however, that labeling of this sort has advantages that outweigh the disadvantages. The view that patients have an illness decreases the tendency to become emotionally reactive and assign negative meanings to symptoms. If families can believe that patients are ill rather than malingering or purposely attempting to upset others, they are less likely to become angry at patients or the treatment team. Furthermore, helping patients recognize that their symptoms are behavioral manifestations of an illness gives them greater understanding of the purpose and need for treatment.

PREPARATION FOR THE WORKSHOP

In preparing for the workshop, there are a number of important points to consider that will help to plan the day and make it comfortable for all concerned. While the format of issues discussed (Table 3-1) has remained the same for both morning and afternoon sessions over time, great flexibility characterizes the order of themes presented as well as the intensity and depth of the discussion around a given issue. Frequently the composition of the group (e.g., the education level or age of participants, families of first vs. multiple episode patients), feedback, and intervening questions from family members dictate the educational process. Thus, the *themes* are more strictly adhered to than their order, depth of presentation, or discussion.

Furthermore, the information provided is also flexible and dynamic. The scientific and clinical understanding of schizophrenia is *not* a static process. It is continually being developed, expanded, and qualified. Presenters and clinicians must keep up with current developments, if for no other reason than to maintain credibility. As staff members, we routinely use the *Schizophrenia Bulletin* and its annotated bibliography as a current source of information, together with interim articles of interest that appear in journals such as the *Archives of General Psychiatry* and the *British Journal of Psychiatry*. If one has an operational "model" of schizophrenia in mind, the task of identifying and integrating relevant new information is much less difficult.

Presenters must also become comfortable with the information to be presented. As simple as this might sound, it is very easy to get in over one's head in such areas as biochemistry, genetics, and psychopharmacology. It is best not to pretend to know what is not known. It is more appropriate for presenters to say that they don't know and will try to find an answer from the relevant authority on a given topic. No one in this profession can be expected to be equally well informed as scientist, scholar, clinician, administrator, and public speaker.

It is also true that little has been "proven" in psychiatry. Professional maturity, after all, is a continuing state of suspended doubt. As the field advances in wisdom and understanding, practitioners must take a chance. Having evaluated past attempts at understanding the nature, treatment, and outcome of schizophrenic disorders, as well as the principles of psychotherapeutic practice and psychodynamics, we feel that the benefits that accrue to families by this approach far outweigh the risks involved.

There is another practical issue faced by presenters. An audience of relatives will most often be entirely comprised of nonprofessionals. They will not be taking professional competency examinations at the end of the workshop. Thus, the precision of definitions, sophisticated qualifications of the studies cited, and the like is not as important as the goal of providing a *cognitive restructuring* of the family's understanding of schizophrenia; a model in which their own behavior, the patient's behavior, and the behavior of professionals make sense. Follow-up interviews with relatives have convinced us that most do, in fact, achieve some cognitive mastery of schizophrenia as an illness with its biological and environmental components. They rarely remember the details of neuro-transmission. We feel that information is best assimilated by family members when the workshop presenters are able to maintain a personable style. Although schizophrenia is a very serious illness, we use humor appropriately as a way not only to rob the reality of unnecessary threat, but to instill hope and confidence. The treatment of schizophrenia and life with a schizophrenic patient is, after all, a human experience, and a smile is the property of our nature as well.

It is important to know that everyone who attempts to provide this kind of information to families is uncomfortable initially. The anxiety does not disappear completely even in subsequent workshops. Many of us have been trained, overtly or covertly, that "advice giving" is both superficial and antitherapeutic. This message has been communicated to us in various ways: "Families will not understand"; "information is not what they need, exploration of feelings, attitudes, and behaviors toward the patient is what is required to bring about more appropriate coping styles"; "families will rationalize their own behavior given the tools of unproven theory"; "information will provide the relative with a justification to reject the patient." Although these attitudes may at times be valid in looking at the experiences of individual cases, the evidence available regarding the effectiveness of a psychoeducational approach argues against these concerns. Exploration of feelings and improved coping skills are, obviously, legitimate objectives, but they do not preclude the dissemination of accurate information.

Thus, our recommendation is to take a chance. Most families are desperately anxious and willing to share the consequences of receiving information, good and bad. However, if a workshop presenter has not resolved a personal ambivalence as to whether families, in some way, "cause" schizophrenia or deliberately "need" to keep a member of the family "crazy", then our advice is *not* to get involved in this process. Not only will families be sensitive to these latent feelings, but attempts to provide management techniques, coping skills, and a knowledge base will make no sense unless presenters subscribe to those basic underlying theoretical assumptions that do *not* blame families for schizophrenia.

INTRODUCTION

Family members are greeted, thanked for coming, and offered coffee or tea and doughnuts by the workshop presenters. Name tags are provided to make it possible for people to interact in a personal way. An introduction to the day's format is presented by the moderator who next suggests that all present introduce themselves and their relationship to the patient or program. Staff participants at the workshop frequently include a moderator, the morning presenter (who might be a psychiatrist or other professional versed in the psycho-social-biological aspects of schizophrenia), and the afternoon family expert. Other primary clinicians who are involved in the aftercare of the patient may be invited to attend, such as the patient's nurse and family clinicians, behavior therapists, or rehabilitation specialists. When a program is new, there are frequent requests from other professionals to sit in. This might become a source of distress for the presenters since a workshop offered to professionals is very different in terms of the language used and details provided than one offered to families. We recommend not inviting other professionals from outside the program until the workshop organizers have a reasonable amount of experience with the workshop process. This way, they are less likely to be oversensitive to potential criticisms and less likely to become frustrated by attempting to respond to all suggested revisions. Later, simply ignoring visiting professionals during the workshop and focusing on the needs of the relatives is the most helpful posture to adopt.

After general introductions of the participants, the moderator then introduces the principal workshop presenters, giving some information about their backgrounds and credentials. The important task here is to establish the legitimate authority and experience of the presenters. (If the workshop organizers are the *only* professionals available or willing to conduct these sessions, then by definition, they are the legitimate authorities.) Nevertheless, it is important to give family members some reason to listen to what the presenters have to say. Knowledge, training, and experience regarding schizophrenic disorders are, in the end, the principal qualifications of an expert for this kind of endeavor.

HISTORY OF SCHIZOPHRENIA

The formal didactic session begins on a historical note to place the experience of patients and families in some perspective. Behaviors that resemble schizophrenia have been found as early as the 12th-century B.C., for example, in the Indian text *Carka Samita*. Most of what we understand today regarding schizophrenia, however, has its origins in 19th-century European medicine (see, e.g., Alexander & Selesnick, 1966; Mora, 1980). In 1801 the French physician Pinel coined the term *"démence"* and, when referring to the behaviors of schizophrenic patients in the same year, the English physician Haslam described a state of "insanity without furious or depressing passion."

It was not until 1845 that the German psychiatrist Griesinger (1867/1965) began to speculate that the most aberrant forms of human behavior represented a singular "disease of the brain." As so often happens with human reasoning, a bold statement stimulates others to consider alternative explanations. Indeed, the Belgian psychiatrist Morel and the French physician Falret argued the existence of a *separate* disease (*démence précoce*) which had the characteristic signs of an early onset (*précoce* or adolescence), a "march of symptoms" that included deterioration of self-care and social withdrawal, and a "course of symptoms" that ultimately led to a loss of intellectual capacity (*démence*). These are the themes that have been attributed to the German psychiatrist Kraepelin who, in 1896, changed the French term to its Latin equivalent, "dementia praecox." But Kraepelin's actual contribution was his distinction between this illness and "manic-depressive insanity" which, he said, tended to appear later in life, did not lead to ultimate deterioration and, between episodes, left patients in a more functional state (Kraepelin, 1896). As it turns out, recent epidemiological studies of manic-depressive disease, now called "bipolar disorder," indicate that this illness does not always appear in later life, does not always permit the patient to return to an adequate level of functioning, and does not necessarily guarantee an immunity from further deterioration (e.g., Angst et al., 1973).

These very early attempts to divide aspects of human behavior into discrete diagnostic categories have greatly influenced our current attempts at diagnosis, as represented in the third edition of the American Psychiatric Association's (1980) *Diagnostic and Statistical Manual of Mental Disorders* (DSM-III). Even prior to 1896, contemporaries of Kraepelin had already started to categorize mental illnesses and were labeling variations of the psychotic process as paranoia (Sander, 1868), hebephrenia (Hecker, 1871), and catatonia (Kahlbaum, 1876). In 1911, the Swiss psychiatrist Eugen Bleuler examined the extensive spectrum of these variations on "dementia praecox" and labeled them the "group of schizophrenias" (Bleuler, 1911/1950), a term that we continue to use today, even though the understanding of schizophrenic disorders remains largely based on the conceptual ideas of Kraepelin and his colleagues. We remind relatives of schizophrenic patients that the tendency to become enamored of fancy sounding Greek words such as "schizophrenia" occurred in a time and place that represented a medical "renaissance" of sorts, where sophistication in the use of language tended to impart an aura of validity to the terms. Bleuler himself struggled with the words "amblythymia" and "dysphrenia," for example, before settling on the name "schizophrenia."

Bleuler, however, drew attention not to the age of onset, or to a course that he argued was not, inevitably, a deteriorating one, nor to the presence of such pronounced symptoms as hallucinations and delusions. Rather, he focused on what has come to be called his four A's:

- a loosening in the *Associations* among otherwise logical or coherent ideas
- an inappropriate, flat, or blunted *Affect* or "feeling" level
- an *Autistic* or private preoccupation with fantasy
- a disturbing *Ambivalence* or conflicting uncertainty.[1]

The naming of discrete behaviors as distinct diseases did not end, however, with Bleuler. In the mid-to-latter part of this century, attempts to focus on the manifestations or the course of the "group of schizophrenias" have given rise to such terms as "simple schizophrenia" (Diem, 1904), "schizo-affective disorder" (Kasanin, 1933), "schizophreniform disorder" (Langfeldt, 1939), "pseudoneurotic" schizophrenia (Hoch & Polantin, 1949), "cycloid psychosis" (Leonhard, 1961), "first rank" schizophrenia (Schneider, 1959), and more recently "Type I" and "Type II" schizophrenias (Crow, 1980). Yet, in spite of the proliferation of named subtypes, there is still scant evidence that different types have different onsets, treatment responses, courses, and outcomes.

We spend time on these issues because it is this labeling process that has tended to confuse families and "turn off" many professionals who were trained outside medicine. Some of these professionals are either uncomfortable with or actually refuse to use a term that has no "real" basis. In fact, we have actually seen clinicians work with

---

1. Ironically, modern diagnostic systems have largely abandoned these Bleulerian ideas, not because they are necessarily invalid, but simply because most professionals, it seems, have a hard time agreeing on what the terms mean.

schizophrenic patients for many years, yet, tragically, never even say the word aloud in the presence of patients.

Once an appreciation of the arbitrariness and limitations of an historical, human process is achieved, an attempt is made to develop an understanding of the utilitarian value and *purpose* of a classification system. When we use the term schizophrenia, we *define* it, and hence we provide a common basis for communication among ourselves, patients, and families. Schizophrenia becomes the symbolic term reflecting a defined cerebral process—no more and no less. It is not a pejorative weapon, nor is it an indictment of despair and poor outcome, nor an exercise in name-calling or social distancing.

The point of all this discourse surrounding the history of schizophrenia is for the family to learn that classification is not diagnosis. Classification is a useful *aid* to diagnosis. Diagnosis in the last analysis remains the artful exercise of understanding the individual variation regarding the past, illness onset, treatment needs and response, course, and outcome. We point out to relatives that there is no litmus test, no laboratory procedure, no x-ray, or biological probe at the moment, by which we can absolutely "diagnose" schizophrenia. The term, after all, reflects a classification system of convenience, and when its meaning is shared and agreed upon by professionals, patients, and families, then there is, indeed, a common ground for communication and understanding. Classification schema, we note for relatives, are as old as mankind. Ancient Chinese, for example, had literally thousands upon thousands of classifications of dogs: those with short tails; those with long tails; those that hopped on three legs; those that chased butterflies, and so on. The bishops of 15-century Cologne, in their infamous *Malleus Maleficarium*, listed on a single page the categories of behavior useful for identifying the "male witch." (The remaining pages were, of course, used for diagnosing female witches. See Springer & Kramer, 1928.) Their description of the "wizard archer" looks like a page from DSM-III.

As such, when we say that a member of a family is suffering a schizophrenic disorder, we are aware of the limits of classification. In fact, we readily admit to families that in our own studies an average of 10% of patients will ultimately have a *change* in diagnosis, particularly if evidence of an underlying organic brain syndrome or a more specific affective disorder, requiring a different treatment, becomes apparent. Nonetheless, every patient under our care and every patient whose family is in attendance at the workshop has shown signs of psychosis, at least at the point of entry into treatment, signs resembling those that are universally agreed upon as fundamental to our definition of schizophrenia.

We also talk about what schizophrenia is not. Schizophrenia is not "split personality," despite the misinformation perpetuated by the media, popular novels, or the movies. Dual or multiple personality disorders, we say, are as rare as hen's teeth. The "split" in schizophrenia, if anything, is a discordance between the thinking life and the feeling life of a *single* personality. Schizophrenia is not demonic possession, nor willful behavior, nor moral shortcomings secondary to spiritual failure, theological determinism, or childhood masturbation. Schizophrenia, we believe, refers to a disease process that has its origins in the brain and its course influenced by experiences.

Our belief in schizophrenia as an "illness," however, while shared by many others in the past, has not always had benign consequences for patients. We remind relatives of the very sordid, but well-intended "treatment" history of schizophrenia throughout the centuries as described in the Preface. In our own lifetime, professionals have used medication to put these patients to sleep and to keep them awake. They have plunged them in tubs of cold water or wrapped them in ice packs, and in other times submerged them in the swirling pools of the pre-Jacuzzi. They have attempted to cleanse their blood, bowels, or mouths. (In the 1920s, for example, the best clue to a diagnosis of dementia praecox, as one strolled the grounds of public asylums, was a toothless smile.) Patients have been shuffled from the fields and sundecks of the rural countryside, to the inner-city squalor of their own "community" or "catchment area."

This contrast between the desperation of past therapeutic attempts and the reason and effectiveness of current therapeutic interventions is not lost on relatives and goes a long way toward reassuring them that they are at a special, evolving point in history where the understanding and treatment of schizophrenia has improved, but nonetheless remains incomplete. Hope is instilled, but *not* the unreasonable expectations of a cure.

EPIDEMIOLOGY OF SCHIZOPHRENIA

The next step of the program is the presentation of information to relatives regarding the epidemiology of schizophrenia in terms of its incidence (the number of new cases appearing in a year) and its prevalence (the number of both new and old cases in the population at a given point in time). Schizophrenia, even if not universal among primitive man, has at least been recognized consistently among people known to western man. This part of the "cognitive scaffold" surrounding schizophrenia is put in place for the purpose of reinforcing the now

growing belief among workshop participants that they are not alone
in their experiences.

In the early years of our own training, over 500,000 people occupied
mental hospital beds in the United States. This represented one half
of all hospital beds, both medical and psychiatric, in this country. In
the late 1950s, at least one half of these patients carried a diagnosis
of schizophrenia and a large number had been hospitalized continuously
for many years (Yolles & Kramer, 1969). It is primarily modern treatment,
principally the introduction of antipsychotic medication in the mid
1950s, that has kept the number of these chronically hospitalized
patients from rising into the millions. Hospitalization for schizophrenia
is now measured in days rather than years. But new cases have continued to appear at a constant rate in spite of the fact that reproduction
is less among schizophrenic patients (males tend not to marry) and
that high rates of early mortality (e.g., suicide) continue to characterize
the disorder. Unfortunately, at least in North America, an increase
in the number of schizophrenic patients has been observed among
subsamples of the population with the highest birth rates (Kramer,
1978). Incidence rates worldwide are generally less than 1 case per
1,000 in the population. But period (1 year) prevalence rates are higher
and vary from 1.5 per 1,000 to 5.1 per 1,000, internationally (Jablensky
& Sartorias, 1975). In the United States, an average of 3 persons per
1,000 can be observed to have schizophrenia at any given time (Yolles
& Kramer, 1969). Thus, schizophrenia is a disease with a low incidence
rate. However, once it appears, it is likely to stay around, thus giving
rise to a relatively high prevalence rate.

From the prevalence rates available, we would conservatively
estimate (depending on definition) that between 4 and 6 million people
in the United States, within the age of risk, have experienced an
episode of schizophrenia. There are, if one includes episodes treated
in the private sector of general medical practice, over 1 million schizophrenic patients under care in this country annually (Kramer, 1978).
Between 1 and 2% of the entire population will sometime in their life
experience a schizophrenic episode (Yolles & Kramer, 1969). By illus-
tration, schizophrenia is three times more prevalent over a lifetime
than illnesses such as multiple sclerosis or muscular dystrophy and
has about the same lifetime risk as diabetes mellitus (Beeson,
McDermott, & Wyngaarden, 1979).

Only in recent years have support groups of patients, families,
and their friends begun to go public in the important exercise of
consciousness raising, fund raising, and "ire" raising of legislators
who control funds and influence policies. Support for the research
and treatment of schizophrenia is but a fraction of that provided for
equally or less prevalent illnesses. Yet, schizohrenia is very expensive

both in treatment costs and in lost income, amounting to nearly 20 billion dollars annually in this country by one estimate, based on data that are now over 10 years old (Gunderson & Mosher, 1975). The cost of a single case of schizophrenia has been calculated to be six times that of a myocardial infarction, a leading cause of death and disability (Andrews et al., 1985). Schizophrenia accounts for about 2% to 3% of the Gross National Product.

Schizophrenia has an early onset, very often in those years when one is just becoming a person of hope and promise: late adolescence and early adult life. *Peak* onset years occur somewhat later, in the late 20s for men and early 30s for women (Lewine, 1981; Loranger, 1984). This sex difference (an illness onset 1 to 10 years earlier in men) is puzzling and many answers have been offered, ranging from the antipsychotic properties of naturally occurring estrogens in women, to earlier detection among men, to a greater vulnerability among males regarding all diseases that affect left cerebral hemispheric functioning (Lewine, 1981; Seeman, 1982). Whatever the reason, the differences do seem real. By the time the age of risk is past, however, women have caught up to men in terms of the number experiencing schizophrenia. It would be unusual to experience a first episode of schizophrenia after age 35 and rare indeed, to see schizophrenia for the first time in someone over age 40. The DSM-III (1980) precludes the diagnosis of schizophrenia in a first psychotic episode over age 45.

SCHIZOPHRENIA: THE PERSONAL EXPERIENCE

With the history and epidemiology of schizophrenia presented, the process of demystification and deisolation should have begun. But an understanding of schizophrenia is still beyond the grasp of most family members. A description of what it is like for the patient to go through the first encounter with schizophrenia facilitates this understanding. To make this description more relevant, it is often helpful, prior to the workshop, for presenters to be made aware of the particular symptomatic and behavioral characteristics of those patients whose families will attend the workshop so that these factors can be explained in greater detail.

The first indicator that something is wrong is often a decline in the person's ability to select "relevant" aspects of the environment to "attend to" while, at the same time, ignoring or inhibiting irrelevant cues. Patients might feel that their minds are "playing tricks" on them. Table 3-2 lists a few of the deeply personal phenomena that patients in the throes of an early schizophrenic episode might experience. There are literally scores of autobiographical reports which attest to

TABLE 3-2
Schizophrenia

The personal experience	The public manifestation
Distraction	Thought disorder
"Overload"	Delusions
Sensitivity	Hallucinations
Misperceptions	Withdrawal and reduced feeling

the early disturbances in attention among "becoming" schizophrenic patients (e.g., Freedman, 1974). Presenters can borrow liberally from these published reports and from the examples we offer below. "Attention," it should be pointed out, is the most fundamental human capacity required for the process of learning, and hence for the formation of one's sense of person. Without an intact attentional capacity, we could not record or respond to the experiences of daily living, nor could we place such experiences in memory. There would not be available for recall those important bits of information that provide us with a continuing sense of who we are. People with a serious disturbance of attention would likely leave this workshop at 4:00P.M. with no more information conceptualized and stored than they had at 9:00A.M.

McGhie and Chapman (1961) described this disturbance in attention and its sequelae. The disturbance tends to make perception more "global" and "undifferentiated." Sensory perception becomes more diffuse. "Willed action" is less controlled and is subject to an increased awareness of bodily functions. Finally, concentration and thinking (in the face of distraction) become more impaired as patients struggle with and often fail to abstract those "internal associations" from incoming stimuli which are necessary to maintain logical thinking.

Distraction

Utilizing examples of distraction from McGhie and Chapman, and other sources as well, we provide examples of what patients have actually said about this early disturbing process.

> I couldn't read the newspaper because everything I read had a large number of associations. I mean, I just read a headline and the headline would have much wider associations in my mind. It seemed to start off everything I read, and everything that sort of caught my attention seemed to start off . . . Bang! Bang! Bang! . . . like that, with an enormous number of associations. . . . (Freedman, 1974, p. 335)

Another patient remarked:

> I jump from one thing to another. If I am talking to someone, they only need to cross their legs or scratch their heads, and I am distracted and forget what I was saying. (McGhie & Chapman, 1961, p. 104)

We point out to relatives that the competing sounds in the room during the workshop (cars and buses going by in the street; the hum of the air conditioner or heating system; the drone of a flourescent light) are representative sources of distraction. Instead of the voice of the speaker becoming the principal stimulus, a schizophrenic patient, in the midst of an episode, might allocate equal "attention" to all these sources of competing information.

> I am speaking to you just now, but I can hear noises going on next door and in the corridor. I find it difficult to shut these out and it makes it more difficult for me to concentrate on what I am saying to you. Often the silliest little things that are going on seem to interest me. That's not even true; they don't interest me, but I find myself attending to them and wasting a lot of time this way. (McGhie & Chapman, 1961, pp. 104–105)

Overload

We share with relatives that stimuli are generated internally as well. Past events and experiences, memories of people, places, conversations, music, photographs, and so forth, all compete with externally impinging stimuli. The onslaught can be devastating. Even Freud himself reminded us that above the reception of stimuli, the human organism more likely required protection from too much stimulation. Many patients describe this process as an "overload." We use the analogy of a telephone switchboard operator, perhaps on the day that the *Steelers* won their first Super Bowl: Phone calls would all come in at once, needing to be sorted out and directed to their proper source. The calls would overload the switchboard—and the operator. One patient, describing this process, remarked:

> It's like being a transmitter. The sounds are coming through to me but I feel my mind cannot cope with everything. It's difficult to concentrate on any one sound. It's like trying to do two or three different things at one time. (McGhie & Chapman, 1961, p. 104)

Another patient described the overload as a broken "filter":

> At first, it was [as] if a part of my brain "awoke" which had been sleeping and I became interested in a wide assortment of people, places and ideas which normally made no impression on me. I think that the mind must have a filter that functions without our being aware of it, sorting out things and allowing only those that are relevant to a situation to come into consciousness. I guess that this filter must have to work at maximum efficiency at all times. (MacDonald, 1960, p. 219)

And she later concluded:

> My brain after a very short time became sore trying to handle all this
> information with a real physical soreness as if it had been rubbed with
> sandpaper until it was raw. It felt like a bleeding sponge. I had very
> little ability to sort the relevant from the irrelevant. The filter had broken
> down. Completely unrelated events became intricately connected in my
> mind. (MacDonald, 1960, p. 219)

Sensitivity

In the midst of this bombardment by stimuli, many patients will
often comment that the "quality" or properties of sensory stimuli
have changed: colors may be brighter, sounds louder, sensory images
more detailed and vivid, and familiar objects more ominous and
threatening.

> I have noticed that noises all seemed to be louder to me than they were
> before. It's as if someone had turned up the volume . . . I notice it most
> with background noises, you know what I mean, noises that are always
> around, but you don't notice them. (McGhie & Chapman, 1961, p. 105)

> Colors seem brighter now, almost as if they are luminous. When I look
> around me it's like a luminous painting. I'm not sure if things are solid
> until I touch them. (McGhie & Chapman, 1961, p. 105)

Misperceptions

With the sensory presentation of the external and internal world
now dramatically different, relevant and irrelevant cues equally worthy
of attention, "too many balls coming over the net," sounds, colors,
shapes, experienced in an unfamiliar manner, it does not take much
to appreciate the fact that patients will make "mistakes" in perceiving
reality. In many ways, the perceptual distortions that occur are similar
to the more familiar psychedelic drug experiences (LSD, PCP or "Angel
Dust," "Speed"). Some researchers, in fact, have suggested that perhaps
the acute psychotic process might follow upon the human body actually
producing its own "toxic chemical substance," although no definitive
proof for this theory is yet available (for a review see Iversen, 1978).

For one patient, the misperceptions rest between the realms of
illusion and reality:

> If I am looking at something and there's a sudden noise, perhaps an
> airplane passing or a bus, what I am looking at seems to swing or move
> in front of me although I know it's stationary. (McGhie & Chapman,
> 1961, p. 106)

For another patient, it is more real:

> Everything is in bits. . . . It's like a photograph that's torn in bits and
> put together again. . . . If you move it's frightening. The picture you

had in your head is still there but it's broken up. (McGhie & Chapman, 1961, p. 106)

And for yet another patient, the misperception *is* the reality:

Everything [is] a jumbled mess. I have found that I can stop this happening by going completely still and motionless. When I do that, things are easier to take in. (McGhie & Chapman, 1961, p. 106).

Sometimes the misperceptions can fill the patient with a morbid fear:

That's the horror! That's the horror of the great big open space! It's like something gone mad about the place. I could never walk in the streets. Never! It's a terrifying place, isn't it? Soon as the houses lift off buildings on both sides of the road, as if it's flat and you could see right over it like a mad horse or something . . . it would look mad and terrifying, like it would hurt something. (Strauss, 1966, p. 78)

Or fill the patient with dread:

I went to my teacher and said to her, "I am afraid. . . . " She smiled gently at me. But her smile, instead of reassuring me, only increased the anxiety and confusion for I saw her teeth, white and even in the gleam of the light. Remaining all the while like themselves, soon they monopolized my entire vision as if the whole room were nothing but teeth under a remorseless light. Ghastly fear gripped me. (Sechehaye, 1951, p. 22)

Obviously, these problems in perception and information processing must be terribly upsetting to patients, making them more anxious, nervous, and excited. In medical terms, one would say that patients are increasingly "aroused." Later in the workshop, we demonstrate that increased arousal, in fact, contributes very much to the growing problem of disattention and misperception.

SCHIZOPHRENIA: THE PUBLIC EXPERIENCE

Once the presenter feels that family members have an appreciation of the disordered process of attention and arousal, the rhetorical question is asked: "How would *you* act if this were happening to you?"

The differences in individual response to this process have contributed greatly to the difficulties in diagnosis. It would be convenient if everyone responded in the same way. Unfortunately for diagnosticians, human beings insist on being individuals, yet, there are commonalities in the *process* of responding, even though the *content* of the patient's explanations might differ widely. In order to make the following more relevant, presenters might want to use actual behaviors which the families present at the workshop have witnessed.

Thought Disorder

Considering all that is going on in the patient's head, attempts to explain the experience often don't "hang together." A single word of explanation might start off indirect associations to other words or ideas. (When asked if he felt concerned that he would be deserted by his friends, one patient responded: "I wonder what's the dessert today?" [cited in Spitzer, Endicott, & Robins, 1978]) This aspect of thought disorder is referred to as *"loose associations,"* one of the cardinal Bleulerian hallmarks for diagnosing schizophrenia. Patients will sometimes stammer or halt in their speech. The loosely associated ideas, when strung together in sentences, make little or no sense to the listener. The meaning attached to words sometimes seem very personal and very private. It is hard, at times, for family members to follow the patient's conversation. The diagnostician, when listening to such speech, might characterize it as "illogical" or "incoherent" or "private," all of which are signs of a thought disorder.

Delusions

At times when patients' explanations are even understandable, family members can become terribly upset when they believe that such explanations are simply untrue. When patients are convinced of ideas that most people around them feel are untrue, the ideas are called delusions or false beliefs. Unfortunately for families and friends, the patients' explanation of what is going on often does contain a "kernel of truth." Frequently, the psychotic process might go on for weeks or months before family and friends are convinced that, in the long run, the seemingly valid explanations just don't make sense. If patients, for example, have had a rough time with their employers or co-workers, they might be convinced that it is these persons who are "doing it" to their mind. If family relationships have become stressed and strained, patients might seize on the disrupted relationship and begin to blame and accuse the family members for their problems. Public and international events involving spying, espionage, counterintelligence, and other sinister forces frequently provide the explanation and justification for the disturbing personal experience of schizophrenia. These types of false beliefs are called *paranoid delusions* or *persecutory delusions*. The content or reasons often change with the times. Decades ago, God was most often given as the source of the problem, later, satellites and color television. Today, "sex" is often identified as the culprit. In some cultures, "spirits" do it to the patient and in others, the patient's "ancestors." No matter what the source, it is the falseness of the belief that makes it a delusion.

At other times, the personal experience of schizophrenia might be so frightening or recognized as so bizarre and unusual that patients become convinced that someone or something (e.g., television or a satellite) must be putting these disturbing thoughts and altered perceptions in their heads. *Thought insertion* is a frequent characteristic of severe psychosis. At other times, the personal sensory horror of schizophrenia might be so real, so vivid, so loud, and tumultuous that patients become convinced that others can "hear it," "see it," and "sense it" as well. *Thought broadcasting* and *reading one's thoughts aloud* are equally severe aspects of psychosis.

Hallucinations

One of the frequent and tragic consequences of a breakdown in the "inner filter" of the brain may be that sensory stimuli are generated internally. In other words, there is no apparent *external* source of stimuli capable of accounting for the experience. This phenomenon is called a *hallucination*. Sounds, particularly "voices," are the most common internally generated stimuli and are labeled *auditory hallucinations*. The voices might be familiar or unfamiliar, one voice or a number of voices. They are frequently threatening and terrifying in the early stages of the illness. Sometimes after recovery, a friendly voice or two might persist, especially when patients are alone or given to fantasy and rumination. We sometimes will show relatives a PET scan picture of the "brain in action," with the auditory centers of the brain "lit up" in activity, even though the patient's ears are plugged! Such examples serve to impress upon the relatives the fact that these altered perceptions and sensory images are *real*, not "made up," and not to be dismissed or argued as "imaginary."

Withdrawal and Reduced Feeling

Many times in the face of the personal living nightmare of schizophrenia, patients will develop ways to "block it all out." Many patients, even through the long period of recovery, will learn to avoid these sources of stimulation (e.g., heated conversations, the demands of school or work) and take to their rooms or "travel alone." Some appear emotionally paralyzed by the inner turmoil as well. Social withdrawal, and a "flattened" or "blunted" affect or feeling level are important distinguishing characteristics of schizophrenia, especially when they occur in the context of thought disorder, delusions, and hallucinations. It must be pointed out, however, that the world is filled with people who are shy, socially uncomfortable, and have a reduced feeling level, but who are not suffering a schizophrenic illness.

THE PSYCHOBIOLOGY OF SCHIZOPHRENIA

With the private experience and public manifestation of schizophrenia thus described, the important task of the presenter now is to explain the process as it is currently understood in the psychobiological sciences. Many "theories" are available, but we utilize the evidence outlined in Chapter 1 when presenting this information, albeit in a more simplified manner. It is this theory which will provide the cognitive mastery desired, an understanding of the subsequent treatments to be recommended, and the principles around which the months and years of family therapy will be organized.

Attention and Arousal

We utilize a schema (see Figure 3-1) loosely referred to as the "attention–arousal" model of schizophrenic pathophysiology. As internal and external information in need of processing impacts on the person, the "wheel" begins to turn. Increased demands for processing lead to increased levels of arousal, to further distraction and disattention, then to further arousal that in turn stimulates distraction and around again. The wheel, which represents the inner life of patients, begins to turn faster and faster, making it impossible for patients to control their thoughts. This image allows everyone in the workshop to physically sense the inner chaos of the schizophrenic process as truly a "vicious cycle."

We point out that attention, during this process, can be conceived of as a beam from a large spotlight (Wachtel, 1967). If it is broadly focused so that it illuminates all the aspects of a scene, then too many

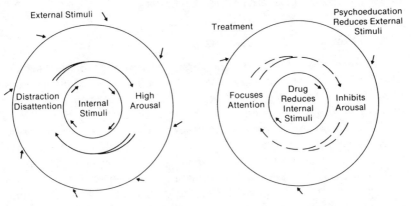

FIGURE 3-1
The attention–arousal–disease model of schizophrenia. (Adapted from Tecce & Cole, 1976.)

demands are placed on the organism's ability to sense, integrate, and understand either the "picture," or the separate pieces. Sometimes patients will "narrow" the beam of light as a way of coping. But then attention becomes focused on single bits and pieces and the larger picture is often lost. Learning and processing become serial (a bit at a time) instead of simultaneous (a lot of information at one time), deliberate instead of automatic, with arousal increasing continuously. A good analogy to explain this process is the student who tries to "cram" for an exam. Bits of information which must be learned are focused on until the student becomes increasingly anxious. Discrete parts of the problem are memorized but the pieces are not logically integrated into a whole picture. Thus, the information learned is quickly forgotten once the examine is over, much to the dismay of the student's teachers (not to mention his or her parents who probably have been footing the tuition bill).

The "wheel" analogy, however, also provides us with cues as to how the brain might be acting and how the "spinning" can be slowed down. Families can be helped to see that the external arrows or sources of stimuli, for example, could be "blocked" or weakened in their intensity by modification of the environment, while medication might help to internally regulate arousal and attention. These interventions provide a way out of the psychotic episode, as well as the means to avoid another.

The Brain's Message System
(see Frazer & Winokur, 1977)

The processing of any piece of information, even the automatic pulling of one's hand away from an open flame, involves a complex system of messages being transmitted from a sensory organ to the brain and in turn back again to the organ in the form of a response. Families are told that the regulatory "box" in the brain which sets the general tone of emotional response, is well hidden and protected in the middle and lower section of the brain (the *mesolimbic system*), located near the base or *stem* of the brain itself. These structures are believed to be the oldest evolutionary sections of the human brain. Many important nerve cells (or *neurons*) are found here. These are composed of a main branch (*axon*) from which numerous fibers, called *dendrites*, extend upward, sideward, and forward, like branches of a tree, to the important centers of the brain which regulate our "thinking" and "feeling" life. These structures are called the *frontal* and *temporal lobes* and their surface is called the *cerebral cortex*. Information is transported along nerve cells by electrical energy and the message is carried by chemical messengers from neuron to neuron. These chemical messengers are called *neurotransmitters*.

On every neuron that contains neurotransmitters (not all neurons do) there are as many as 250 or more "message transmission centers" or *synapses* (another Greek word that simply means "bound tightly together"). These message centers tend to act like continuously busy traffic cops; some of them containing chemical messengers that slow the flow of information down, and others that speed it up according to the needs of the person. At this point, we actually pass around pictures of the brain, neurons, and dendrites, derived from such popular sources as *Newsweek Magazine* (Begley, Carey, & Sawhill, 1983) and *Scientific American* (Hubel, 1979). Critical brain structures and their function are described and identified. As this material is shared in order to appreciate the complexity of this process, we further indicate that this wonderful brain of ours contains over 100 billion neurons, hundreds of synapses on a neuron and many, many neurotransmitters. For example, before we started our family program, eight chemical messengers were well known and studied. Now there are at least 50. If certain neuropeptides eventually prove to be chemical messengers themselves, the number of neurotransmitters will rise into the hundreds. A quadrillion or more neuron centers and messengers might thus be involved in processing a complex piece of information.

Relatives are told that in spite of the mystery and complexity of our brain, much of modern psychiatry has come to focus on the small space within the synapse in order to better understand the process of neurotransmission, the source of schizophrenic symptoms, and the means to treat them chemically (Frazer & Winokur, 1977). These synapses were, for many years, thought to be physically joined together—dendrite to dendrite, neuron to neuron. The development of the electron microscope, however, made it possible for us to see that there is, indeed, a space between one half of the synapse (the presynaptic membrane) and the other half (the postsynaptic membrane). Modern psychiatry has attempted to find out how the message gets from "here to there," from the presynaptic membrane across the space to the postsynaptic membrane.

An electron microscopic picture of one human synapse is shown and what is thought to be the process of neurotransmission is described (Frazer & Winokur, 1977). Electrical energy coming down the axon stimulates the "action potential" of the resting neuron and starts the storage vessels of these chemical messengers (located in the presynaptic neuron) moving toward the edge where they open and release their chemical messengers into the space itself. This complex process is called *exocytosis*. The messenger then seeks out a specific receptacle at the entry point on the surface of the postsynaptic membrane or *receptor*. A specific chemical messenger will only "fit" into a specific receptor especially designed for it. The analogy is offered that a neurotransmitter is very much like a key and the receptor is its lock; certain keys fit only certain locks. Once the chemical messenger is received at the postsynaptic receptor, it induces the neuron to either increase or decrease the rate at which it responds or "fires." Any amount of a messenger that is not needed is either reabsorbed into the storage vessel or "chewed up" and "destroyed" by chemical enzymes, or "Pac-Men" of sorts, called *MAO* (monoamine oxidase) and *COMT* (catechol-3-O-methyltransferase). These processes occur almost simultaneously, and most often in an orderly process of speeding up or slowing down the message. Various chemical messengers act in harmony. When this harmonious interaction falters, problems arise.

It is the disturbance in neurotransmission that has given rise to many explanations of severe mental illness such as schizophrenia. While neurotransmission is influenced by many things, from poorly functioning glands that secrete the hormones that regulate neurotransmission (e.g., the pituitary gland), to problems in the supply of food to the brain which helps to manufacture neurotransmitters (e.g., reduce cerebral blood flow or cerebral spinal fluid reflux), to the loss of important neurons themselves (cerebral atrophy [see Chapter 1]), many researchers have focused on the process of altered neurotransmission itself, independent of its cause. For example, many theories of schizophrenia mention the neurotransmitter *dopamine*, a particularly important messenger (Meltzer, 1979). While we *never* say that dopamine causes schizophrenia, we do suggest that too much dopamine or too many receptors might lead to disturbances in attention and arousal, and subsequently to such behaviors as thought disorder and hallucinations. Drugs such as amphetamine ("Speed") or LSD, which cause "schizophrenic-like" symptoms, stimulate the release of large stores of dopamine and *other* neurotransmitters from their presynaptic storage vessels. Other important neurotransmitters such as *serotonin* and *norepinephrine* (which often serve to inhibit neuron activity) have been implicated in the process of altered transmission. Too much or too little of a good thing, and particularly disturbances in the *balance* among these neurotransmitters, can have profound behavioral consequences, such as schizophrenia.

At this point, one explanation for schizophrenia has been given, and aspects of the psychobiological processes underlying normal and abnormal functioning and behavior have been described and illustrated. Whether the details of this material are understood or not, workshop attendees become visably less anxious as they hear it. The next portion of the day concentrates on how modern treatment capitalizes on this psychobiological process, but first, there is a break for coffee and snacks. During the break, an attempt is made to answer specific and personal questions which workshop attendees might not have been able to ask in front of the group. Sometimes it is necessary to assure relatives that the complicated material they have heard was simply to lay the groundwork for the next section regarding the treatment of schizophrenia and not a list of facts that must be memorized.

ANTIPSYCHOTIC MEDICATION

One of the truly momentous, yet serendipitous discoveries of this century—or any other—was the finding in the early 1950s that a rather unassuming chemical molecule (*chlorpromazine*) could often undo the ravages of the psychotic process. Modifications of this chemical have led to a proliferation of similar drugs and knowledge of its "mechanism of action" has led to the development of structurally dissimilar drugs, which nevertheless have similar behavioral effects.

All of the antipsychotic drugs currently available in the United States today do certain things in common. At the postsynaptic receptor, they all initially "block" the action of certain naturally occurring neurotransmitters, particularly dopamine (Snyder, Banerjee, Yamamura, & Greenberg, 1974). Utilizing the earlier analogy regarding keys and locks, this theory is described in the workshop as follows: The antipsychotic drug molecule looks like dopamine, gets into the synaptic space and takes its place at the postsynaptic receptor like dopamine, but it *does not* pass the message along like dopamine. It is a *phony* neurotransmitter. By taking the place of the real neurotransmitter, the subsequent effect is to slow down and block the process of neurotransmission. More importantly, the blockade of these postsynaptic receptors or regulation of the presynaptic neuron appears to have crucial behavioral effects through a complex "feedback" mechanism that slows down the firing rate of certain neurons. The description of this process gets us back to a discussion of the attention–arousal model. Study after study has documented the two important, consistent effects of receptor blockade: (1) the normalizing of arousal (where excited patients can be calmed down and underactive patients can be livened up a bit) and (2) the more correct deployment of *attention* to relevant environmental cues (Spohn et al., 1977).

The result for the majority of patients, depending upon the type and severity of symptoms, is a reduction and often disappearance of the most serious forms of psychotic symptoms (Cole & Davis, 1969). For this reason, we call these medications "antipsychotic drugs" and not "tranquilizers." They are as likely to activate patients as to calm them down. They are not (as many professionals have told family members) drugs that simply "cover-up" symptoms and the underlying problem. But neither do they cure the chemical imbalance. As such, they are not curatives as are the antibiotic drugs for bacterial infections, nor are they simply symptom covers, as aspirin might be for an underlying illness presenting with fever. Rather, these drugs act like many others that influence a disease process (helping patients become well, but not curing them) such as antihypertensives in the treatment of high blood pressure, and insulin in the treatment of diabetes.

At the present time, many attempts are being made to help those few patients who do not respond to antipsychotics alone. Such mood (and electrical potential) regulating drugs as *lithium*, anticonvulsants such as *carbamazepine*, the supplemental use of drugs that stimulate "inhibiting" receptors such as the *benzodiazepines*, as well as other compounds that influence the presynaptic release of neurotransmitters are under investigational study as possible adjunct medications.

Side Effects

As with all medications, these antipsychotic drugs are not without their problems. Too often families are loathe to support the need for continuing maintenance medication because of bad experiences with these drugs. "I brought you a normal boy," one mother remarked, "and you gave me back a zombie." Unnecessary tragedies such as this occur because often clinicians don't know how to use these drugs. They seem, at times, to subscribe to the belief that if a little good, a lot must be better. Many patients can recover from an episode, given time, with very low doses of antipsychotic medication, without the disabling side effects that follow upon higher doses (J. McEvoy, personal communication, 1985). In fact, one of our ongoing aftercare investigations has demonstrated to us that we are able to maintain patients who *recover* from their acute psychosis on very low doses of medication (e.g., 4 mg of fluphenazine decanoate every 2 weeks).

In another theory of how antipsychotic drugs work, chronic low dosages, for example, might lead to a down regulation in the electrical potential (*depolarization*) of the neuron and hence impede the release of "too much" neurotransmitter (Bunney, 1984) with the effect that the patient can remain well—and comfortable. As such, disabling side effects may not be the inevitable price patients have to pay in order to remain well. In fact, sometimes side effects even can be used to advantage. For example, an antipsychotic drug with a sedative side effect can be used for patients experiencing sleepless nights, thus avoiding the need to use an additional hypnotic.

Describing the biological mechanism of side effects often helps relatives to understand their appearance and the efforts necessary to control them. When one "fools Mother Nature" by dopamine receptor blockage or depolarization, she, in her marvelous compensatory manner, sends out yet another neurotransmitter (*acetylcholine*) with a message that not enough dopamine is being produced, telling the brain to "crank it up," so to speak. It is the relatively greater ratio of this chemical messenger (acetylcholine) that is responsible for the most frequent side effects of antipsychotic drugs: slowness, stiffness, tremors, eyes rolling up into the head, or the inner restlessness of akathisia (Synder *et al.*, 1974). In fact, these are called *pseudoparkinson symptoms* because the process is much like that seen in true Parkinson's disease. But rather than blocking dopamine receptors, in Parkinson's disease the dopamine containing neurons are actually destroyed and the resulting accumulation of acetylcholine leads to the disabling symptoms of this disease. Fortunately, we have available "anticholine" drugs that serve to block acetylcholine receptors, thereby giving symptomatic relief from these side effects. In some patients (about 14% according to one ongoing prospective study [Kane, Woerner, & Weinhold, 1982]) a persistent movement disorder will be observed, generally involving an involuntary movement of the mouth and tongue, which is called *tardive dyskinesia*. About one half of these involuntary movements will go away or lessen over time if the drug is discontinued. However, a small number do persist in a moderate or severe form and are the basis for considerable research today both here and abroad. Further, many compounds are being tested internationally that do not appear to produce tardive dyskinesia. Nevertheless, given the benefits of these medications, the costs seem far less than those routinely associated with drugs used for the treatment of other severe illnesses in other areas of medicine.

EFFECTS OF DRUG AND PSYCHOSOCIAL TREATMENT

Much of what is known about the long-term efficacy of antipsychotic medication in the treatment of schizophrenia is summarized in Chapter 1. With the mechanism of drug action and its relationship to the schizophrenic process already described, "hard data" on drug effects seem to have a visible and enduring impact on the relatives of patients. Many patients have little insight into their illness or their need for medication. This fact, combined with the impact of side effects, makes drug noncompliance by far the most serious obstacle to the health maintenance of these patients. Knowledge of drug efficacy contributes greatly to engaging families as allies in treatment. When families understand and support the rational use of medication, their efforts not only sustain drug compliance over time, but they can also become a source of information regarding the often subtle behavioral side effects of medication that might be easily missed by the supervising clinician. The beginning of an ongoing and necessary dialogue between the family and nurse clinician, for example, is often facilitated in the workshop.

We present data on rates of therapeutic response to medication during the acute episode. Seventy to more than 90% of patients will resolve their active psychosis with these antipsychotic medications, with a larger number responding who manifest more classical, positive signs of the illness such as hallucinations, delusions, and thought disorders. As one encounters less typical features and "negative" symptoms of schizophrenia, response rates appear lower. Nevertheless, it takes time for these drugs to manifest their effects. An optimal blood plasma level must be reached and maintained, a process that often requires days or even weeks. Many studies have shown that "sloshing the brain" with high doses of antipsychotics in order to speed up antipsychotic effects simply does not work (Davis, 1976; Donaldson, Gelenberg, & Baldessarini, 1983). Unfortunately, rather than the 6 to 12 weeks of inpatient care often needed to bring about a more complete remission of symptoms, patients now are frequently hospitalized for 3 to 4 weeks, or even less. As a result, a good number of patients are still actively psychotic when discharged, which adds not only to the burden of the family, but to the problems of the usually understaffed ambulatory care clinic as well. Because treatment decisions are not always made in the best interests of the patient, we point out to relatives that it is extremely important for them to determine the basis of treatment recommendations made in behalf of their ill family member. Are these recommendations based on misinformation, politically motivated, fiscally determined, clinically expedient, or fadish? Or are they drawn from a wellfounded clinical and research base taking into consideration the patient's response to treatment interventions?

Many of the positive effects of inpatient care probably can be traced to the provision of chemotherapy and a supportive, controlled environment. Too often, however, inpatient units themselves can be sources of "overstimulation" in the form of individual and group therapy sessions designed to unveil, explore, analyze, and interpret the nuances of "intrapsychic conflict" during an acute psychotic episode. We suggest to families that if they are to be used at all, these intensive treatments are best postponed until the patient has been stabilized and is functioning well in the outside world.

Families are also told about patient response to ongoing outpatient drug treatment. For instance, upon discharge, about 20% of the first episode patients appear to be able to recover without continuing treatment, but as mentioned in Chapter 1, it is unfortunate that no one at this time can predict who these patients will be. First episode patients who are maintained on medication for a year, have an extremely low risk of relapse. Sometimes first episode patients who are doing well on medication might be gradually withdrawn from drugs in the second year of treatment. If a relapse then occurs, it is best to continue them on maintenance antipsychotic drugs indefinitely, on as low a dose as possible.

Prior to modern treatment, 10% to 20% of patients would have had a catastrophic and deteriorating course after the first episode; one that would often have required continuing inpatient care. It is clear that the number of these patients has dramatically decreased internationally in the last 30 years (Hogarty, 1977). Today, we most often encounter patients who show intermittent or periodic episodes of schizophrenia. *The frequency and the number of interim psychotic episodes is most strongly associated with the absence of maintenance treatment, particularly with the absence of maintenance antipsychotic drug treatment* (see Hogarty, 1984). On average, 68% of all patients, and from 80% to 100% of chronic schizophrenic patients will experience a relapse within a year following their discontinuation of medication. Eighty percent or more of the patients "off medication" will experience a relapse within 2 years of hospital discharge. Maintenance chemotherapy alone can reduce these relapse rates to 35% in the 1st year following hospital discharge and to 12% to 15% in subsequent years (see Chapter 1).

Nevertheless, the reality that large numbers of patients continue to relapse even on antipsychotic medication has led to an increased recognition of the need to continue to develop psychosocial strategies of intervention. We inform relatives that our type of family intervention, as well as other psychosocial attempts to manage the patient, when used in combination with medication have greatly reduced relapse at least in the first year following an acute episode. As hoped, these effects appear to be accomplished through the selective management of internally and externally derived stimulation and stress. In general, however, psychosocial treatments, by themselves, in the absence of a medication program, seem no more effective than no treatment. In fact, in past studies, certain patients were seen to have a relapse or deterioration in adjustment that could be attributed to psychosocial therapies when used in the absence of medication (Hogarty, Goldberg, Schooler, & Ulrich, 1974).

At this point in the discourse, we review the nature of stress which has been associated with schizophrenic relapse. It is made clear that stress alone, particularly the stress associated with becoming an adult, going to and getting out of school, finding employment, or establishing a family, is not the cause of schizophrenia. If it were, the world would be overwhelmed with psychotic individuals. The stress–diathesis model is discussed (Figure 3-2), reinforcing the family's role in helping to manage stress.

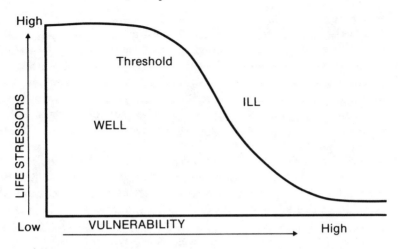

FIGURE 3-2
Stress-Vulnerability Model. (Adapted from Zubin & Spring, 1977.)

Unfortunately, forestalling relapse is only part of the problem in the treatment of schizophrenia. Seemingly less amenable to treatment are the residual effects of the illness which take the form of problems in motivation, social judgment, interpersonal effectiveness, and vocationally appropriate choices and behaviors. To improve upon these areas of adjustment, while not exposing patients to additional sources of symptom-provoking stress, the careful management of all systems appropriate to the patient's life must be accommodated, such as: the inner feelings and concerns of the patient, family life, prevocational and resocializing experiences, and job or school involvement.

Finally, we reemphasize the crucial importance of moderation during the "first year out." The patient has suffered a profound and serious illness, which requires time to heal. Lethargy, indifference, social withdrawal, and, at times, an inordinate need to sleep will be characteristic of the life styles of many patients for at least the first 6 to 12 months following discharge. The process of rehabilitation will be slow. Periodic setbacks will be encountered, but the goal of achieving maximum health and performance will be maintained even though the process will be something akin to playing 78 rpm records at a 33⅓ speed.

Other Treatments

The field of mental health is, has been, and undoubtedly will continue to be characterized by periodic claims of cures (followed by bouts of hopelessness) quickly seized upon and promoted by the popular press. Antipsychotic drugs, for example, are routinely "bad-mouthed" or exaggerated in the media, as reporters focus upon patients who have been victims of the profound misuse of antipsychotic drugs.

Before endorsing any new treatment, it is crucial to review the recommendations of national scientific committees, primarily those formed under the guidance of the National Institute of Mental Health, for current information on alleged alternative treatments to schizophrenia. Megavitamin therapy, for example, had been widely heralded in the 1960s and 1970s as a more effective treatment of schizophrenia. While vitamin deficiency in some few patients might indeed contribute to their schizophrenic-like illness, the results of carefully controlled studies have generally demonstrated no specific advantage for megavitamin treatment (Autry, 1975). The same might be said for the proponents of diets low in wheat glutten as a treatment. Patients, like everyone else, must maintain a balanced and nutritious diet.

Most families have questions about treatments their particular patient has been given, or about which they have read. A number of specific topics are raised in almost every workshop. For instance, in more recent years, the filtering of alleged "psychotoxins" by means of renal dialysis has captured the attention of many clinicians worldwide. Families are told that while certain individual patients appear at times to respond positively to this most difficult and unpleasant procedure, controlled studies of real and "sham" dialysis have produced no convincing findings in favor of dialysis (Schulman et al., 1984). Claims of efficacy for therapy based on "screaming" and "ridicule" are also without any empirical support. Lobotomy, because of better alternatives and the irreversible consequences of severing brain connections has been largely abandoned.

Sometimes, even today, electroshock treatments might be used for schizophrenic patients who do not respond to more conventional treatments, particularly those who have an abiding and severe depression associated with their schizophrenia. Advantages and disadvantages of various "group" versus "individual" psychotherapies also are discussed. The need to avoid "overstimulation" is the principal concern in evaluating any of these approaches.

Interwoven in this discussion of alternative treatments are comments on "consumables" which should be avoided. Caffeine, particularly in the form of colas and coffee *must* be limited. "Caffeinism" is extremely difficult to separate from the anxiety, nervousness, and excitement which could be part of the schizophrenic process itself. It is also difficult to separate from *akathisia*, a feeling of internal restlessness, which is often a side effect of antipsychotic medication.

Alcohol consumption should likewise be limited. Since a requirement of complete abstinence sometimes creates more problems for patients and families to negotiate, we tend to be flexible about this issue. Nevertheless, in light of the fact that alcohol frequently potentiates or enhances the effects of concurrently used psychotropic medication, we strongly suggest the patient avoid drinking alcohol if at all possible. Further, alcohol is a central nervous system depressant, even in moderate doses, and might exacerbate the depression which is frequently observed during the recovery phase of schizophrenia. Most important, alcohol and illicit drug use have become the overwhelming obstacles to maintaining patients at work or in vocational rehabilitation programs. Soft drugs, such as marijuana, should not be used by schizophrenic patients. Many studies indicate an enhanced vulnerability of schizophrenic patients to a further episode if they "smoke dope."

Tobacco, on the other hand, is a more complicated problem. While it is not as obviously toxic as other drugs, it is a physical health hazard. Cigarette smoking is also a constant source of concern for families who fear that patients whose judgment is impaired, might set fire to their beds, or cause some other disaster. On the other hand, some in the field believe that the pharmacological effects of cigarette smoking on nicotine receptors might have beneficial consequences. On balance, however, the costs of cigarette smoking seem to outweigh the equivocal benefits claimed.

At this point in the discussion, if one of the medication clinicians who actually sees the patients is present at the workshop, it is often useful to have this individual discuss other aspects of diet and substance abuse as they relate to assessment, drug maintenance, drug side effects, and clinical course of patients. Because this person is responsible for the management of individual patients, specific concerns of each family member can be addressed, and the family's relationship with the patient's clinician can be reinforced.

GENETICS AND OTHER POSSIBLE CAUSES OF
SCHIZOPHRENIA

The morning session concludes with a comment on etiology, that is, the "causes" of schizophrenia, particularly the contributions of genetics. If any doubts remain that schizophrenia is a psychobiological illness amenable to chemical intervention and modification of the environment, these are discussed at this time. It is most important to touch on causes that directly or indirectly "implicate" the family. Once again, the purpose is to alleviate the unjustified guilt that often follows the family's "search for meaning" as they attempt to understand the reason for schizophrenia in their own family.

We begin this discussion with a return to the stress–diathesis model (see Figure 3-2). According to current thinking, the diathesis or "vulnerability" contribution to schizophrenic illness can either be "acquired" or "inherited," but to date, no one can talk with much authority about the cause or causes of schizophrenia *per se*. The description of the psychobiology of schizophrenia offered earlier documents the seriousness and complexity of the "cause" issue. It thus becomes quite clear to relatives that earlier scoldings, or the fact that they deprived Johnny of his bicycle at age 5, could not have produced such a profound cerebral disruption. Falling off his bike and sustaining a severe head injury, however, could represent a contributing cause, but again, given the number of bike accidents young children have, such an event would not necessarily represent the definitive or necessary cause of schizophrenia. All serious infectious diseases that affect the brain could ultimately predispose a patient to schizophrenia, including bacterial infections or perhaps "slow viruses." Birth trauma, particularly those involving brain impairment or lack of oxygen, might represent important contributing preconditions (Schulsinger *et al.*, 1984). Serious or chronic abuse of "mind altering" drugs such as LSD also might influence neuronal functioning in a way that could ultimately dispose a person to a later psychosis, even in the absence of the offending drug. As such, there are numerous possible experiences that could leave an individual more disposed to a later psychotic episode when faced with the difficult adaptive tasks of early adult life.

But clearly there is another source of this vulnerability which, in some patients, seems inherited. It must be remembered that families pass on to their offspring a great deal more than what is in their genes, including characteristic modes of interacting with, perceiving, and responding to the environment. While the "risk" of schizophrenia varies from 1% to 2% of the general population, many studies have shown much higher risk rates for schizophrenia among "first degree" family members of the patient (parent, siblings, and children) (Gottesman & Shields, 1982). These risk rates, it is emphasized, vary widely and seem to be greatly influenced by two factors: (1) whether the definition of schizophrenia is broadly made (higher risk rates) or narrowly drawn (lower risk rates), and (2) the underlying base rate of the general population from which the patient is drawn. For example, a risk rate of 15% for siblings is only five times greater if the norm group has a base rate of 3%, but is 15 times higher if the norm group being studied has a base rate of 1%. It is emphasized that while there are clear associations between family history of schizophrenia and the risk for a schizophrenic episode in an individual member, about 90% of the schizophrenic patients we see have *no* family history of schizohrenia. From twin studies and from other family studies of schizohrenia, it has been concluded that when one identical twin (i.e., a monozygotic twin sharing the same genes) develops schizophrenia, the other has about a 45% chance of developing schizophrenia as well. Between nonidentical twins (i.e., dizygotic twins who share half the gene pool) the rates of concordant schizophrenia are about 13% to 15%, or about the same as the risk rate if one parent had schizophrenia. But if both parents have schizophrenia, the risk rate rises to about 35% or 40%. Brothers and sisters of a schizophrenic patient have about a 10% risk. In general, these estimates of increased risk of schizophrenia have been supported by studies wherein the offspring of schizophrenic parents reared in foster or adoptive homes, independent of the family of origin, were investigated.

As one moves further down the genetic ladder to include aunts and uncles, or nieces and nephews, for example, the risk rate for schizophrenia decreases to about 3 or 4%, a low risk rate but still somewhat higher than that found in the general population. One investigator who had the unique opportunity to study the rather closed society of Iceland has argued from his intergenerational studies that his data support the theory that as many as one out of six individuals "carry" the genetic predisposition to severe psychosis, but that only a small fraction of these ever manifest the disorder (Karlsson, 1973). This is known as the "single, dominant gene with incomplete penetrance" theory. Other theories have also been proposed, particularly those citing multiple genes, (i.e., the individual at risk must have the presence of a unique combination of genes which, in turn, often need to be exposed to selected life experiences before they express themselves as psychosis). Quite interestingly, an ongoing adoption study in Finland, in which adopted children of schizophrenic and nonschizophrenic mothers were studied, reveals that the experiences of family life might indeed be related to the ultimate manifestation of psychosis among genetically "loaded" children (Tienari, 1984).

As such, heredity does tell us something about the fact that schizophrenia is not a random phenomenon and that its cause, in some cases, is at least partly linked to one's biology. But the larger number of cases of schizophrenia cannot be explained at this time on the basis of human genetics. We must look to other sources, including birth trauma, infectious disease, and so on. Finally, even if one were "loaded" for schizophrenia either by nature or nurture, the positive management of one's life obviously seems to go a long way toward avoiding or minimizing the schizophrenic experience.

To sum up: The misperceptions, the competing stimuli, the feelings of "overload," and the terror that they produce all have a basis in altered brain function, particularly alterations in the "chemical messengers" and their neuropathways. These alterations occur in the important structures of the brain responsible for the primitive and basic functions of information processing (attention) and the regulation of our readiness to respond (arousal). Behaviorally, they interfere with a person's thinking and feeling ability, the signs of which we call "schizophrenia," for lack of a better word. Such signs have been observed and recorded for centuries, in different parts of the world, and at a fairly constant rate throughout history. The sources of these problems are many and the subject of considerable debate. They are not willed or voluntary. In fact, nearly the same symptoms can be induced in "normal" persons by certain chemicals. Fortunately today, we have other drugs that can help to influence the chemical message system. But sometimes these drugs are not enough. Either the sources of stimulation (stress and life epochs) or the underlying brain dysfunction itself can be so severe that these drugs, though essential, are unable to prevent another episode. The efforts and skills of family, friends, clinicians, employers, teachers—in fact all who are involved in and concerned about the patient—are needed. Based on the knowledge of what is going on in the brain of the schizophrenic person, all of us can better learn how to help the patient sustain a recovery, how to identify and handle potentially harmful stress, how to negotiate change, how to pace the rate of growth, and how to steer an even course between "too much" or "too little" stimulation. *This* is the purpose of psychoeducational family therapy.

INFORMAL INTERACTIONS

If, as in this program, a day-long workshop format is used to provide information to families, the material about the symptoms, possible theories of causality, treatments for the illness, and the philosophy of the program should take most of the morning. Before beginning to share information about family coping, which takes most of the afternoon, it is very important to allow, and even encourage, informal exchange between workshop participants. Therefore, in addition to the questions and answers that occur during the formal didactic sessions, informal interactional times should be built into the program. These informal breaks (two coffee breaks and lunch in our program) provide important opportunities for families to interact with one another and with staff; for family members to ask questions that they would not ask in front of the group; and for individual family members to compare their personal experiences. The breaks also generally help to facilitate a more relaxed and open climate between family members and professionals. The role of all staff members during these times is to circulate and encourage conversation among people who seem uncomfortable or reticent. It is vital that the staff does *not* use these times to congregate together to discuss professional issues or to review the workshop. These activities can be saved until the workshop is over.

THE FAMILY AND SCHIZOPHRENIA

Coping

The afternoon portion of the workshop begins by providing a bridge between the available data about the possible pathogenesis of the illness and what might be possible for families to do about it. To build this bridge, it is helpful to provide a summary of the main points about the illness discussed in the first section of the workshop, particularly as they relate to the goals of psychoeducational family treatment. Thus the family coping section of the workshop begins by reemphasizing the following:

1. Schizophrenia is a serious illness that is likely to be chronic. While approximately 20% of those who have an initial episode will not have another, most patients will have multiple, acute episodes over the course of many years, with varying levels of functioning between these events. Currently, it is prospectively impossible to identify those patients who are likely to have only one episode.

2. While no one knows the cause of schizophrenia, the best current explanation suggests a disturbance in brain functioning of unknown origin which leaves patients vulnerable to internal and environmental stimulation. Thus they may react badly to any situation involving intensity (both positive and negative), including many situations common to family life.

3. Neither the positive symptoms of schizophrenia, (i.e., hallucinations, delusions, etc.) nor the negative symptoms (i.e., withdrawal, lethargy, amotivation) are willful misbehaviors, but are rather manifestations of the illness.

4. There is no evidence that families cause schizophrenia. The earlier theories implicating families (schizophrenogenic mothers, marital schism or skew, the double bind hypothesis, etc.) either have not been supported by subsequent research or are identified family patterns that may exist independently or that may have occurred as a result of the illness.

5. While there is no cure for schizophrenia, in many cases it is possible to bring it under reasonable control, or at least to minimize

the number or intensity of crises that patients and families experience as a result of its presence. A sizeable number of patients do improve considerably and some recover fully.

At this point in the workshop, family members occasionally will ask why it is necessary to involve them in a treatment program if the professionals conducting that program do not believe families play a causal role. Three main reasons are given for soliciting family cooperation in the patient's treatment. First, emphasis is placed upon the fact that schizophrenia inevitably has an impact on everyone in a family. Although most family members readily acknowledge this fact, quotes from other family members struggling with the illness are used to emphasize that other families have gone through similar experiences. The following quotes are shared to give just a few examples of statements made by family members about the impact of the illness:

> Since he's been sick, I've had to do everything. I work, I take care of the kids. It's been so frustrating. The kids don't bring friends home. I think they're embarrassed. One of them isn't doing well at school. We all pay a price.

> He's our only son. He won't let anyone help him. Our hearts are breaking. When he suffers, we suffer. We don't go out anymore. We can't enjoy ourselves knowing he's sick.

> Our entire family life has been devastated. The other kids don't get our time or attention. We can't think of anything else; it's been a nightmare.

Second, the point is made that when a family experiences the severe and chronic stress associated with living with this illness without receiving help and support, its members will be less able to continue to help the patient effectively. Even worse, it is possible that they may begin to develop problems. It is common to see marital conflict between parents, acting out in siblings, and depression or physical symptoms in just about everyone. These potential difficulties are mentioned at this time to underscore the importance of all family members developing and maintaining a healthy concern for themselves, not only for their own sakes, but also for the sake of the patient. Thus, it is emphasized that their presence in treatment helps them to learn to protect themselves.

Third, family members are told that we believe there are specific things they can do that may make things better for the patient. It is stressed that the suggestions which will be made are not necessarily the natural responses anyone would have to someone who is ill. Nor are the suggestions meant to imply criticism of the ways family members may have coped in the past. If common sense solutions worked, neither patients nor families would need to seek help. Families also are told that while the staff of the program are experts on schizophrenia, and on patients and families in general, *they* are experts about the patient in *their* family, and experts on the way *their* family operates. It is emphasized that while the workshop will provide many coping techniques, some will not be appropriate or possible to use in their particular situation. They must be the final judges of which ones they will attempt to use.

Before providing specific coping techniques, it is also important to let families know that the program's staff have some understanding of the experiences they have been through. As was mentioned in Chapter 2, family members are less likely to accept any suggestions if they do not believe the staff understand the difficulty of following these guidelines. For this reason, common emotional responses of other family members to the illness are reviewed, along with common behavioral responses. Although no active attempt is made to encourage discussion of these issues, this review often stimulates considerable sharing of personal experiences by family members. Discussion is allowed at this point based on the belief that this sharing can help everyone begin to feel less isolated and more willing to accept support both from other families and from the professionals in the program. The following specific emotional behavioral responses to the patient are touched upon.

Common Emotional Responses

Anxiety, fear: Since the onset of schizophrenia involves significant behavioral, emotional, and cognitive changes, family members often will have become anxious and fearful even before it is clear that the patient is seriously ill. Watching a loved one develop strange, inexplicable behaviors is incredibly upsetting. Fears and anxiety about the cause or meaning of these behaviors, as well as about the patient's future, are inevitable. In general, professionals will have done little to alleviate these feeings since, if family members are seen at all when patients are treated, they are unlikely to have been given much information or reassurance.

Guilt: Lack of knowledge about the possible causes of this illness has led to a proliferation of theories, many related to the pathological impact of the family. Even those families who have not encountered these theories tend to fear that the patient's problems were caused or exacerbated by something they did or did not do. When something goes wrong, most people look to themselves to see what they could have done differently, and most people find something that they can worry about. These concerns tend to be reinforced by the messages of the popular media (magazines, TV, and radio) that emphasize the connection between good parenting and a child's success. Thus, a certain amount of guilt seems to be inevitable.

Stigma and embarrassment: People with mental illness are among the most stigmatized groups in our society. Much of this is due to fear, society's lack of understanding of mental illness, and the disproportionate publicity given to those few patients who are disruptive, violent, or criminal. Understandably, when patients behave in an unusual manner, they often cause pain and embarrassment to their family members.

Frustration: When someone in a family becomes mentally ill, other family members usually try every possible way of helping that person, while also trying to keep family life stable and predictable. Because so many common coping mechanisms either produce minimal results or fail altogether, most family members become increasingly frustrated.

Anger: Anger is a normal response to chronic frustration. Even when family members realize that the patient is ill, it is impossible to avoid feeling angry at behaviors that are thoughtless, inconvenient, or irritating. Anger is particularly prevalent when family members believe that patients could control their behaviors if they only tried harder, or if they were not lazy or manipulative.

Sadness, mourning: Most family members experience, at one time or another, a sense of sadness about the loss of their hopes and dreams for the patient. These feelings are particularly acute when family members first realize that the patient will never be the same as he or she was before the illness. Giving up hopes and dreams is particularly sad for parents, and even worse for parents when the patient is an only child. Nevertheless, it is also sad for spouses of patients when they must mourn the loss of a partner who was genuinely responsive to them and learn to cope with the self-preoccupation or diminished capacities of their loved one.

Common Behavioral Responses

Adapting and normalizing the situation: The most common initial response of family members to behavioral changes in patients is to adapt their routine to incorporate the behavioral patterns of the patient. If the onset of the illness is slow and insidious, there is usually a slow, continuous adaptation by all family members that allows the patient to maintain a role in the family and "get by" in the world. As the patient becomes more dysfunctional, however, it becomes difficult to constantly and increasingly adjust to the home environment, and this coping mechanism loses effectiveness.

Coaxing and rational persuasion: The natural instinctive response of family members when a loved one begins to behave or think strangely, is to try to convince them that their unusual ideas and belief systems are not true, or to coax and persuade them to behave in a different, more acceptable manner. Early in the course of the illness, the lack of any overt physical disability often leads to the assumption that it is possible for patients to have control over their symptomatology. Thus, family members often continue to try to coax and convince patients long after it has become clear that this method of coping is an ineffective one.

Making sense out of nonsensical communications: As it becomes more apparent that the patient does not make sense, family members often try to discern the meaning of the patient's bizarre or nonsensical statements. They search for the core communicative message or some element of reality in the patients' irrational ramblings or statements. This, of course, is both frustrating and exhausting, and over time might also cause other family members to develop habits of communicating in unusual ways.

Ignoring: When the patient's behaviors do not demand a response, family members will often try to cope by ignoring them, hoping they will go away. Family members may even express the hope that the patient "will grow out of it," but more likely they will try to deny the significance of the symptoms, focus on other aspects of their lives, and try not to think about it. Again, ignoring the illness only works for short periods of time, or when behaviors are not extreme.

Taking on extra responsibilities themselves: As patients become increasingly dysfunctional, family members often attempt to be supportive by assuming more of the patients' tasks and roles. This coping mechanism often allows patients to survive outside an institution even when they are quite dysfunctional since this way of coping usually reduces the amount of dissension about the patient's failure to perform even minimally. There is, however, a limit to how much and how long family members can tolerate these extra burdens.

Providing constant supervision: As the patient becomes more disturbed, the fear and anxiety of family members often leads them to try to monitor the patient's actions on a minute-to-minute basis. Since there is a strong sense of unpredictability, continued supervision provides some protection for the patient and gives the family some sense of having control over a potentially chaotic situation. Ultimately, however, most families cannot maintain this state of hypervigilance, and this coping mechanism breaks down.

Curtailing their own activities to care for or support the patient: As in any crisis in any family, family members tend to plan their routine and activities so as to be able to care for or offer maximum support to the member with a problem. It is easy to see how the chronic problems of a patient slowly cause all family members to begin to base their schedules and routines on his or her needs. Either they must actually take care of the patient, providing supervision in the home for fear of harm to self or others, or family members find themselves too exhausted and overextended to use what little free time they have to do anything but the minimum tasks necessary to maintain a home.

Ignoring the needs of the other family members: As the patient increasingly becomes the focal point of the family's energy and attention, the emotional and functional needs of the rest of the family almost automatically become secondary. This does not mean that the needs of others lose their importance, or that other family members do not care about one another, but rather that caring for the patient ultimately becomes a fulltime job. Over time, this can mean that other family relationships deteriorate, or that others will come to feel uncared for or neglected, because there just isn't enough time and energy to go around.

These are just a few examples of the emotions and behaviors that family members may develop in response to the patient's mental illness. When reviewing these responses for the group, it cannot be overstressed that they should be framed as appropriate and normal for any family coping with a difficult situation and a confusing illness. The pain associated with the gradual realization that most of these coping mechanisms are futile must be addressed before moving to the specific recommendations of the treatment program. If family members do not perceive that the workshop staff appreciates the difficulties they have experienced, and that they have done their best considering the overwhelmingly difficult circumstances, they will be more likely to be defensive and unreceptive to trying new ways of coping.

Suggestions and guidelines are given to family members to prepare them for working with the staff of the program on an ongoing basis. Over time, these suggestions can be modified and adapted to specific plans for specific family situations, based on the individual strengths and problems of the patient and the family system. All suggestions are based on the assumption that a family can positively influence the course of the patient's illness.

The stated overall goals for patients are reviewed: A return to as normal functioning as possible over time and breaking the cycle of repeated psychotic episodes. The working premise presented is that if patients can be maintained on medication and not overstimulated during the time of highest vulnerability (the first 12 to 18 months postepisode), it may be possible to avoid the full-blown recurrence of overt psychotic symptoms, leaving more time and energy for patients to enhance problem-solving skills and develop ways of protecting themselves. While it is never implied or suggested that this delaying tactic will cure the illness, it is suggested that there is genuine hope for improvement. Families are told that some patients will eventually be able to look and act like anyone else, others will have occasional problems but still be able to function effectively, and some will require ongoing or periodic intervention. Few, however, need to be either in constant crisis or continually disruptive to their families.

WHAT THE FAMILY CAN DO TO HELP

The theme of the entire treatment process is explained to families as one of maintaining a delicate balance between too much and too little stimulation. Family members are asked to help by providing a relatively low-key, but not permissive, environment for the first several months after an acute episode. This low-key environment is framed as a way of "buying time" during which the patient may be able to become more tolerant of stimulation and the normal demands of life.

More specifically, it is emphasized that the goals of the first year following an episode are primarily the avoidance of another episode or hospitalization and the gradual assumption of basic roles within the family. Anything else achieved is regarded as a bonus. The goal of the second year is to begin the gradual process of starting or returning to work, school, and social functioning. The following general suggestions are given to families to help to achieve these goals.

Revise Expectations, at Least Temporarily

Temporarily modified or decreased expectations of patients enables families to be less surprised or "let down" by inevitable patient behaviors. The first half of the workshop, which described the symptoms, course, and treatment of schizophrenia, usually helps to facilitate the development of more realistic expectations. Nevertheless, the need for revised and diminished expectations is reinforced and made explicit as part of the guidelines given to relatives for coping effectively.

For families who are experiencing the patient's first episode, the point is made that, because the hospitalization may have been brief, this does not mean that the patient's illness is not a very serious one. It is suggested to family members that it would be useful to regard patients as if they had a very serious physical illness, one which required a long process of recuperation. After the initial stabilization of the patient's psychotic symptoms, a period of inactivity, amotivation, and excessive sleep is common. Even if patients do not experience these negative symptoms, they tend to have restless energy, with little ability to follow through effectively on even small tasks. Thus, the need for increased rest, sleep, withdrawal, and limited activity for a period of time is predicted in advance. It is important to stress the fact that these patterns are a natural part of the course of the disorder since some family members will otherwise tend to assume that patients are healthy but lazy when overt symptoms have subsided. If families can be helped to understand that this apparent laziness merely represents another stage of the illness, they may be better able to tolerate the inactivity and amotivation that can otherwise be extremely irritating. In fact, it may be helpful to label these negative symptoms as the body's adaptive response to a debilitating stress, since this provides some sort of explanation for a level of inactivity that seems inexplicable. Whether these symptoms are actually adaptive or not is less important than the fact that they are predictable and difficult to influence. Most patients do become more active and interested over time. However, to aid in coping with these symptoms while they persist, the family clinician is established as someone who will be available to offer support and to help family members make specific judgments regarding the symptoms of the illness as opposed to possible malingering.

To enable family members to tolerate the slowness of change during this period of low expectations, the idea of using an "internal yardstick," is presented. As patients begin to recover from an acute episode, both family members and patients are encouraged to compare the patient's current behaviors to those of a month ago, rather than to someone else's current behavior. This yardstick concept was, in fact, generated by a patient to help herself. She was a very bright young student who was extremely frustrated after hospital discharge because, although she did extremely well, she found she couldn't keep up with the other people in her class. She was unable to do the very things she used to be able to do with ease. After spending months getting repeatedly depressed and furious because she didn't have the control or ability she once had, she learned on her own how to gauge change. She said, "I have to compare myself to where I was 6 months ago, not to where my brother is today, not to where my peers are today, but to where I was 6 months ago. I have to ask myself 'Am I better now than I was then?'" If patients and families, and even the professionals treating these patients, can learn to use this way of measuring success, they can develop a greater tolerance of the slow progress inherent in the recuperative process. The idea is to help people to see and appreciate the "inches" of movement as they occur, thus decreasing feelings of discouragement and hopelessness. The appreciation of very small positive changes may also eventually help patients to have more appropriate expectations for their own behavior.

Create Barriers to Overstimulation

Families are helped to see that they can influence the course of schizophrenia by learning to modulate the level of stress within the home (Brown & Birley, 1968; Brown et al., 1972; Goldberg et al., 1977; Torrey, 1973; Vaughn & Leff, 1976). Decreasing stimulation and stress is labeled as central to an eventual decrease in patient vulnerability. The family is told that the diminished stress tolerance of the patient includes a diminished tolerance for the interpersonal stresses common to family life. The results of studies of the posthospital adjustment of schizophrenic patients (mentioned in Chapter 1) are shared. These results have demonstrated that relapse is often related to the amount of stimulation in the patient's environment, including the amount of intense affect or conflict within families. While the details of these studies need not be shared, it is suggested that conflict, simultaneous and multiple interactions, unclear power structures, and diffuse generational or interpersonal boundaries will be difficult for patients with schizophrenia to manage. Thus, decreasing stress implies decreasing the emotionality and intensity of family life.

Families are helped to see that certain instinctive behaviors common to all families in crisis are generally not helpful in dealing with schizophrenia because of the particular nature of the disorder. Generally, these less helpful behaviors can be put into three categories:

1. Conflict and criticism between family members in general and toward the patient in particular.
2. Extreme involvement with the patient, (whether positive or negative).
3. Decreased involvement with each family member's own social network or other potential supports or gratifications beyond the nuclear family.

Thus, a series of suggestions are given to help family members to limit interactions that could constitute overstimulation for schizophrenic patients. Much like the Muzak heard in department stores and dentist offices in which the range of tones is compressed, family members are told that they will be asked to modulate the highs and lows of their family interaction, to create a family attitude of "benign indifference." In other words, they are encouraged to minimize the negatives of nagging, rejection, fights, and conflicts, as well as the positives of extreme concern, encouragement, and enthusiasm. An example of the upsetting nature of both of these extremes, provided by a patient early in the project, is shared. He described his upset when his mother would continually nag him to take out the garbage. He also described at least as much upset, however, when she not only stopped berating him, but rewarded him excessively ("That was wonderful") when he did carry it out. As he stated, "I knew it was no big deal to carry out the garbage. I just knew how much I had been letting her down when she made such a big deal over nothing." These examples are used to underscore the importance of benign, relatively neutral responses, however difficult they may be. The idea is to create distance without rejecting the patient.

It is also suggested that families allow patients to withdraw when they seem to need to do so, and learn to recognize which patient behaviors signal the need for "time out" from interaction or activity. Operationally, this may mean simply allowing patients to keep the doors to their rooms closed, to have a room in a quiet part of the house, to eat dinner away from the rest of the family, to know in advance when company is coming, and so on. To help avoid complete withdrawal of patients during this phase, families are encouraged to offer patients opportunities to engage in activities, such as going to a movie or going bowling, but to accept patient refusals if they seem unable to participate or need to be by themselves.

It is emphasized that this sort of attitude may initially seem artificial, difficult to implement, and unfair to both family and patient so soon after an acute episode, but that it is of great help to patients. In general, messages demonstrating an awareness of the difficulty of all these suggestions are important since they reinforce the notion that the staff truly appreciates the problems families will have in operationalizing these principles. These messages also allow the staff to emphasize that suggestions are only made if they are considered extremely important for the patient's recuperation or the family's survival.

Set Limits

Another method of decreasing the likelihood of overstimulation of the patient and overextension of family "coping resources" is the creation of reasonable rules for living together and the reinforcement of them through setting limits. Families are instructed not to confuse the need for low stimulation with permissiveness. Because patients are sick does not mean that families can or should do whatever they ask. The emphasis placed on creating rules and limits often confuses family members who are still attempting to assimilate the concept of "benign indifference." Thus, time must be taken to explain how limits can help to maintain a low-key, predictable home environment, and how they can be set without increasing stimulation or conflict.

Families are helped to understand that external limits are reassuring to patients who are feeling overwhelmed by the chaos in their own minds, and that these limits also are crucial in preparing patients to live in the real world, a world that will be less tolerant of bizarre or symptomatic behaviors. It is also emphasized that limits are important in helping to keep the level of stress placed on other family members within tolerable bounds. It is never helpful to permit patients to engage in unusual rituals or strange, irritating behaviors if they unduly upset others in the family. The following guidelines are given to help families to set reasonable and effective limits on most behaviors.

1. Decide ahead of time on the minimal conditions or rules necessary for the patient to come home to live with the family. In making these decisions, try to separate behaviors that are just irritating from those that are intolerable, and establish priorities based on a concensus about what upsets the patient and other family members the most. Family members should never tolerate abuse, but other behaviors can be left negotiable dependent on the family's reaction to them. For example, one patient required his entire family to remove their shoes when entering the house. For his parents, this was a tolerable, if somewhat inconvenient request. For his adolescent brothers and sisters, who had to explain the ritual to friends who visited, this was very irritating and extremely embarrassing. Considering the needs of these siblings, then, this ritual became a priority for parental limit setting.

2. Set limits clearly and without detailed discussion. It is best to avoid discussions of why a limit is being set or how everyone feels about it. A direct statement such as "that's not acceptable" is preferable to a detailed explanation since it is both more clear and less stimulating. For example, Naomi and her parents typically engaged in long discussions about why she played the stereo at night. She would describe her need to interrupt the voices she otherwise would hear while her parents would stress its disruptiveness to other family members. There was no visible resolution after months of negotiation. When her parents were able to clearly state that the stereo had to be off by midnight, period, Naomi complied, and in fact, seemed reassured and less anxious. Later they were able to buy her a miniature tape player with headphones, a solution which addressed her needs as well.

3. Keep request specific. Try to avoid asking the patient to follow general guidelines or multiple suggestions given simultaneously. For example, don't ask patients to "help out more." It is better to say, "Your job is to carry out the garbage twice a week." Since lack of initiative is a common problem, when the time comes to carry out

the garbage, another specific reminder is in order. One family was becoming increasingly angry at what they perceived to be the patient's continual refusals to help out around the house. During a family session, however, they became aware that Tim did not know what they wanted him to do. Making a list of specific tasks, with Tim's input, eased the conflict considerably.

4. Set limits before the tension builds. Excessive anger is much worse than limit setting in terms of undermining a low-key environment. Thus, when possible, rules should be established beforehand, or limits set as soon as something begins to brew. Emily's mother was becoming increasingly upset by Emily's "playful" way of hitting her. She did not express her growing anger at this behavior because she felt Emily was sick and was therefore unable to respond to limits. Her failure to set limits on this behavior only made things worse as it contributed to the growing tension in the household. A pattern developed in which Emily's mother would tolerate the behavior as long as she could, then "blow her stack." Unfortunately, she would then feel guilty and return to tolerating the abuse again. The relationship, and the home environment in general improved vastly when she began to simply stop Emily *each* time she engaged in such inappropriate behaviors.

5. Don't be guided by the patient's chronological age. It may seem unreasonable to establish rules and chores for someone in their 20s or 30s. Nevertheless, if patients are not behaving as adults, it is important to supply the structure they need rather than to wait for them to "grow up." For instance, Amanda's father was very upset when she stayed out until 3:00 A.M. and then slept until noon the next day. He worried about her judgment, which seemed impaired, but felt he had not right to set limits as though she were an adolescent when she was almost 30. Amanda reinforced this view as well by telling him he had no authority. It wasn't until he was given support for his right to establish the rules for her living in his home, whatever her age, that he was able to establish a firm curfew and consequences related to breaking it. Despite her complaints, Amanda accepted this structure that she was unable to provide for herself. It also provided the beginnings of some motivation to eventually become independent.

6. Avoid threats. Before setting any limit, family members should ask themselves, "Can I follow through on this?" They should never set a limit or consequence if they are not prepared to insist on compliance. If what is being asked of the patient is impossible to enforce, then it should be put aside for the time being. Eventually, the treatment team will attempt to find ways of helping family members deal with these more difficult issues. This policy is important in that it serves

to avoid struggles that cannot be won, thus decreasing the likelihood of frustration, anger, and eventual burnout.

7. Expect limits to be tested. Establishing reasonable control of a patient's negative behaviors takes a while, especially if the behaviors have existed for a long time. Many families too soon give up a stand they have taken, feeling it has failed because they tried it once and it didn't work. It is important for family members to be able to take a consistent stand and give it some time before deciding it failed. For instance, Mike had an elaborate ritual he would go through before he felt he could enter a room. The ritual included interrogating members of his family in a way they found offensive. It took weeks of consistent limit setting by all the family members before Mike gave up expecting their cooperation in this process.

8. Admit it when limits are primarily for the needs of other family members. Don't try to convince patients that everything that is said or done in the family, especially in the areas of limits, is exclusively for the patients' own good. Sometimes limits are set on the patient because it is important to consider the needs of others in the family. Patients must learn to live with the fact that they and their needs cannot always be the center of family life. For example, Duane's parents had a long-standing rule against using the kitchen after 10:00 P.M. Their bedroom was right next to the kitchen, Duane's father had to get up for work at 4:00 A.M., and the noise in the kitchen disturbed his sleep. However, they were very uncomfortable asking Duane to obey the rule since he often got hungry late at night. It wasn't until they were reassured that the father's needs were very important and not selfish, that they were able to enforce this limit.

9. When in doubt about whether or not to set a limit or in need of support in doing so, use the clinical team. The setting of comfortable and effective limits should be as much a collaborative effort as other aspects of treatment. The treatment team is available to help in this process.

The topic of limit setting is given a good deal of time since limits are so crucial in providing structure, maintaining a low-key environment, and establishing a home atmosphere everyone can tolerate. Particular emphasis is given to setting limits on psychotic, violent, or bizarre behaviors since these behaviors are not only the most upsetting, but also the least accepted by society. The only exception to setting limits on these kinds of behaviors has to do with paranoid delusions. It has been our experience that if family members attempt to *directly* confront or limit a paranoid idea, patients tend to become more agitated and may even begin to believe that particular family members are a part of whatever plots they believe exist against them. In these situations, it is suggested that the family respond to the anxiety beneath the statement rather than the statement itself. For instance, they might respond to a patient by saying, "That doesn't make sense to me, but I can appreciate how upsetting it must be to you if you believe it," or just, "It sounds as though you're really feeling like it's you against the world. It must be tough."

Selectively Ignore

Not focusing on everything at once is an important guideline in determining what limits to set and what goals to strive for. Without carefully established priorities, it is extremely difficult to maintain a suitable environment. No one can change everything at once, and attempting to do so only makes everyone feel overwhelmed and hopeless. Thus, family members are encouraged to choose one or two issues as their initial focus, with others to be selected after these first issues are managed successfully. While ignoring negative behaviors is almost always difficult, most families are able and willing to do so if they have established their own priorities, if they can see progress in other areas, and if they can believe that the other issues will be addressed eventually.

It is important, however, that families never be encouraged to ignore violent or psychotic behavior. Inevitably the question of what to do if violence is threatened arises during a workshop, more frequently stimulated by media representation of mental illness than by personal experience. In response to questions about violence, families should first be reassured that the incidence of violence among schizophrenic patients is not great. The majority of schizophrenic patients are, in fact, remarkably unassertive. However, in the event that particular patients have threatened to be or have been violent, families are given a number of suggestions. First, because violent acts may be precipitated by delusional thinking or hallucinations, rational discussion rarely is effective in toning things down. Rather, a good deal of violence can be avoided by establishing and maintaining a structured environment and agreeing in advance on the limit-setting procedures already described. Patients who are not overwhelmed by stimulation are less likely to react catastrophically. Families who *have* experienced violence are asked to review the precursors of these past experiences in an attempt to identify precipitants. Signals of impending violence, as well as events that touch it off, differ in every case, so it is important to be very specific in reviewing these events.

When it is possible to identify precipitating behaviors and events, plans for dealing with it can be made *well in advance* of a crisis. For example, if the beginning indicators of potential violence are at all predictable, a cooling-off period can be planned in advance and instituted at the first sign of trouble. As a first resort, the family can ask the patient to go to his or her room. If this is ineffective, it may be possible to have the family member directly involved go to another part of the house or leave the home for a brief period, just to give time to reestablish some sense of control. In order to work, however, this maneuver must be implemented early, before either the patient or family member has become agitated beyond the point of control. If patients tend to be responsive to clinician influence at such times, families are encouraged to call the clinician (see Chapter 4).

Once a patient actually has lost control, however, very little can be done unless someone in the family is sufficiently larger and stronger to either intimidate or physically restrain the patient. This is not particularly desirable, and in most families, it is also not the case. Therefore, if extreme behaviors cannot be avoided by the techniques discussed, it is important that family members get help as quickly as possible. If immediate harm seems a possibility, the family is encouraged to call the police. In smaller communities, it is sometimes possible to develop a positive and collaborative relationship with police, who come to know these patients over time. In some communities, however, police avoid contact with mental patients or give these calls a low priority. In such cases, it may be easier to get police to respond to a request for help if the caller reports "an assault in progress," rather than asking for help with a psychiatric patient (Kanter, 1981). Finally, in situations where there is the potential of sudden or unprovoked violence (based on past history), family members are asked to take preventive measures such as removing or locking up obvious weapons such as guns and knives. While this does not offer total protection since almost anything can become a weapon under the right circumstances, it sometimes decreases the seriousness of spontaneous outbursts.

Suicidal threats or behaviors also cannot be ignored. Since suicide is a genuine risk with these patients, if family members are concerned about this issue, they are encouraged to call the treatment team immediately, and to directly supervise patients until arrangements can be made that will keep them from accidentally or intentionally hurting themselves. Although suicidal talk or behavior is frightening, families are given the message that a calm response is likely to have better results than intense reactions that could trigger an impulsive gesture.

Keep Communication Simple

Specific advice regarding a limited number of communication skills may be given. The philosophy of providing these suggestions is based on the belief that the content of family interactions matters less than the clarity and simplicity of the messages sent. Thus, family members are asked to keep their communications simple with an appropriate amount of detail and a moderate level of specificity. Rigorous training in effective communication skills is avoided since such a task is thought to be too ambitious, frustrating, and anxiety provoking for both family and clinician at this point in time. Thus, only three themes relating to communication skills are emphasized:

1. *The ability to acknowledge the statements of others and to accept responsibility for one's own communications.* In any family, a certain amount of "mindreading" occurs. That is, family members make the assumption that someone else's thoughts are known even if they are not expressed. These assumptions can cause particular difficulties and create distorted communications. Thus, family members, and eventually patients, are not only encouraged to speak for themselves, but also to avoid assuming they know what others want or need, and to accept and respect what others say even if they don't agree with it. This communication skill, once learned and practiced, helps to reinforce interpersonal boundaries.

With patients who have difficulty in processing incoming stimuli, pauses and delays in communication responses are common. Family members therefore often develop a habit of speaking or responding for the patient. Unfortunately, this not only allows patients to become less and less responsible for their own messages, but it also undermines their sense of being separate, autonomous adults. Thus, it is important to help family members learn to wait and to respect the patient's ability to contribute to the conversation.

2. *The ability to keep things at a moderate level of specificity, avoiding excessive detail or too many abstractions.* When families are experiencing times of crisis, it is not appropriate to discuss highly charged and rarely resolved issues. The meaning of life, sexuality, religion, or politics are issues that tend to be highly emotional even when things are going well. Thus, families are encouraged to avoid topics such as these while the patient is ill.

In addition to these upsetting topics, some communication styles can be particularly confusing or misleading for patients. For instance, some family members tend to have an obsessive style, frequently becoming involved in detailed discussions about even neutral topics. Such a style would not be likely to cause problems in other circumstances, but schizophrenic patients are more likely to find detailed discussions stimulating or confusing.

Problems can also occur if family members get involved in inappropriate conversations with patients as they search for a core element of sense in a patient's delusional statement. In general, it is best to encourage family members not to attempt to discern the hidden meanings of bizarre communications. Others in the "real world" will not take the time to translate strange communications, thus patients should be helped to make themselves clearly understood.

The following brief conversation took place between a patient and his wife early in treatment. It can be shared with families to help them understand how to handle unusual or unclear messages while the patient is still acutely disturbed.

NAOMI: I'd love to get out to a movie with him.
CLINICIAN: What do you think about that, Art?
ART: The force will control the scene and laser radiate animals.
NAOMI: Huh? Oh, he must be talking about when we saw *Star Wars*. We really liked that. I guess he wants to go.
CLINICIAN: That's incredible. To be honest, Art, I didn't understand what you said. (*To Naomi*) Did you really understand him?
NAOMI: Well, I guess not. It's just easier sometimes to try to make sense out of it than to ask.
CLINICIAN: I'm sure it is. Art's comments must be tough to follow sometimes. But, I think it would help Art if we both ask him to answer more clearly. Not everyone he talks to is going to have your patience.

In the discussion of communication issues, the staff reinforces the need to limit psychotic communications and to help patients to be more clear, while at the same time offering understanding about the frustration families experience when they must deal with such strange messages on a day-to-day basis. These instructions give the implicit message that patients are capable of communicating more appropriately, given support, structure, and time.

3. *The ability to express and emphasize positive messages and supportive comments.* Over the course of the illness, family members are likely to become increasingly sensitized to problems or potential cues that difficulties are developing. This sensitization can lead to a focus on the negative aspects of the patient or the home situation as positive interactions and accomplishments are minimized or ignored. Thus, helping family members to focus on and reward small, positive behaviors is an important goal. Examples of what other families have learned in this regard can help to make this point. For instance, Laurie's father has learned to look for and value small gains. The following quote describes the importance he attaches to a small piece of positive behavior from his daughter.

You know, the other night I was just talking to Maureen [his wife] and I mentioned how some ice cream would be nice. . . . You know, kind of hinting and hoping she'd volunteer to get some for us. Anyway, I kind of forgot about it and then, 5 minutes later, Laurie came in with a bowl of ice cream for me. Wow, you could of knocked me over with a straw. I mean she hasn't done something like that for years. Finally, I said, "thank you." Later, I started thinking. I mean it was such a small thing and nothing important. But it *was* important to me, and made me feel . . . just a little bit, that there was a ray of hope.

The ability to recognize small steps of progress and to appropriately reinforce (but not overreinforce) them is an important skill for both family members and professionals to nurture. Recognition of these accomplishments offers hope to the family and courage to patients to continue to expend the energy and commitment necessary to attempt positive steps.

Support the Patient's Medication Regime

Because families can facilitate or impede the implementation of a medication program, information about the benefits and risks of drugs is shared early in the workshop, with the goal of increasing the likelihood of the family's support for medication compliance. At that time, the use of medication is explained as one way to decrease the patient's vulnerability to stimulation. At this point in the workshop, it is emphasized that most patients are ambivalent about taking medication. Some are uncomfortable with the side effects, while others wish to stop medication as soon as they begin feeling better, since taking medicine is associated with being sick. Unfortunately, or fortunately, the positive effects of medication can take several weeks or even months to fade after the medication has been discontinued, while the negative side effects diminish more rapidly. This leaves the *appearance* that medication is no longer needed. Without this understanding, it is often very hard for either patients or family members to appreciate the connection between medication and well-being. For this reason, time must be devoted to help each family member to understand the way these drugs operate (particularly the time delays between initiation or cessation of drugs and the effect of these steps), and the possible benefits of a medication regime. In this regard, statistics demonstrating the relationship between medication compliance and community tenure are reemphasized.

When patients are resistant to taking medication, the support of family members is often necessary to avoid noncompliance with the drug program. Nevertheless, families must also be helped to weigh the possible costs and benefits of a drug program (including the possibility of tardive dyskinesia), so that they can make a truly informed decision about whether or not they wish to support the role of drugs in the patient's treatment program.

Normalize the Family Routine

During this portion of the workshop, discussion should also focus on the need for family members to normalize their own routine as much as possible in preparation for the demands of long-term care. It is suggested to family members that they not center their lives around the patient. During an acute illness in any family member, of course, it is necessary for the rest of the family to focus their attentions and their energies on the patient. However, in any long-term illness (like diabetes, heart disease, *or* schizophrenia), patients must learn to live with their limitations and life must go on for those around them. If this does not happen, the impact of illness can become debilitating to families. In fact, family members may experience so much stress that they will be unable to offer ongoing support to patients, and may even incur additional problems of their own. Good parenting, as one of our colleagues says, begins by taking care of ourselves. This is also true in marriages: Being a good spouse begins by taking care of your own needs. In any family then, enlightened concern for self is a core part of each individual member's ability to care about others. Obviously, self-concern is difficult when a family member has this illness. Nevertheless, it is vital to the preservation of everyone's emotional and physical health. Furthermore, if other family members begin to be negatively affected by the patient's illness, patients can come to feel guilty and responsible, thereby experiencing their family as a burden, not a support.

Since most families with a schizophrenic member become increasingly isolated over time, family members are encouraged to see the importance of maintaining a support system beyond the nuclear family. Originally, the need for a well-maintained support system was stressed in the belief that those families with fewer or less available social supports outside the immediate family probably would have a lower tolerance for stress and deviance within the family (Brown *et al.*, 1972; Vaughn & Leff, 1976). Thus, family members without social supports were assumed to be family members who were also high in expressed emotion. As it turned out, data from our project suggested that while there was a connection between the length of the patient's illness and the increasing social isolation of family members, there was no connection between the number or quality of social supports and the expressed emotion of family members (Anderson, Hogarty, Bayer, & Needleman, 1984). Thus, our original efforts to have family members talk about their difficulties to friends and extended family, and engage such people in psychological support services were modified based on these data and clinical experience. We came to believe that family members, extended family, and friends were not those most likely to be most helpful in actually dealing with the impact of illness.

Nevertheless, the importance of maintaining contacts outside the immediate family continues to be stressed for three reasons. First, social contacts can be useful as temporary distractions from experiencing the pain of the illness, as well as being of possible use in providing general support and recreation to help occasionally relieve the tensions of family members. Second, having social contacts can make it easier to divert the concentration of too much energy and attention on the patient. Third, social contacts can help family members in times of crisis by providing instrumental and practical support. Unfortunately, making time to see people outside the immediate family requires motivation, time, and effort. Over time, coping with this illness tends to decrease the motivation necessary to maintain these contacts. Giving encouragement and providing these explanations may help to motivate family members to reestablish some of these vital links.

It remains difficult for many family members, however, to concentrate on meeting their own needs and establishing their own social network. Many consider their own needs as minimally important when another is in crisis. Therefore, it is essential to emphasize that family members must consider their own needs for survival *so that they will be able to help the patient.* The point is made that if they deplete themselves, in the long run they will be less able to help one another or the patient. For instance, the need to attend to other children in the family is emphasized. The disproportionate amount of attention needed by the patient in a chronic illness often occurs at the expense of the needs of other children. Siblings of patients frequently complain that their parents side with the patient no matter how unreasonable he or she is, while they always are expected to understand and avoid conflict.

In general then, while ongoing familial, social, and work activities are often impossible to maintain during the acute phase of the illness, family members are encouraged to see the need for an expanded repertoire of management techniques for the "long haul." These management techniques must include a life style that does not entirely center on the patient and his or her needs. In this regard, the need for each family member to find time away from the tension within the family is stressed.

It is also common for patients to have become socially isolated and devoid of any activities or support systems outside of the immediate family, especially those who have been ill for a long period of time. Family members often point out that it is the absence of friends that forces the patient to spend an inordinate amount of time at home, thus increasing the likelihood of family conflict. It certainly is possible that patients with fewer or less available social supports outside the immediate family are more vulnerable to family intensity and family stress since they are more involved in and dependent on their families to meet their multiple needs. At this time, therefore, family members are told that the staff eventually will initiate attempts to decrease the intensity of family relationships by distributing this intensity throughout a larger network, not only for other family members, but also for the patient.

During the latter part of this section of the workshop, the issue of the vocational and social potential of patients is discussed. Although no promises are made, the success of the program in helping some patients to develop vocational skills and even to attain employment is shared. It is made clear, however, that these goals only can be achieved after the patient's illness has been controlled, and only then after a good deal of time and hard work. While many patients probably will never be able to work in an unsheltered setting or develop independent social networks, it is important to provide hope that patients will develop an increased ability to function more normally, even if at a relatively low level, at some future date.

Learn to Recognize Signals for Help

The family is asked to develop an awareness of those behaviors that tend to signal the experience of increased stress or difficulty for their ill family member. Over time, when possible, the family and the patient together will be helped to identify which behaviors require the family's help or support, and which behaviors simply signal the patient's need for increased psychological space. The family is told that the staff will help both patient and family to become as aware as possible of any early indications of decompensation, and will help them to mobilize their resources to modify the environment and/or control symptoms. To decrease family anxiety and overresponsiveness, emphasis is placed on the fact that some signals, such as withdrawal, are not always negative, but at times are the patient's adaptive response to the threat of being overwhelmed. A review of the significance and meaning of possible signals helps family members to avoid the tendency to respond to every symptom as if it meant a patient was getting sick again, or conversely, to "keep the peace" at all costs by ignoring potentially vital messages.

Although these "signals" differ from patient to patient, and must be further defined during future family sessions, the message given to family members is that there may be a number of warning signs that could allow early intervention, and thus the avoidance of a major psychotic episode. This, in itself, can decrease anxiety in family members by giving them a better sense of having some control of the situation. It should be noted, of course, that some patients do not have definable early warning signs and that the symptoms of the illness in such patients can arise suddenly. Whether or not signals exist, family members are taught to initiate fast and appropriate contact with professionals as soon as trouble occurs in an attempt to avert a full-blown psychotic episode.

Family members are specifically advised to use professionals when they have questions or concerns. A lifeline must be established because the progress of the patient is likely to be very slow. In our particular program, we have found it most beneficial to limit actual family sessions to once every 2 to 3 weeks except during times of crisis (see Chapter 4). Therefore, it is important that family members be assured that they can reach their clinicians between sessions should they be uncertain about the appropriate response to a given situation. Some families require encouragement regarding the use of this resource, since they have learned not to alienate clinicians by imposing on their time. Thus, workshop time is used to stress the availability of the family clinician and other members of the treatment team for emergency phone and in-person contacts, as well as the clinician's desire to continue to play the role of ombudsman for the family in relation to other therapeutic and rehabilitation systems, services, and personnel. It is particularly important that family members be able to use staff for frequent consultation early in the course of treatment. Until family members feel they understand the principles of the program and how to handle the crises that occur, it is better that they check things out. This policy of "as needed" contact may mean a little extra work for clinicians initially, but over time it establishes a good treatment relationship, a better home environment, and fewer crises for clinicians to deal with in the long run. To avoid the creation of inappropriate dependency or the unnecessary depletion of staff, families are helped to differentiate between the kind of questions that can be saved for family sessions and the kind they should regard as emergencies.

Finally, the importance of every family member's constant input into the patient's treatment is stressed repeatedly. It is predicted that some stages of treatment will seem slow and painful, causing both patients and family members occasionally to wish to discontinue treatment. The role of preventive and maintenance work in avoiding future episodes and crises is stressed, as is the importance of an ongoing commitment.

The final section of the workshop is left open to allow family members to bring up questions that may not have been covered during the formal presentations. Most family members use this time to ask about specific ways of handling situations that have troubled them for some time. Others again raise questions about possible causes or treatments after they have had time to think about the morning presentation. All questions are dealt with as honestly and clearly as possible. At the end of the day, families are asked to evaluate the workshop and make suggestions for future workshops.[2]

REACTIONS OF FAMILIES TO THE WORKSHOP

Family members are usually very positive about receiving the information given at the workshop. Many claim that they have begun to understand the patient for the first time in years. The following are just a few verbatim comments from family members about their previous understanding of the illness and their responses to the events of the day.

The mother of a patient, talking about her understanding of schizophrenia before the workshop, stated:

> To me, schizophrenia was something like I'd seen in the movies, something like a split personality or a paranoid that would cower in cupboards and be afraid to eat food for fear that it was poisoned. . . . I mean it just covered all kinds of things like you would find in a snake pit and it was a very bad impression of a mental illness. . . . The very worst thing you could say about a patient would be that they had schizophrenia.

The mother of another patient described the benefits of seeing other families at the workshop:

> The big thing we came away with was hope . . . and knowing that we're not the only ones with the problem. That there are other people going through the same situation was a revelation to me. And you sort of hope that you can handle it a little better. . . . After the workshop, you take a different view toward the illness. With more education, you learn that there are people who have it a little worse than you. They need more compassion because their problem is greater.

The wife of a patient described the impact of the information itself:

> We never had an idea about his illness, and you know, I always thought secretly, deep down inside, well, you know, if he has any "calmies" at all, he can control this (*Laughs*). He really, we found out that day, they really cannot control it. It is something that you have no control over and that was a rude awakening for me. But, it helped a great deal, it really did, to know that he really has no grip on reality, and it's something he cannot control. That reality never hits until it's explained to you. Then you can go on. You can build from there. If you have that fact

---

2. A copy of the workshop evaluation form can be found in Appendix B.

right in front of your face, "You know, this is a chronic illness; it's not going to go away. It's like having cancer, or liver disease or heart disease, this is the way we will help you to deal with it." And, that's what you people did. Before, I would look at him when he was getting sick and say, "Oh boy, we have to go through this again," and that was selfish. I learned not to be selfish. It was always from my point of view, you know, "I've got these kids to take care of and he's laying up there," and it was just frustrating. That's what I thought, but when I came away, you know, when I came home from the workshop, I took a long look at my husband and for the first time in a long time felt sympathy and understanding because I was made a little aware of what went on inside his head when he got ill. You don't know how I appreciate that.

SUMMARY

In this chapter, we have described a psychoeducational "Survival Skills Workshop" for the families of patients with schizophrenia. Using a multiple-family format, this workshop involves a day-long session during which attempts are made to share with families what is and is not known about this illness. Theories of etiology, the impact of various treatment approaches, and suggested strategies for coping are reviewed, with ample time allowed for family members to ask questions and to raise issues of concern.

There are specific reasons for giving families information beyond our obligation to offer it and the fact that they are requesting it. Considering the overwhelming nature of most mental illnesses, it would not be surprising to find that what looks like antagonistic, disturbed, or irrational behavior in some family members is simply caused by excessive anxiety. People fear and resist the unknown and are made anxious by what they do not understand. Excessive fear and anxiety can interfere with any individual's ability to cope, and can impede the incorporation of new learning. Arietti states that psychotherapists of schizophrenic patients should "at least in the first and middle stages of treatment not only aim at causing very little or no anxiety, but also at diminishing the anxiety already present" (Arieti, 1980, p. 464). It makes a good deal of sense to extend this principle of treating schizophrenic patients to the treatment of patients in any serious crisis, and to treatment of their families as well.

Thus, basic to this method of intervention with families of schizophrenic patients is the diminishing of the fears and anxieties of family members, and increasing their sense of being able to predict and control their lives together. The connecting process (described in Chapter 2) is a beginning attempt to decrease anxiety. The process of providing information described in this chapter continues our work toward this goal. Specifically, connecting with family members allows them to hear information that helps them by decreasing their concerns about having caused the patient's illness, by creating more realistic expectations, and by providing a basic rationale for the incorporation of effective ways of living with and managing the patient. The provision of information by professionals also sends a metacommunication of respect and reinforces the message that the therapeutic team and family must be regarded as partners in the treatment process. While there are many things we do not know about mental illness, there is evidence that telling family members what we *do* know may be of some help.

Whether it is the information itself, the decreased sense of blame and guilt that is communicated by the absence of an emphasis on family etiology, the conveying of respect and equality, or the increase in hope generated by a new approach, the response to these workshops has been dramatic. The climate between staff and families seems to become less polarized, less tense, and resistant family members become more cooperative. Families and professionals both become less isolated, and thus less subject to "burn out." Finally, with the nature of schizophrenia explained, the principles of treatment and management become better understood and accepted.

CHAPTER FOUR

REENTRY: THE FIRST YEAR OUT

It was hard to back off. I didn't want to leave him alone. If we were invited to go out without him . . . I really didn't want to go. At first, I would make myself go and worry about him the whole time I was there, but I finally got over that.

I don't think you should put them under a microscope. You say, "Well, how are you doing today?" Kind of always looking at it, lifting the scab up to see if it's healing. I think that prolongs the whole thing.—*Parents of a patient*

During the initial connecting sessions and especially during the educational workshop, family members receive a significant amount of information about schizophrenia and its management. They also receive a great deal of support to help them to deal with the acute stage of the illness and the problems inherent in the patient's hospitalization. Once the connecting and information phases of treatment have been completed, families and patients are ready to participate in the next phase of treatment of the patient.

The purposes of ongoing treatment are multiple, but all relate to the themes that were established during the initial sessions and the survival skills workshop. Primarily, these sessions are designed to help patients to survive in the community by: (1) helping families to apply the principles outlined at the workshop, offering support and suggestions about how to do so over the "long haul," and (2) beginning a gradual process of reintegration of both patients and families into a normal work and social world.

This phase of treatment begins immediately following the patient's discharge from the hospital and lasts until the patient is ready to focus on work and social functioning. For some patients and families, this phase may last only a month or two, but more likely it will last as long as a year or more. The length of time is determined by the patient's ability to resume responsibility within the family. This ability is measured by the performance of small tasks agreed upon by the clinician, the patient, and the family. The patient's ability to do these tasks consistently, without increases in symptoms, is a prerequisite for moving on to the next phase of treatment.

132

GOALS AND METHODS

To accomplish the goals of this phase, the family clinician must deal with issues that seem common to most patients and families dealing with schizophrenia: the patient's vulnerability to stimulation; the patient's tendency to discontinue medication; the prevalence of negative symptoms; the tremendous frustrations inherent in living with the ramifications of a debilitating chronic illness; and the tendencies of family members to center their lives around the patient. At the same time, however, the clinician must remain aware of the issues, perceptions, and problems of other family members which may or may not be related to the patient's illness. Treatment goals and interventions are individualized, taking into consideration the needs of each family and the ways in which its members are able to cope. Successful negotiation of these issues is primarily accomplished by careful attention to the themes of gradual resumption of responsibility by the patient and appropriate maintenance of interpersonal, generational, and family–community boundaries.

Type and Frequency of Contact

During this phase of treatment, contacts with patients and families may occur in three ways: regularly scheduled family sessions, phone consultations, and crisis contacts. The frequency of sessions is determined by clinical experience and an understanding of the illness. In many aftercare treatment settings, the severity of schizophrenia has given rise to the notion that the more treatment the better, particularly during the early phases of aftercare. After all, most of these patients have just been released from a hospital where they have had 24-hour-a-day access to professionals. Also, it is well documented that the early months following an acute psychotic episode are the time of greatest risk of relapse (Hogarty, 1984). As in other areas of medicine, it seems only logical to most clinicians that a correlation should exist between the severity of the illness and the intensity of the treatment approach.

However, with this particular patient population, there seems to be a paradoxical relationship between the amount and/or intensity of interventions and the amount of patient progress (Goldberg *et al.*, 1977; Hogarty, Goldberg, & Schooler, 1974; Linn *et al.*, 1980). The nature of the illness, especially the patient's vulnerability to intensity and overstimulation, requires a slow treatment pace. Frequent meetings also appear to give the metacommunication to the patient and the family that rapid progress should occur between sessions, thus intensifying expectations. When such progress is not forthcoming, frequent sessions may increase, rather than decrease, the anxiety and stress of the patient, the family, and the clinician. Following the workshop, therefore, sessions with families are generally scheduled at two week intervals—a frequency which we believe provides the optimal pace and intensity for treatment. The clinician establishes a flexible agreement in this regard, allowing for more sessions if a crisis or major change takes place, as well as allowing for a decrease in the frequency of sessions as the patient stabilizes, and the patient and the family display progress toward their goals.

The infrequency of sessions requires that help be available to both patients and family members when needed. For this reason, the treatment team must clearly communicate a willingness to be available by phone, should either questions or crises arise at any time. Early in treatment, most families tend to need and use this resource. They are unsure of the skills they have learned at the workshop and uncertain as to whether they are doing the right thing. Furthermore, because of the brief nature of most hospitalizations, patients often have psychotic symptoms after discharge. They may continue to hear voices or have active delusions, either regularly or when feeling stress. In any case, their anxiety level is likely to be high and their trust in the clinician low.

Being available by phone to both patient and family during these times allows clinicians to help in a number of ways. They can insert structure into potentially chaotic situations and decrease the likelihood of intense interactions between family members by listening, giving advice, and/or affirming the appropriateness of the family's coping skills. Finally, the immediate availability of the clinician can, in itself, add to the rapid development of the therapeutic relationship.

In the following example, the clinician is able to reassure a mother who is concerned about her daughter, Sandy, and the way she and her husband are handling Sandy's behavior.

MOTHER: Thank you for returning my call so quickly. I wanted to check with you about something Sandy is doing. I know you told her she should try to get some exercise. Well, she's been swimming at the spa a few times a week and that's fine. But now, she's taken to going for long walks. My husband and I are worried because she goes alone into the park, even at night. We think it's dangerous, but in the past, she's gotten very angry when we tell her we're worried. We don't want to get her agitated. I know they said at the workshop to keep things cool.

CLINICIAN: I'm glad you called. You're right to be concerned, that park has a pretty bad reputation. Exercise is good for her, but I wouldn't want her to get hurt.

MOTHER: Exactly. So what do I do?

CLINICIAN: It's fine to tell her she shouldn't walk there alone. Remember, limits are good, just don't go into a long involved explanation of why.

MOTHER: So, just say, "you can't go."

CLINICIAN: Yes, or offer an alternative—like suggesting she go with a friend.

MOTHER: (*Reluctantly*) She still may get angry with me.

CLINICIAN: That's normal. No one likes to be told what to do, but it's in her own best interests. Would you like me to talk to her and take some of the heat off?

MOTHER: Would you? She's here now.

CLINICIAN: Sure, put her on.

SANDY: Yeah?

CLINICIAN: Sandy, your mother and I have been talking about your parents' worries about your going for walks in the park alone.

SANDY: I know. She worries too much just because I've been sick. I'm better now, and it bothers me that she butts into everything.

CLINICIAN: I know you're better and I'm glad you're exercising. But to tell you the truth, I agree with your parents. I don't think you should walk in the park alone, especially at night. It has nothing to do with your being sick. It just isn't safe. *I'd* be uncomfortable walking there at night.

SANDY: You mean you agree with her?

CLINICIAN: On this one, yes. I told her she should tell you not to go. I know she gets overprotective, but I don't think she is in this case. I think it's a good idea. Can you think of a compromise?

SANDY: (*After a pause*) I guess I could go swimming instead.

CLINICIAN: Or go for a walk *with* someone.

SANDY: I don't want to go with my mother.

CLINICIAN: Fine, but someone else?

SANDY: I guess so. Maybe it is bad to go alone.

In this example, the clinician reinforced the mother's use of a phone consultation to check out a way of handling a problem that had caused stress in the past. He affirmed the legitimacy of the parents' concern and of their right to set limits on behavior that could get their daughter into trouble. When the mother expressed some fear of her daughter's response, he offered to diffuse the potential argument by talking to Sandy directly. When he did so, he again reinforced the mother's position but emphasized the reason for this limit as one of general safety, not illness. Since both Sandy and her mother seemed to accept this compromise, no further intervention was made. In general, phone calls are kept brief and problem focused so as to encourage the use of sessions for the major work of treatment and to discourage unnecessary dependence on the clinician. If the situation is one which is serious and not easily resolved, a crisis session is scheduled, as in the following example.

MRS. A: Jack, I'm sorry to bother you, but I'm really worried about Sam. He's staying in his room almost 24 hours a day. I know they said at the workshop that he might sleep a lot, but this seems too much. Then when he comes out, just the past few days, he looks at us really funny. He seems very agitated.

CLINICIAN: Have you tried asking him about it?

MRS. A: Yes, but he won't say much. Just that what he's doing is for our own good . . . whatever that means.

CLINICIAN: But you definitely get the sense he's feeling worse?

MRS. A: Oh, yes. To tell you the truth, I'm a little scared of him.

CLINICIAN: Could you ask him if he'll talk to me now?

MRS. A: Well, I'll try. I'm not sure he'll come to the phone.

SAM: (Some minutes later) Hello.

CLINICIAN: Sam, it's Jack. How are you doing?

SAM: Not so good.

CLINICIAN: What's going on?

SAM: (Long pause) I've got these funny ideas. Someone is telling me what to do.

CLINICIAN: What are they saying?

SAM: (Pause) I don't want to talk about it. I'm scared though.

CLINICIAN: Scared that something might happen to you?

SAM: More scared that something might happen to my family. Like someone might kill them.

CLINICIAN: That's a serious worry. Tell you what, would you be willing to come in and talk about it, see if we can do something to make you feel better?

SAM: I guess so. When?

CLINICIAN: Right now. If it's okay, I'll talk to your parents and ask them to bring you down.

SAM: Okay.

In this phone conversation, the clinician determined that both Sam and his mother were aware that things were not going well, and that both were also worried that Sam was losing control. Sam directly implied that voices were telling him to hurt his family. In such cases, adding structure to the family environment is usually insufficient, so a crisis session is scheduled.

Crisis sessions are scheduled whenever there appears to be a risk of things getting out of control. Reasons for such a session might include the threat of violence (on the part of patients or family members), the risk of suicide, or reports of major increases in psychotic symptomatology. These sessions are scheduled immediately and focus only on the presenting issue. During such sessions, clinicians take an even more directive stance than usual by reinforcing rules and boundaries, and taking all the steps necessary to defuse the crises as simply and directly as possible.

The following example came from a crisis session that was called by the clinician following a phone call from a mother saying that her son, Tom, was significantly symptomatic and had broken into the store downstairs from their apartment.

CLINICIAN: Your mother told me over the phone what she felt happened, Tom, but I'd like to hear from you also.

TOM: (*Agitated*) I had to get rid of the spirits. They were getting worse. Thought they were smart—hiding [in the store], but I found them.

MOTHER: (*Upset*) Now they'll ask us to move. I can't stand to think about it.

CLINICIAN: (*Firmly, but calmly*) I understand that everyone is upset and concerned about different things. Right now I'd like to help calm the situation down and help Tom to feel better. If there are any legal problems or landlord hassles that come from this, we can deal with them as they come up. Tom, I'd like to help you feel better. Can you tell me how many days you've been feeling this upset?

TOM: For a few, but it's been getting worse.

CLINICIAN: How do you feel right now?

TOM: A little better—now that I found them [the spirits].

CLINICIAN: How have you been sleeping?

MOTHER: Not good. I hear him pacing all night.

CLINICIAN: Is your mother right?

TOM: Yeah, I haven't been able to sleep. I'm too worried.

The clinician continues to discuss Tom's worries for a few minutes, and then sums things up in the following manner:

CLINICIAN: All right. Let's do three things. First, I want you to see Mrs. J [Tom's medication clinician] with me as soon as we're done here to see about possibly changing your medication to make you feel more comfortable. You look pretty tired and strung out.

TOM: Okay.

MOTHER: Good.

CLINICIAN: Second, let's try to meet a little more often for a while and see if we can figure out when you get most worried about the spirits. Maybe we can find some ways to get things under a little better control.

TOM: The spirits aren't bothering me too much right now.

CLINICIAN: Good, it sounds like you believe you've taken care of the "spirits." But in case the feelings come back, I'd like us to be ready to deal with them. The third thing I'd like us to do is to try to figure out the times when they seem better or worse.

A discussion ensues which indicates that Tom's worries about spirits get worse if he watches highly exciting television programs late at night. After making this determination, the clinician sums up again:

CLINICIAN: Okay, let's agree on two things for the time being. One, Tom, you'll try not to watch television late at night. Two, you'll promise to call me before you do anything about the spirits.

TOM: Okay.

CLINICIAN: In fact, I'd like you to call me each day for the next couple of days just to let me know how you're feeling. If I don't hear from you by, say, 3:00 P.M., I'll call you because I'm concerned.

MOTHER: Can I call, too?

CLINICIAN: Absolutely. In fact, I want to hear from you too, even if Tom's fine.

In this example, the clinician behaved in a highly directive way. She attempted to introduce control and structure into a potentially chaotic situation by speaking clearly and defining courses of action in a step-by-step manner. She stressed the importance of medication and arranged to work cooperatively with the professional responsible for Tom's medication regime. She did not leave making an appointment to Tom's initiative and even arranged to physically accompany Tom to the medication clinic to insure that he got there. She repeatedly stressed her availability and the appropriateness of using her during this time of symptom exacerbation.

While some professionals have expressed concern about this kind of availability (feeling it would encourage undue dependency, and/ or be infeasible on an ongoing basis), it is important to emphasize that patients and families rarely misuses this resource. With the inclusion of an educational component to treatment, families learn the principles of managing the illness early on. In ongoing treatment, they seem well able to use this knowledge to handle most situations, using professional help only when appropriate and necessary.

STRUCTURE OF REGULAR SESSIONS

Every session in this stage of treatment has four basic components: the social contact, a discussion of tasks assigned at the last session and/or any other issues that are causing current concern, the creation of resolutions to problems, and task assignment. Conducting family meetings with a regular format gives a predictable structure to the sessions and further helps to maintain a low-key therapeutic environment.

Phase I: The Social Contact

Beginning each session with a social phase serves a number of purposes. One, it reconnects clinician, patient, and family in a comfortable way. It reminds all that, while the relationship is a professional and problem-centered one, everyone involved has other interests that are appropriate and important. It models the necessary skills of social interaction and "small talk" that are often lost in coping with chronic illness. It also enables everyone to settle in before more serious issues are addressed. Finally, it allows the sessions to highlight the family's qualities of strength, knowledge, and competence rather than emphasizing their difficulties.

To be able to facilitate the social phase of each session, clinicians must know something about the interests and problems of all family members. They can then bring up these topics regularly. These might include such topics as work, hobbies, politics, even the weather. For instance, if family members have an interest in sports, a discussion of the latest football game might lead off the session:

CLINICIAN: What did you think of the *Steelers* last night?
FATHER: I can't believe they lost. I'm really disgusted!
CLINICIAN: (*To patient*) Did you watch the game?
PATIENT: I watched part of it, but then everyone was yelling so much, I went to my room.
CLINICIAN: Sounds like a good idea. I'm glad you stayed for part of it. Your family gets pretty excited by the games?
PATIENT: My father goes beserk when they're losing. (*Laughs*)
MOTHER: That's for sure. Of course, he had a few dollars on the game. (*Everyone laughs*)

CLINICIAN: (*To mother*) What about you?
MOTHER: Oh, I watch, but I don't care all that much.

At this point, the clinician might spend a few minutes exploring the mother's interests and reactions or move into the work of the session by further reinforcing the patient's way of responding to an overstimulating situation, exploring the family's response to this behavior or reviewing the tasks assigned at the previous session. These discussions may be short or long, depending on the topic and the family. The important thing is to involve everyone in some sort of positive social interaction that is important to them.

Phase II: Discussion of Assigned Tasks and Other Issues

The second part of each session focuses on the review of how the tasks assigned at the last session were accomplished (or not accomplished) as well as checking on other issues or events of concern that have arisen. The review of the task assignment serves to accomplish several things. First, it provides a continuity between sessions. Second, it communicates to patient and family that the clinician takes the tasks seriously and gives them priority in the session. Third, information about whether or not the task was completed, and how well it was done, provides the clinician with valuable feedback about the patient and the family's current level of functioning. This, in turn, gives information about the appropriateness of the pace at which treatment is proceeding. In conducting task reviews, clinicians always assume responsibility for tasks that have failed. This allows discussions to take place about the problem task without increasing patient or family feelings of inadequacy and defensiveness. The following two examples demonstrate the review of, first a successful task, then an unsuccessful one. In the first example, the patient, Millie, was in her early 20s and living at home with her parents.

CLINICIAN: So, how did the tasks we assigned last time go?
MOTHER: Well, we're doing the dishes every other night. That's working out okay, no problem with that. Right?
FATHER: Right.
MOTHER: Tonight was my turn, right?
FATHER: Right.
CLINICIAN: (*Smiling*) Sounds like Mr. D is the supervisor.
MOTHER: Yeah.
CLINICIAN: Sounds like things went well with the dishes. What about the other tasks that you've been doing?

MILLIE: Setting the table? Sometimes she does and sometimes I do.

MOTHER: Your job was to do the living room furniture and run the sweeper.

MILLIE: I *did* the living room furniture.

MOTHER: But Sunday, I ran the sweeper.

FATHER: Yeah, but she has to do that this week.

CLINICIAN: Well, I'm very pleased that you carried those out. With three adults in one house, it's important to get the chores worked out. Do you feel it's been helpful?

MILLIE: Oh, yeah.

MOTHER: It's good to have her doing things.

In the following review of a task that didn't work, the patient was a young man in his mid-20s who also lived with his parents. The clinician takes responsibility for the failure, but does not allow the patient and family to lose momentum. She rapidly refocuses on a more "doable" task.

CLINICIAN: How did the task go, Sam?

SAM: What task?

CLINICIAN: If I remember correctly, last time we talked about you getting up every day before noon without your mother having to yell at you.

SAM: (*Defensively*) Oh, yeah. Well . . . I did the first 3 days, honest. Then I just didn't feel like it. Why should I anyway? There's nothing to do.

CLINICIAN: I can understand your feelings. I guess I'd have trouble getting up every day if I had nothing to do. I think the task was a little off base. That's my fault.

SAM: (*Visibly relaxing*) That's okay.

Later in the session after more discussion:

CLINICIAN: I'll tell you what. I missed the boat last time with the task. How about if we plan a task that will give you something to look forward to?

SAM: Okay.

CLINICIAN: I was thinking . . . a couple of sessions ago, you talked about enjoying that task where you did something with your father. How about you and he planning something now—preferably something that would mean you'd have to get out of bed before noon.

SAM: Yeah, I'd get up for my dad, but not every day.

FATHER: Fine with me.

CLINICIAN: Good, I'm not talking about every day right now. What would you two like to plan?

The session continues with Sam and his father deciding on a task they will do together: in this case, washing the family car Saturday morning. The clinician recognized that Sam's complaint about the first task had validity. It isn't easy for someone struggling with lethargy and amotivation to get up in the morning without a good external reason. She assumed responsibility for the failure of the first task, and gave one which built on more desirable areas, that is, Sam's relationship with his father and his interest in cars.

Phase III: Creating Resolutions to Problems

During the task and issue review phase, problems are defined by failure to accomplish tasks, by the success of tasks (indicating readiness for a next step), and by the raising of other issues and concerns by any member of the family. These data establish the basis for the next stage of the session. Clinicians ask family members to discuss the situation, as they see it, to gain an understanding of what happened. Anything that interfered with task behaviors or with following the general guidelines for living together is examined to determine what might be blocking satisfactory performance. This review often reveals other issues or resistances on the part of the patient or the family, but often also reveals errors on the part of the clinician (i.e., moving too quickly, implying the family is to blame, failing to attend to the needs of other family members when assigning a task to an individual, etc.). Once clinicians feel they have an understanding of an issue or problem that is interfering with a task, they ask families to participate in deciding what should be done about it, always retaining the final authority in the decision-making process. Clinicians should make the problem and its resolution explicit so that family members can generalize learning to other situations. The following two examples give an idea of how to begin to generate a solution to a failed task, and how to generate a solution to an issue raised as a problem.

CLINICIAN: (To husband of patient) I understand your concern. When Susan goes back to bed after you leave for work, that leaves Jimmy [their 5-year-old son] to fend for himself. However, I think I overestimated your wife's readiness to get up by herself so early and take care of your breakfast and then be with Jimmy until it's time for school.

SUSAN: I want to do these things . . . but I can't seem to do it.

RON: That's a wife's job.

CLINICIAN: It sounds like Susan agrees that's her job, but she needs a little help right now to get back on track. I wonder if the two of you can discuss this with me and come up with a temporary solution.

SUSAN: If Ron could just help a little bit with Jimmy in the morning, I wouldn't feel so overwhelmed.

CLINICIAN: How do you feel about that, Ron?

RON: I guess it's okay, as long as it's not permanent.

The clinician and the couple continued to explore Ron's helping as a temporary arrangement. Ron discussed his concerns about how this plan would work in the morning and how Jimmy would react. During this discussion, the clinician explored issues that would interfere with the new task of shared responsibility. He was careful to keep the task small and specific since the last week's task had not gone well. If too many tasks fail, family members begin to feel badly about themselves and/or the clinician begins to lose credibility.

In the following example, Paul's family reported that the task assigned last week had gone well. After a discussion of the task, during which the clinician rewarded everyone for their accomplishment, the family began to raise other concerns.

MOTHER: As I said, the task went fine, but we have another issue.

CLINICIAN: What's that?

MOTHER: Paul has been drinking 4 or 5 quarts of tea everyday. I don't think it's good for him. If it isn't tea, it's soda.

PAUL: I'm just very thirsty.

FATHER: We think the caffeine is making things worse. He paces all the time, and smokes cigarettes constantly. He's up half the night. I can hear him moving around in his room. I can't sleep.

MOTHER: I'm worried about the smoking, too. He smokes in bed. I'm afraid of fire. We'll all be burned in our sleep.

PAUL: Aw, come on. . . .

CLINICIAN: So you're really raising three issues: (1) the caffeine, (2) smoking in bed, and (3) disturbing the family all night. Let's take them one at a time.

Providing structure and breaking larger problems down into manageable issues allows the clinician to explore concerns and mutually agreeable solutions. Dealing simultaneously with all three areas (caffeine, smoking, and disturbing the family in the middle of the night) would probably be too much. The clinician starts by focusing on the most dangerous or upsetting issue, moving in later sessions to the ones that are just disruptive or unhealthy. In this case, since Paul's behavior constituted a fire hazard, she first worked to get some agreement about a plan that would encourage the development of careful smoking habits. A compromise was reached in which the family agreed to get Paul a comfortable chair for his room, if he would agree to stop smoking in bed.

Phase IV: Task Assignment Phase

Each session ends with a task assignment, even if the task is small or the same one as was given at a previous session. The creation of tasks helps to prolong the impact of sessions and gives the patient and family a focus and a sense of progress over time. Tasks are related to the work of the session and the phase of treatment. In the following example, a task discussed earlier with Sam is assigned as the session ends.

CLINICIAN: So, let's agree here. Sam, you're going to wash the car with your father on Saturday. When do you tend to feel best?

SAM: I guess around lunch.

CLINICIAN: (To father) So that's a clue for you. You have the best chance of getting him involved if you don't try too early in the morning, but it should be before lunch. Don't ask him though, because he's already told us he isn't going to feel like it. Just say, "Come on, Sam, it's time to wash the car."

FATHER: Okay. Is that okay with you, Sam?

SAM: Yeah.

CLINICIAN: (To mother) Now, one thing Sam mentioned is that he feels more negatively if you remind him of these things. So, I'd like you to leave this to Sam and his Dad.

MOTHER: But, they might forget. His Dad can be as bad as Sam. He gets real lazy on weekends.

CLINICIAN: That's okay. If they don't do it, it's between them and me. I want you to take the day off. You've been working awfully hard keeping these guys going. How about getting out shopping on Saturday, so they won't make you nervous about whether they are going to do it?

MOTHER: (Laughs) I guess I could. Do you guys really think this will work?

FATHER: Sure.

SAM: (Just looks at mother)

In this particular task assignment, the clinician paired Sam with his father for two reasons. First, Sam had very little initiative at this point and was unlikely to follow through on any task he was asked to do alone. Second, Sam's relationship with his father was less intense than his relationship with his mother. This pairing, therefore, was less likely to result in emotional interactions that would be over-stimulating or perceived as burdensome. The clinician specifically blocks Sam's mother's input into the interaction in order to avoid the intensity that would be inherent in a three-party interaction; the intensity that would result if conflict arose over whether or not to do the task; and the intensity of Sam's frequent power struggles with his mother.

Tasks are formulated based on where the patient is "at" and vary from patient to patient and family to family. Often the initial tasks focus on the patient taking better physical care of him- or herself. Many times, the patient has totally ignored his personal hygiene and this in itself is a source of conflict within the family as a parent or spouse continually nags the patient to bathe or change clothes. Thus, the task requiring a patient to take three showers a week may have the dual purpose of decreasing the stress of negative family interactions and helping the patient to begin to assume more personal responsibility.

MOTHER: I've tried everything to get him to shave or even take a shower and brush his teeth.

ART: I'm not going anywhere so what's the point?

FATHER: (*Angrily*) Because your mother told you to, that's the point.

ART: (*Interrupting*) Well, that's just—

CLINICIAN: Hold it, slow down and let me get a word in here.

MOTHER: Good.

CLINICIAN: (*To Art*) I know you don't feel like doing much and there doesn't seem much point to it . . .

ART: That's right.

CLINICIAN: . . . but I think we could work out a deal with something for everyone. Would you agree to take a shower three times a week if I got your parents to agree not to mention the whole issue?

ART: Sure, *that* would be worth it. But she'll never do it.

MOTHER: Neither will he. He doesn't even do it when I nag.

CLINICIAN: Well, since it isn't working with the nagging, how about giving it a try my way, just until next time?

ART: Okay by me.

MOTHER: Well . . . I guess so.

FATHER: Why not?

In this example, the clinician sidetracks family conflict, preventing escalation and further polarization of family members on the issue of Art's personal hygiene. He then suggests a resolution that gives Art motivation to wash, that of getting his mother off his back. To cope with Art's mother's skepticism, he simply asks for a trial, rather than attempting to prove his point. After getting this basic agreement from both parties, the session continued with the clinician refining the task with Art, deciding on which days and times he would take the showers. He agreed with the whole family that this issue had been a sore point and that it would be difficult for the task to succeed since it requires everyone to cooperate: Art to shower and his parents not to nag. He ended the session by affirming his belief that, despite the issue, the task could succeed.

The use of tasks also allows clinicians to establish concrete structure and control with overly enthusiastic patients or overly critical families. If clinicians sense that patient enthusiasm is coupled with very low stress tolerance, tasks can be used as a control to slow things down. Some patients are acutely aware that they are not performing as their peers do and thus have the desire to "get back on track" quickly. This is a particular problem with first episode patients, who often push to return to work or school, although they may not be ready to do so. A structured, task-oriented approach allows clinicians to control and delay this process without totally dampening enthusiasm. The major goal of returning to work can be reinforced by clinicians but broken down into a number of steps and tasks that require patients to gradually assume increased responsibility within the family, and then the community. In a sense, small tasks allow patients to demonstrate how well they can do. If they can handle every successive task, so much the better. If they occasionally exceed their tolerance levels, returning to less ambitious tasks need not be a major setback.

In the following example, Stephanie has been out of the hospital 4 weeks, and wants to go to work.

CLINICIAN: I'm glad to hear you want to go to work, Stephanie. Before we discuss it, how about if I find out what's been happening at home?

MOTHER: It's the same. She's sleeping all the time and not doing anything.

STEPHANIE: I'm bored.

CLINICIAN: I understand, but working requires a lot of energy. I think it's a great goal and I want to help you get there.

STEPHANIE: Good.

CLINICIAN: First, then, I think we have to work on your getting energy back and getting used to doing things. How about discussing some things you can do around the house that will help you get ready for the demands of a job?

STEPHANIE: Anything that will help me to work.

In this discussion, the clinician used Stephanie's desire to work to begin to motivate her to do some small task around the house. She made the connection that Stephanie's ability to do these chores would contribute to her ability to function in a more complex setting. The quality of her task performance, then, was established as a way of gauging her readiness for more ambitious work or training.

If patients lack interest or motivation and movement is slow, tasks also offer concrete proof of progress and tend to buy more time and patience from family members who can see the patient at least is trying. In the following example, the clinician attempts to define a task that will be useful to both patient and family in this way.

CLINICIAN: I know you don't feel like doing much these days, but let's try to find some small thing for you to do so you and your family don't feel like you're "vegetating." We need to keep everyone's morale up.

MOTHER: I'd even be happy if he gets up before noon.

FATHER: . . . or has dinner with us instead of waiting until we've finished, then getting food to take to his room.

CLINICIAN: (To patient) Sid, do either of those things sound possible?

SID: Well, I could get up if my mother didn't nag at me.

MOTHER: I nag because if he gets up, he lays down on the couch and watches television. He might as well be in bed.

CLINICIAN: At least it's a start if he's out of bed for a few hours. What about agreeing he'll spend at least a few hours out of his room each day? Later, we'll work on what he does with those hours.

The clinician recognizes Sid's parents' need to see some movement, but also appreciates Sid's problem of low energy. He develops a task that only requires Sid to alter his present routine minimally, but frames it in a way in which success can be viewed as a positive step.

There is an art to assigning tasks in a way that will make them acceptable to patient and family. For instance, however important personal hygiene is, many patients with schizophrenia would consider a self-care task (such as showering) as demeaning. There is no question that performing small household tasks, such as carrying out the garbage, seem demeaning to someone who once functioned independently as a salesman or a computer programmer. Without providing a rationale that ties the task to some larger desirable goal, patients are painfully aware that the prescribed behaviors are not particularly significant ones. Assignment of tasks that either patients or family members feel to be condescending could have the effect of decreasing treatment compliance rather than increasing functional behaviors. For this reason, the purpose of assigning tasks is usually explained in a way that ties them into the overall goals of patients and families as well as into the overall goals of treatment. The need to become reaccustomed to a routine, the need for the body to get used to being active again, the need for increased tolerance for doing boring or unpleasant chores can all be related to the ability to hold down a job or be an integral part of a family. These explanations can give meaning to otherwise mundane tasks. The patient, family and clinician can also use tasks to evaluate readiness to move to the next stage of treatment. With more resistant patients, it is sometimes useful to offer tasks as "suggestions," or to more actively involve patients and families in the development or choice of their own tasks.

During the immediate "recuperative period," tasks for patients tend to relate to learning to recognize and respect their own internal signals. They must learn when they need distance, when they need support, and when they are stressed. Tasks for the family during this phase relate to maintaining the attitude of "benign indifference." Although this concept is explained during the workshop, the slow pace and frustration of the first few months of treatment necessitate continued discussion and support in maintaining a more neutral attitude. Initial tasks in this regard can be geared to help family members to tolerate patient amotivation and withdrawal, in large part by focusing less on the patient and his or her progress. Family members are asked to begin to attend to their own needs and those of other family members as a way of putting this concept into practice. As time goes on, the focus of tasks should shift to the gradual resumption of responsibility by patients. As just mentioned, it may be necessary to begin at the level of physical self-care, but more often it is possible to begin to help patients to assume responsibility for minor household chores.

At any time, safeguards against task failure should be built in if at all possible. There are a number of ways of providing this protection. First, the chore or task given should be one to which the patient and family have agreed. Second, the tasks assigned to patients should be ones that the clinician feels are possible considering the patient's levels of skill, tolerance, and motivation. Third, the needs, skills, and relationships of other family members must be considered when tasks are assigned. Finally, particularly early in treatment, tasks should be assigned that involve patients with another member of their family. There are multiple reasons for this last point. As stated earlier, for an extended period after a psychotic episode, patients often exhibit little internal motivation, even after they appear to be free of major psychotic symptoms and seem capable of functioning. Pairing the patient with a family member to complete a task allows the other person to mobilize the patient by supplying the motivation. This type of task also allows patients and family members to have positive interaction and communication around a joint activity. For some family members, the accomplishment of these early tasks may constitute the first positive experience they have had with one another in years. In the following example, the clinician uses a task to pair Loren with his relatively withdrawn father. Although both father and son had expressed interest in improving their relationship, Loren's father had also complained that he did not know how to relate to his ill son.

MOTHER: If you don't get that car fixed, it will never pass inspection.
LOREN: Yeah.
CLINICIAN: Is that something you can do, Loren?
LOREN: Yeah, sometime.
CLINICIAN: Sounds like it's needed, but you may need some help to get started.
LOREN: I guess.
CLINICIAN: (To father) How about you? You must be pretty much of an expert since you drive trucks for a living. Can you give Loren a hand?
FATHER: Well . . . I'm awfully tired after work, but if it will help, maybe on Saturday?
LOREN: Will you really?
FATHER: Sure.
LOREN: (Beaming) Gee, thanks.

To help in tolerating the slowness of change, it should be remembered that all tasks are designed to lead gradually toward independence. Sudden emancipation could produce stress in and of itself, however. Gradual moves toward independence, while still living in the home, can result in less contact between patient and family, increased differentiation, and decreased interpersonal stress, expressed emotion, and potential for relapse. Therefore, the desire to emancipate as expressed by patient or family is never completely discouraged, but rather framed as an appropriate and achievable long-term goal, as shown in the following example.

JACK: All I want is my own place, the sooner, the better.
MOTHER: Sure, just like the last time you had an apartment. You know, he left the water running in a stopped up sink for 4 hours. You wouldn't believe the damage and we had to pay.
CLINICIAN: It sounds like last time didn't work out so well.
FATHER: That's for sure. We lost the deposit and some furniture.
CLINICIAN: Hm, but it sounds like you were supportive of Jack's move out last time?
FATHER: And would be next time if we thought it would work.
CLINICIAN: I'm glad, and I'm sure Jack is glad to hear that. I'm with all of you. I think it's a great goal to work towards when the time is right.

JACK: How about now?

CLINICIAN: Well, to be honest, I think the time isn't right yet. I think there are a lot of things to work on to make sure the next time goes well. But, I'd really like to work with you on getting ready. Let's talk about some ways to begin. . . .

In this example, the clinician attempts to walk the fine line between accepting the reality that Jack is not ready for independent living and not discouraging Jack's desire and motivation. She offers to maintain the goal as something to work towards, but does not allow herself to be pressured into accepting a plan she does not believe is realistic. The rest of the session is spent in discussing a task that would be a good first step. In this case, it was decided that Jack would take responsibility for managing his own money and begin to pay his parents a small fee for his room and board.

In reviewing all tasks assigned to patients, the responses of clinicians and family members to task accomplishment should be appropriate to the significance of the task. Small successes should be recognized, but not overvalued. This point is particularly important because after months of tolerating patient inactivity, it is common for family members to become overenthusiastic and give too much praise for the completion of the smallest task. In the following example, the clinician attempts to reward task accomplishment while discouraging effusive praise.

MOTHER: I'm *so* happy. Andy did your task, and I didn't have to say one word. It's *great!* He took the garbage out three times. I'm *so* proud of him.

ANDY: (*Looks at the floor and does not comment*)

MOTHER: Really, Andy, it's great!

CLINICIAN: Well, I'm glad that Andy did the task and that you didn't have to remind him. I realize that it's exciting when the first step is taken, but it is only a small step. Maybe the word "good" rather than "great" is more appropriate.

ANDY: *I'll* say.

In Andy's case, it was particularly important that he not be praised more than his efforts deserved since he tended to become irritated rather than pleased in such situations. He knew that taking out the garbage was no "big" thing in the real world. His mother, therefore, was encouraged to modulate her praise and enthusiasm.

Finally, if tasks are kept small, failure when it occurs, can be minimized and patients can be quickly restabilized at the level at which they were once successful. This is easier than dealing with the major sense of failure and stress that occurs when patients quickly return to work but cannot perform because of a return of florid symptoms. In any case, lack of success at any task is never defined as failure or resistance on the part of patients or families. Rather, the onus for noncompletion of tasks is assumed by clinicians who first give the message that the tasks they assigned were either too difficult or given too soon. They can then refocus everyone's energies on less ambitious tasks. In the following example, a clinician goes through this process in a session that occurred the day after a patient, Peter, had moved back home after living in his own apartment for 4 weeks.

CLINICIAN: I understand that you feel quite badly. I think it's my fault though. I should have insisted that we wait a little while longer.

PETER: (*Really discouraged*) It's not your fault. I really wanted to move out. I guess I'll never leave home. I just can't do it.

CLINICIAN: I haven't given up that goal and neither should you. Actually, I think it's really positive you made it a month. It is the first time you've been on your own. I'd like to keep "living on your own" as a goal. You have the strength to achieve it. However, I think we have to plan a step-by-step way to help you to be ready the next time. Let's learn from what happened. What was one of the biggest problems?

PETER: Food. I spent my month's food money the first week.

CLINICIAN: Good place to start. How about if you shop for your own food now while you're at home? Maybe the first few times, you can go with your mother to get the feel for it.

PETER: Fine with me.

MOTHER: Fine with me, too.

CLINICIAN: Good, now let's discuss how much money you'll have for food each week and how to spend it.

Split Sessions

The previous section reviewed the sequence of each family session and its four phases (the social contact, the review of tasks and issues, the development of resolutions to problems, and task assignment). While the structure of each individual session can fluctuate in response to patient, family members, and circumstances, usually everyone in a family meets together with the clinician. This tends to decrease the likelihood of miscommunication of therapeutic messages since misunderstandings can be clarified immediately and family conflict can be defused when it occurs.

However, occasionally seeing various segments of family groups for portions of sessions allows a number of other goals to be accomplished. First, when dealing with two-generational families, splitting sessions along generational lines can be used to strengthen and emphasize the importance of generational boundaries. The mere fact that parents are seen alone lets them know that it is appropriate that they have private issues separate from those of their children. It also stresses that patients and their siblings (especially since they usually are adults or near adults) have issues and concerns that need not be shared with their parents. Thus, each subsystem of the family is given the message that the illness does not eliminate their needs and rights for privacy.

A number of other common problems can be addressed between clinicians and various subsystems of families. For instance, family members sometimes need to express their anger and frustration about the patient or the slow pace of change. Although most common and intense in the sessions during the connecting phase, these feelings can arise in any family member at any stage of treatment. It is important to allow these feelings to be expressed, but often it is better if these expressions can occur without the patient present. Such discussions are intense and can be upsetting to patients without necessarily generating positive results. By seeing other family members alone, clinicians can offer understanding and support, admitting that the process of recovery is painfully slow. Moreover, they can do so without making patients feel bad about themselves. In the following example from a split session including only the parents, Sam's father expressed his frustration with the slowness of change.

FATHER: I do appreciate that Sam is beginning to do things with me or his mother, but just once, I'd like to see *him* suggest something. Just once, I'd like to see him get off his dead ass and start something on his own.

CLINICIAN: I can certainly understand your frustration with the wait and give you a lot of credit for your patience and frustration. It *is* a slow process. I get frustrated sometimes, too.

MOTHER: You do?

CLINICIAN: Yes, I need support from my team sometimes, and a reminder to measure progress along Sam's "internal yardstick."

FATHER: I guess, using *that* yardstick, I do see progress, but it's imperceptible at times.

CLINICIAN: I sense that everyone, including Sam, gets frustrated. It's normal to get impatient. Even a saint would now and then.

FATHER: I guess I never stop hoping. I appreciate your hearing me out. It helps sometimes just to talk about the frustration.

CLINICIAN: I know it's slow, but he is coming along. He's doing chores, he's being more considerate at night. . . .

FATHER: I know. He hasn't been this well in years. It just gets to me sometimes.

As is demonstrated in this example, it is important to allow the expression of negative feelings and to accept them as natural, before offering reassurance. If the clinician had stressed Sam's progress as soon as his father had expressed his frustration, a pointless struggle may have resulted in which the father had to keep emphasizing Sam's deficits and the clinician had to keep stressing Sam's very small gains. As it worked out, Sam's father was better able to see Sam's progress after he had had a chance to air his frustrations.

Split sessions also are helpful when clinicians see patients who adamantly insist that they have no illness and who do not see the need for medication or treatment. The resistant patient will be discussed in more detail later (see p. 163). But for now, it is important to note that occasionally seeing such patients individually will help the joining process by allowing the clinician to empathize with the patient's perceptions without alienating other family members who are often very sensitive about the patient's denial. In other words, split sessions allow the discussion of issues that could otherwise trigger negative family interactions. For instance, family members who have a great deal of difficulty hearing patients deny their illnesses tend to jump in to convince patients they are sick. Patients then respond with increased anger and denial, precipitating a rapidly escalating family conflict. Split sessions allow the clinician to see family members alone in order to discuss nonprovocative ways of getting the patient to cooperate. The clinician can then see the patient alone to discuss ways to behave in order to gain distance from his or her parents. The following example is from a split session, this half with the patient alone.

CLINICIAN: You seem pretty hassled, Hank.

HANK: If I hear my parents ask one more time if I'm taking that stupid medicine, I'm moving out. I don't need it anyway.

CLINICIAN: I understand what a hassle that can be, even when you know that they're asking because they care.

HANK: If they *really* cared, they'd leave me alone.

CLINICIAN: I'll tell you what. I hear what you're saying and I'll do my best to get them to back off. I also hear you don't need to be reminded to take your medicine.

HANK: No, I'll take the damn stuff for now, but not if they keep checking.

CLINICIAN: Fair enough. . . . I'll go along with this if you will agree to let me know if you make a decision to stop the medicine.

HANK: If you can get them off my back. . . .

CLINICIAN: I'll do my best. I appreciate your letting me know how you feel.

HANK: That's okay. I don't mind seeing you by myself once in awhile. It was funny that you threw them out.

As in this case, sessions with patients alone also can reinforce the fact that the clinician respects their right to privacy despite the illness and the treatment contract with the whole family.

Finally, offering a portion of a session to a patient's siblings without either their parents or the patient present makes it possible to head off other potential areas of conflict. Often, with the many crises of dealing with a severely ill patient, the needs of siblings are overlooked and their feelings are minimized. Furthermore, they tend not to express their needs, expecting that they will not be met or fearing that they will be viewed as selfish. Occasional sessions with the siblings of a patient, even of a half-hour's duration, give them a chance to express their feelings more honestly. Once siblings have had this opportunity, it is possible to help them to get more of what they need from their parents; to help them to set reasonable limits on what they can do for or put up with from the patient; and to enable them to proceed with their own normal developmental tasks. Only when their own needs are being met can one expect siblings to offer genuine cooperation in the patient's treatment.

The following example comes from a session with the patient's younger brother and sister, both of whom still live at home.

CLINICIAN: Even though neither of you said much, I got the sense from our last session that you both have a lot of feelings about what's going on.

JERRY: (Blurting out) Things are lousy around the house. We try never to be there. We can't have friends over because he says weird things and makes them all take their shoes off. It's embarrassing. I don't hate him, but he's sure tough to take sometimes.

CLINICIAN: Have you talked to your parents about your feelings?

JERRY: They don't care.

SALLY: They just don't have the time. They're so worried about Mark. It's been that way for years, for as long as I can remember.

CLINICIAN: I guess if I were you, I'd have similar feelings. But, I think you may underestimate your parents' caring for you and willingness to listen. How about if I ask them to come back in and help you to express your feelings so that they do hear?

SALLY: Well, okay, but I don't think it will do any good. They'll just say how sick he is and how he needs us all to be understanding.

CLINICIAN: I know they've said that in the past, but they're trying to change. Remember what we said at the workshop. Both you and your parents have to learn to look out for yourselves, too. Just worrying about Mark won't help you *or* him.

JERRY: Maybe . . . but what can we do?

CLINICIAN: Well, for a start, I think you are absolutely right that your friends shouldn't have to take their shoes off. One of the first things we could try to change is to get Mark to stop asking visitors to do that.

SALLY: That would help for a start. Could you also see if we could have a rule about how he answers the phone? He tells boys who call me that I've gone to Mars.

CLINICIAN: Sure, let's all talk together, and see what we can do.

CONTENT OF THE SESSIONS

As with the frequency and structure of sessions, the content of sessions is also fairly predictable. While differing somewhat from case to case, there are a number of issues that arise so frequently that it is possible to provide suggestions for resolving them.

The Importance of Early Warning Signs

Every family, and every family member, has a different level of tolerance for unusual behaviors. Behaviors that are regarded as particularly irritating by some family members may be insignificant to others. For this reason, it is important that clinicians involve family members in identifying what they consider to be problem behaviors, rather than assuming they know which are likely to cause trouble. Once identified, ways of coping with these issues can be developed. While all upsetting behaviors must be dealt with eventually, it is necessary to give first priority to behaviors that may constitute *prodromal signs* of the illness (subtle symptoms preceding an acute psychotic episode). For some patients, these behavioral changes might be dramatic, while for others, they may be nothing more than a subtle increase in withdrawal. Because prodromal signs differ from patient to patient, family and clinician must work together to identify which signs preceded previous episodes. While these behaviors may not always predict another episode, they can often be used to help monitor the patient's condition and progress (Goldstein, Rodnick, Evans, May, & Steinberg, 1978). Through these discussions, patients and families often recognize that past episodes tended to be preceded by subtle changes in behavior such as increasing irritability, changing sleep or eating patterns, increasing isolation, or reports of vague fears that something terrible might happen. An awareness of the significance of these signs can enable patients and families to get help early before an acute exacerbation gets out of hànd. Patients and their families gain a greater sense of control and structure by knowing that, like most illnesses, the course of schizophrenia often has a predictable pattern. This allows families to be less sensitive to minor changes in patient behaviors, decreasing overmonitoring and tension.

A report of a subtle change in the patient's sleep patterns, for example, is carefully explored in the family session. If sleep problems have usually preceded other symptoms in the past, then this symptom is viewed as an important one. Discussion may reveal that the patient has been experiencing increased stress or making a secret attempt to go without medication, or attempting to experiment with the use of street drugs.

Prodromal signs can alert the clinical team to the need for altering the patient's medication regime or for mitigating environmental stresses early enough to prevent a full blown psychotic episode. Without a thorough discussion of these warning signals, they are frequently overlooked, minimized, or denied. By the time the clinical team becomes aware of them, the intervention required is more intensive and may even necessitate a hospitalization (Carpenter & Heinrichs, 1983). Thus, once the signs are identified, the family and the patient are asked to agree on a set of responses or actions. In the following example, a family and a patient explain how they know an episode is coming on.

MOTHER: Oh, I always know when she's getting sick. She starts having lots of energy—

SANDY: (*Interrupting*) I start feeling real good, and I get interested in religion. I start watching all the religious programs on television and going down to these born again revivals. . . .

FATHER: This is a problem for us because we're Jewish.

MOTHER: Well, it isn't just that, but we know what's coming 'cause then she starts thinking the guys on the television are only talking to her, and then the voices start even when it isn't on.

SANDY: I know now they're voices, and they're in my mind. But at the time, they seem real to me. They tell me things.

CLINICIAN: But before all that happens, are you all saying that you know it will happen . . . how long before?

MOTHER: Oh, several weeks. It starts slow and then snowballs.

SANDY: That's true, I guess. But once I'm hearing the voices. . . .

CLINICIAN: Okay, let's see if we can agree. How about if you all try to let me know as soon as you notice the increased energy and increased interest in religion. Maybe then we can prevent another hospitalization.

SANDY: I'm for that. I hate the hospital, but I do sort of miss the voices.

In this example, the family and the therapist are able to identify one of Sandy's significant prodromal signs. The session continues with the clinician beginning to outline the initial steps that could be taken should the sign appear.

CLINICIAN: If you start getting interested in religion, Sandy, what do you think your family could do to help?

SANDY: I don't know . . . maybe keep me from watching Channel 40 [a religious station].

CLINICIAN: Would you let them?

SANDY: Sure.

MOTHER: You say that now, but once you are really into it, it's hard to get you to stop.

CLINICIAN: That's a good observation, so you'd really have to pick up on this when it first starts?

MOTHER: Yes.

Strategies for Living Together

Although the signs and behaviors that precede the illness are most crucial, any behaviors that are particularly upsetting to family members are also discussed in early sessions. These are identified not because they are predictive of a worsening of the illness, but because they cause stress and interfere with the lives of everyone in a family. The behaviors focused on, however, might involve those of other family members, not just those of the patient. Any issue that is of importance to any family member, be it rights to privacy or consideration, is placed on the agenda.

In the following example, Naomi, who has had schizophrenia for 5 years, voices a complaint about her brother, Nate, who is 2 years younger than she.

NAOMI: He treats me like I'm ten—and he's younger than me! He's always yelling at me and telling me what to do!

NATE: Well, you act like you're ten!

MOTHER: Nate has a quick temper and—

CLINICIAN: I'm sure that it gets frustrating for everyone at home, and everyone, including you, Naomi, loses their cool sometimes. . . .

NAOMI: Yeah, but he shouldn't tell me what to do.

CLINICIAN: I agree. I think you're taking more and more responsibility and don't need Nate as a boss.

MOTHER: I guess that's true. We've let him take over too much.

NATE: If she acted her age, I wouldn't yell.

CLINICIAN: I know it's been tough for you in the past, Nate, and you've done a great job of trying to help at home. Recently though, Naomi has been trying more, too. I wonder if you couldn't try to back off for the next couple of weeks. If you get upset with her, maybe discussing it would be better. I sense that Naomi would be more likely to cooperate if you approached her that way.

NAOMI: That's for sure.

NATE: (*Reluctantly*) Well. . . .

CLINICIAN: Maybe we can spend more time talking about some of the things that create these arguments.

The clinician acknowledged the frustrations of other family members, while at the same time recognizing that Naomi's complaint was justifiable. He emphasized the fact that Naomi was trying to take more responsibility, and then suggested a way of improving communications between the two siblings. Eventually, he asked Naomi and Nate to give an example of a recent argument they had had with one another, helping them to discuss the issue and resolve it within the session.

As far as patient behaviors are concerned, family members are helped to set limits on patient requests if they are unreasonable, and to provide an opportunity for reality testing when possible. By setting limits on behaviors that upset or inconvenience other family members, interpersonal boundaries are also reinforced. These limits can be reassuring to patients, helping them to establish their own limits and provide their own structure as needed over time.

For example, in a situation already discussed, Mark's siblings complained about his "rule" requiring all visitors to remove their shoes before entering the house. This rule was not only upsetting and embarrassing to Mark's brother and sister, but it stimulated anger toward Mark. The clinician handled the situation in the following directive way.

CLINICIAN: (*To Mark's brother*) When we met last time, you mentioned a rule Mark has that is upsetting to some members of the family. I wonder if you'd be comfortable bringing it up now with the whole family here.

JERRY: Yes, he makes everybody take their shoes off in the house. I mean everybody!

FATHER: That's true.

CLINICIAN: How about it, Mark?

MARK: (*Pause*) Yeah, I do that.

CLINICIAN: How come?

MARK: They're made of leather and have germs.

CLINICIAN: I understand you believe that, and it's upsetting to you, but your rule sounds very upsetting to the rest of the family.

MARK: (*Puzzled look*) I didn't know that.

CLINICIAN: In this case, I wonder if you could change your rule. Maybe you could take your shoes off, and if someone else's wearing shoes makes you uncomfortable, maybe you could leave the room.

MARK: Okay.

While not all rituals are as easily interrupted as this one, a surprising number of them can be dispensed with quickly if family members can be firm. While this particular intervention runs the risk of promoting and legitimizing withdrawal, it was made in the context of many others that emphasized an increase in Mark's social contacts within the family.

In some cases it is not the patient who is behaving in an upsetting way. In the following example, a patient's sibling brings up a problem with his mother's behavior.

JOE: You know, Mom, it really bothers me when you let Ron [the patient] push you around.

MOTHER: Does it? I *really* don't mind. I just figure he's sick and he has no one. I think it's his way of getting attention.

FATHER: I agree with Joe. There must be some other way he can get attention without hurting you.

MOTHER: He never *really* hurts me.

CLINICIAN: Whether he hurts you or not, I don't think it's good for him, you, or the rest of the family. He's behaving in ways that upset people, ways that wouldn't be tolerated in the outside world.

MOTHER: Do you really think so? But what can I say to him? I don't want to reject him.

CLINICIAN: I think you can say very clearly that you would be happy to talk to him, to spend time with him, but that he can't hit you. Remember, as we said at the workshop, sometimes love is expressed by setting limits.

Medication Compliance

The best therapeutic programs have a significant chance of failure if patients refuse to take their medication. In ongoing treatment, working with families to gain their support for the patient's medication regime is a major focus since the stability medication provides is a prerequisite for attempting other therapeutic interventions. In general, noncompliance with drugs seems to relate to one or more of the following issues: patient denial of illness or the need for medication; the presence of uncomfortable and/or serious drug side effects; and/or lack of family support for the medication program.

To deal effectively with all of these issues, it is extremely important that the clinician responsible for medication receive accurate feedback about the patient's response to the drugs. The difficulty of achieving a balance between maximum therapeutic benefits and minimum side effects is aggravated when patients fail to report their medication problems and concerns to the clinician. When patients do not complain about their drug problems, they do themselves an immediate disservice by risking being over- or undermedicated. This increases the likelihood that they will eventually feel the need to discontinue the drug altogether. Nevertheless, patients often answer the question, "How are you feeling?" with "Fine," even when they are uncomfortable. For this reason, families are an important source of information about reactions to medications, since they see patients 168 hours a week as opposed to the minutes or hours patients are seen by the nurse or doctor. Prodromal signs, akinesia, akathesia, and pseudoparkinsonism often will be apparent to family members long before clinicians become aware of them.

Lack of support from families for the medication regime is sometimes a sign of resistance, but more often is caused by insufficient information about psychotropic drugs. For this reason, the information about medication and its effects which is shared during the educational workshop is continually repeated and augmented during the course of treatment. Families, as well as patients, are informed of medication changes including the rationale for such changes and the possible consequences. Ongoing feedback is given to family members about the use of psychotropic medication in controlling the positive symptoms of the illness (i.e., hallucinations, delusions) and to alleviate akinesia. They are told that even with medication, the recuperative process is a slow one. Nevertheless, since time tends to ease the intensity of the memory, patients and families must occasionally be reminded of what the acute episode was like. This awareness promotes tolerance of the negative side effects of medication. In the following example, Mike's mother focuses on the negative symptoms that he has been experiencing during the 4 months he has been out of the hospital.

MOTHER: Mike is just laying around the house, not doing anything. That's not like him. Before, he was always out. I think it's that medicine.

I don't think he needs it anymore. He's not doing crazy things now.

MIKE: That's right.

CLINICIAN: (*To father*) Do you agree?

FATHER: I don't know. I still remember what he was like before we brought him to the hospital. I'm scared that without the medicine, the same thing would happen again.

CLINICIAN: (*To all*) What was it like?

FATHER: Frightening. He was acting really crazy for months. At the end, he was locked in his room with a shotgun by the door, petrified that the Communists were coming to get him. When we finally got in, he was hiding under his bed, crying.

MOTHER: It wasn't that bad.

FATHER: Are you kidding?

MIKE: I was pretty scared . . . but I'm not now.

FATHER: We were all petrified. (*To mother*) You were crying all the time.

MOTHER: (*Reluctantly*) Well, I guess it *was* pretty bad.

CLINICIAN: It sounds as though things were rough and I share your concern that without medicine, it is likely to happen again. However, I also hear your frustrations about Mike's lethargy. I don't think it's all due to the medication. It's very common for patients to lack energy following an acute episode. Remember what we said at the workshop? However, I certainly will talk to Pat [Mike's medication nurse] about your concerns and report back to you as soon as possible. How about if I call you tomorrow?

As in the example above, the family clinician must work closely with the family and the patient, monitoring their reactions to the drugs and sharing their reports with the medication clinician to help to keep the patient's drugs at the lowest possible therapeutic dose. Family perceptions of patient states are an aid in making decisions about adjusting dosage levels or even about changing medications altogether. If side effects cannot be controlled, or if they are potentially permanent (e.g., tardive dyskinesia), then the family and patient must be helped to make an informed decision regarding the advisability of drug therapy. Occasionally, patients and families are put in the bind of choosing between tolerating the positive symptoms of schizophrenia or the unpleasant side effects of the medication. Before they make this choice, both patient and family are helped to clearly understand the risks and benefits involved in either choice. Not all patients and families with the same dilemma arrive at the same decision. In the following example, Frank and his family discuss their feelings about the side effects of Frank's medications.

FATHER: His mouth movements could drive a normal person crazy. I just wish the doctor could come to our house for dinner and see what we're putting up with.

MOTHER: It really is pretty bad. It doesn't bother me as much, but I'm worried about what other people will think.

CLINICIAN: Frank, what do you feel about what your parents are saying?

FRANK: The side effects don't bother me that much. Anything's better than going back into the hospital.

FATHER: How can this be better?

FRANK: (*Looking down*) I need my medication.

CLINICIAN: This is a real dilemma and there's no easy answer. The treatment team is really concerned with the side effects, too, but everytime we change the medication, Frank gets symptoms.

MOTHER: That scares me.

CLINICIAN: As I said, it's a dilemma.

FATHER: What's the solution?

CLINICIAN: No simple one that I can think of. What I'd like to do is arrange a meeting with Dr. Cooper, Ellen [nurse clinician], and all of us to spell out the pros and cons of staying on or stopping the medication. After that, perhaps we can reach a decision about what to do. Is that okay with you folks?

MOTHER: Yes.

FATHER: Yes.

FRANK: I need my medication.

During this session, the family was able to verbalize their frustration and concern about Frank's illness and his response to drug treatment. As in many cases, the symptoms of tardive dyskinesia were more upsetting to those around the patient than to the patient himself. The clinician reaffirms the difficulty of any decision about this important issue. She offers to arrange a meeting with the other clinicians directly involved in prescribing the medication so that a final decision can be based on as much information as possible. In this case, because of Frank's own awareness of his tendency to rapidly decompensate following medication reduction, it was decided to maintain the same level for 3 months before attempting a decrease in medication. This coincided with a period in which both Frank and his family did not anticipate any other major changes, thus providing a better time for a trial at a lower drug level.

In the next example, both patient and family are more ambivalent about whether the benefits outweigh the costs of the present medication regime.

MOTHER: I've been noticing little movements around David's mouth, and I remember them saying at the workshop that that could be a sign of tardive dyskinesia. I'm really worried.

CLINICIAN: I've noticed some movements, too. What have you seen?

MOTHER: Well, it's not really bad, but little twitches in his jaw—like back and forth. I would hate to think he was going to have to live with that forever.

CLINICIAN: David?

DAVID: I haven't really noticed, but I don't think I need medication anyway.

MOTHER: Maybe he should stop it.

FATHER: I'm not so sure I want to put up with that.

MOTHER: Well, at least decrease it.

CLINICIAN: That's a possibility. However, changing or stopping the medication may lead to the risk of having symptoms reappear.

MOTHER: I *want* it decreased, if not stopped right now. I don't want him to look like some of the people you see from state hospitals.

FATHER: Well, that really would be bad. Maybe it should be stopped.

CLINICIAN: I certainly understand your concern. However, I'd hate to "throw the baby out with the bath water." The medications are helping to stop the schizophrenic symptoms. Let me suggest that I discuss the situation with the treatment team. I'll be your advocate for a change of the medications. We can then see if we can reduce the side effects without losing the positive benefits. Is that all right with you?

In the two previous examples, the clinicians attempted to help the patient and family to make their decisions based on an overall appreciation of the risks and benefits of medication. Since they do not prescribe the medication themselves, they also attempt to incorporate the appropriate members of the treatment team in the decision-making process. Unilateral decisions by either the family or the team are avoided.

The most common problem precipitating medication noncompliance is related to a lack of acceptance of the illness itself. Because of the peculiar nature of schizophrenia, some patients do not believe that they are ill. They have no cognitive distance from their symptoms, accepting as fact their hallucinations, delusions, or perceptions of reality however unreasonable or nonsensical they may seem to others. Patients who never achieve any distance from their illness are difficult to maintain on medication or even in treatment. Clinicians or family members who attack these beliefs can lose both the patient's trust and their own credibility. Some of these patients have entered treatment only because of pressure from their families or the legal system. Over time, their resistance to intervention may increase, eventually becoming a major roadblock or leading to total noncompliance and relapse.

A number of specific techniques can be used with such patients. In some cases, through negotiation, patients can be encouraged to give treatment and medication a fair trial to see if it can help. Even if they do not accept their delusions as a problem, they may still appreciate that medication may "decrease anxiety" or make them "more comfortable" with themselves. Some patients will agree to a trial of medication to humor their parents or to obtain freedoms or privileges. Thus, clinicians can emphasize the benefits of a medication regime without directly confronting the patient's denial of illness. Sometimes, however, it may be necessary to ask families to take a hard line, that is, to insist that patients must take medication and maintain a minimum level of appropriate behavior, or they cannot live at home. For instance, when patients terrorize their families or behave in ways that are unwittingly dangerous to the well-being of other family members or the home itself, this sort of ultimatum may be needed. It is a last resort because it can create other problems such as increased family conflict. Nevertheless, if the choice is between relapse or forcing compliance to treatment, the use of a familial ultimatum may be necessary.

In the following example, Elaine is refusing medication, and attempts to gain her compliance by less extreme methods have met with failure. Her parents have had difficulty setting firm and consistent limits and the clinician has come to believe that doing so was crucial to Elaine's survival.

CLINICIAN: We've discussed this before and I'm aware that this has been a problem in the past.

FATHER: Every damn time. This was her fourth hospitalization and every damn time she's gone off her medication right after.

ELAINE: I don't need it.

CLINICIAN: We all agree, except for Elaine, on the importance of medication in decreasing the chances of another episode. Let's review again what you have done in the past to keep her on it.

MOTHER: We've threatened her and cajoled but she just makes up her mind. . . . We've said we won't give her money. We've even said she can't live with us. What else can we do?

CLINICIAN: Have you ever carried out your threats?

MOTHER: How can we? She's sick.

CLINICIAN: I understand, but without medicine, I don't think we have a chance of breaking the cycle of Elaine going in and out of hospitals. Based on past experience, it seems obvious that if Elaine stops her medication today, she'll be in a hospital within 2 months.

FATHER: Yes, but what can we do?

CLINICIAN: I think you may have to make a very painful decision. Elaine must take responsibility for herself and for taking her medication. If she doesn't then she has to live with the consequences, even if they're painful for her and everyone else. How about giving her the choice. Either take the medicine or find another place to live?

ELAINE: They wouldn't make me move.

CLINICIAN: I don't know if they can, but I think that if they care enough and have enough strength to do it, it would help you *and* them. I think it's too painful for them to stand by and watch you continually fall apart.

FATHER: Isn't there any other way?

CLINICIAN: You've tried being supportive, taking away privileges, nothing seems to help. The choice now is to leave things as they are, knowing she'll get worse, or. . . .

FATHER: (*Long pause*) We'll do it if you say so, but we're going to need a lot of support.

CLINICIAN: You'll get it. I know how hard it will be for you. In the long run, though, it will be better than this never ending cycle.

FATHER: (*Taking a deep breath*) Okay, Elaine, that's it. Either take it or you'll have to move out.

MOTHER: (*Starts to cry*)

CLINICIAN: (*To mother*) I know it's painful, but are you with your husband on this?

MOTHER: Yes . . . yes . . . Elaine?

ELAINE: (*Sullenly*) I'll think about it . . . I'm angry.

CLINICIAN: I don't blame you for being angry, but your parents are trying to do what they think is best. I'm with them on this one.

ELAINE: Well . . . okay, I'll take it for a while, but I won't like it.

CLINICIAN: I understand.

In this example, the clinician supported Elaine's parents in making a difficult decision, insisting they unite to make it together. In so doing, she strengthened the generational boundary and reinforced the rights of the parents to establish the rules for their home. At the same time, she recognized and respected Elaine's resentment at being coerced in this way. It is best to avoid these extreme coercions if at all possible, particularly when clinicians do not know the patient or the family well enough to predict how they might respond. In this case, the clinician believed that Elaine would cooperate if the message was strong enough, and that the threat would not have to be operationalized.

Although it is usually advisable to continue drug treatment for an extended period, sometimes patients, or family members, decide they want to see whether the patient could get along without drugs. When this decision is unavoidable, the clinician attempts to negotiate three agreements with patient and family: (1) They will allow medication to be gradually discontinued by the clinician rather than stopped unilaterally and abruptly by the patient, (2) the patient and family will remain involved in family sessions and report any changes in the patient to the clinician, and (3) the patient will agree to go back on medication if things worsen or if prodromal signs occur. If the patient and family agree to these terms, a working relationship can be maintained. In working together, it must be stressed that while going without medication is not the clinician's first choice, everything possible will be done to see if this plan can be made to work. Unless patient and family believe that their clinicians are genuinely willing to assist them in their efforts to go without drugs, they will not trust the interventions that are suggested and they may not even report symptoms when they occur.

In the following example, Larry has decided to stop his medication after 9 months of treatment. His father is supportive of the decision, while his mother is ambivalent.

CLINICIAN: It sounds like your mind is set. You're going to stop the medication no matter what I say.

LARRY: Yeah.

FATHER: As I said, I know he'll do fine, maybe even better since he has no energy now.

MOTHER: I can't help being frightened. I couldn't stand it if he started acting like he did. And he's doing *so* good now.

CLINICIAN: I agree. I think Larry is doing much better now, but we've been saying the same things for an hour now and Larry and your husband are standing firm. I truly hope that we can continue to stay on the path of progress without the medication.

MOTHER: By the "we," does that mean you'll continue to see us?

CLINICIAN: Absolutely, if you'll agree to come. I think it's going to be very important now to stay in touch and continue to monitor Larry's progress. In fact, I'd like to discuss three things with you.

The clinician continued to negotiate the agreements related to stopping medication, continually reiterating his hope that a decompensation would not occur. After considerable hesitancy, Larry and his father agreed to all three conditions.

More difficult to handle, simply because it is harder to detect, is passive resistance to the medication program. For example, patients may claim they are taking their medication when they are not, or when they are taking it only sporadically. Unfortunately, it may be too late to discuss risks and benefits of medication by the time everyone finally becomes aware of the patient's noncompliance. In general, the establishment of an open climate and some of the basic rules and guidelines of this program diminishes the likelihood of this occurrence.

Another way of dealing with noncompliance is to replace oral medication with medication given by injection. Switching to long-acting injectable medication with patients who have past histories of noncompliance helps to avoid the issue of medication becoming a power struggle between patient and family members or between patient and treatment team. It also helps to remove families from the role of having to monitor patients by counting their pills or continually asking them whether they took their medication that day.

The following example was taken from a crisis session which followed a phone call from Len's father. At that time he told the clinician that Len was showing an increase in symptoms.

CLINICIAN: You seem very upset, Len. What's the matter?

LEN: (*Mumbling to himself and glancing furtively around the room, does not answer.*)

CLINICIAN: (*To father*) How long have you noticed the symptoms you mentioned on the phone?

FATHER: For the last few days, bad. But a little for about 2 weeks, but only a little at first so I didn't make much out of it. Then it got worse over the weekend. Now, he talks to himself about devils, all the same stuff.

CLINICIAN: Has anything stressful been happening that I don't know about?

FATHER: (*Slowly*) No. . . . (*Len glares*)

CLINICIAN: If I remember, Len has stopped his medication without telling anyone in the past. Len are you taking your medication?

LEN: Yeah

FATHER: No way. I grabbed his bottle before coming. It doesn't look like he's taken any since he got his last "script," 2 weeks ago.

CLINICIAN: Is that true Len?

LEN: No.

CLINICIAN: Well we have a big problem with no easy answer. Len, I'm really concerned that you're upset. I want to help you to feel better. I have to admit that I tend to believe that you probably haven't been taking your medication even though you say you are. I don't want to argue, but I'm concerned you'll have to go back into the hospital. I also hate to have your dad checking up on you all the time.

LEN: I don't like him watching me. You, either. And I'm *not* going into the hospital.

CLINICIAN: At least we agree on that. I'd like to see you stay out of the hospital, too. There is one way out so that nobody has to fight about the medication at all and that's to switch to getting a shot. We talked about this briefly before but now I think it's more important than ever.

LEN: I don't know. . . .

CLINICIAN: Well, I'll tell you what. How about if I call Ann [Len's medication nurse] and see if she's available to stop up and join us now to explain about that kind of medication and to answer any questions you might have. If you agree, we can then arrange for your first shot.

LEN: I'll talk to her, but I'm not promising. . . .

In the above example, the clinician was prepared to deal with medication noncompliance based on Len's past history and his father's feedback. She was thus looking for a way to move to injectable medication to guarantee compliance *and* to tone down the negative interaction between Len and his father. The clinician went with the smallest sign of willingness (Len's "I don't know"), believing that if she gave Len more time to think about it, Len's resistance might escalate. She followed this by appealing to Len's ambivalence and suggesting a positive solution to it.

Patient Resumption of Responsibility

Most families require frequent feedback from clinicians about what they can reasonably expect of patients (and *vice versa*). Without direction, many families tend to react in one of two ways following a hospitalization or an acute exacerbation of symptoms. They can become tolerant of all behavior exhibited by patients regardless of how bizarre or negative it is for fear of even greater upsets. At the opposite extreme, families can show a total lack of acceptance of any behavior that could serve as a reminder that the patient was once or is now "crazy." Either of these reactions can escalate stress for patients since the first response creates an unstructured environment and the second creates one which expects too much, too soon. In either case, patients must overmonitor themselves often creating a paradoxical effect of prompting an increase in symptoms.

A major theme of sessions during the first year is to encourage patients to gradually assume more responsibility for themselves, but at a comfortable pace. During this time, the family clinician must help the patient and the family to accept that schizophrenia is an illness, and that this illness will interfere with the patient's ability to function for an extended period. The clinician must support families in tolerating this prolonged period of diminished functioning while at the same time helping them to put limits on those behaviors that are significantly disruptive to family life. The clinician must gradually, but consistently, promote moves towards health.

If the psychiatric hospitalization or the patient's period of dysfunction has been long-term, family members may have reorganized to form new patterns of interaction that do not include the patient. A sibling may have assumed more authority or a spouse may have developed new social supports during the prolonged crisis. These revised roles may lead to conflict when the patient reenters the home. It is the clinician's job to facilitate the patient's return without unduly upsetting healthy, newly formed roles and alliances. This can be done by defining the patient's reintegration into the family as a difficult and slow process that requires time and patience on the part of both the family and the patient.

The following excerpt came from a session 6 weeks after John's discharge from a 4½ month hospitalization. During this time, his wife had finally managed to get involved outside the home after years of isolation.

CLINICIAN: You say that things are different now?

JOHN: She's like a new person. She's not home as much, and I need her. I don't like her going out. I never know when she's coming or going.

ANNE: I have more things to do. For the first time in years, I have friends. That self-help group was a great idea. I have needs, too.

CLINICIAN: I agree that you both have needs. I wonder if we can't come up with some ways in which they're both met?

In this case, the solution negotiated by the clinician encompassed Anne having one day and one evening to herself to do what she wanted, but that these would be announced to John well in advance. In return, she would spend 3 days and nights with him. In addition, Anne agreed to have John occasionally accompany her to the group so he could meet some of her new friends and supports. By keeping the activities predictable, Anne was able to continue to develop outside relationships, John was able to feel there would be time "just for him," and both were able to begin to go out as a couple.

In the above example, John wanted to begin to socialize with his wife and others. However, it is more common that patients do not have the desire or the ability to resume prehospitalization activities this quickly. Frequently, the most difficult problems for both families and professionals are the so-called "negative" symptoms of schizophrenia, including excessive sleep, lethargy, amotivation, and blunted affect.

Families and professionals often react to these negative symptoms with frustration. A complaint commonly heard is that "He seems normal now, but all he does is sleep." It seems impossible that anyone could be capable of sleeping 22 hours a day. Since the patient is no longer overtly psychotic, it is only natural that many families come to believe that the patient could do more if he tried. If only the patient would get active and busy, they say, he would feel a lot better. If family members or clinicians maintain a covert assumption that the patient's lethargy and amotivation are voluntary and destructive, they will place increasing pressure on the patient to perform.

At such times, clinicians must reemphasize the messages of the workshop by stressing the near inevitability of decreased functioning during this phase of the illness and the need for a *gradual* return to the normal demands of life. Reminding family members of the information that has been provided about the illness helps them to use their understanding to increase their tolerance and control during these difficult times. Early family sessions in this phase are used to work on scaling down goals and expectations that are too ambitious. Repeatedly, the immediate priorities of treatment are emphasized: first, the need for an extended period of recuperation to avoid precipitating relapse and, following that, the need for patients to gradually resume roles and responsibilities within their families. Only after both of these processes are well under way does the resumption of social and work roles outside the home become a focus. Again, these themes are put into action through the use of tasks that gradually increase in difficulty over time.

The process of gradual resumption of responsibility by patients generally begins by assigning tasks that attend to small issues of personal hygiene, moving to assigning tasks that involve small chores around the home (first, tasks with a nonconflictual family member, then moving to independent tasks), and finally moving to assigning tasks and activities that take patients outside the home. It is important that each new task build on previous tasks, and that patients be helped to see the relevance of these small tasks to their own desires and goals. Family members, too, must be helped to see the logic in and importance of these small tasks and the importance of the step-by-step sequences in which they occur, or they will have tendencies to ask too little or too much of patients at these crucial times.

In this entire process, it is the clinician's responsibility to set a pace that minimizes the stress level of patient and family, yet that never completely accepts the status quo. The clinician continually makes probes to gauge patient readiness to assume some responsibilities, testing this readiness out by making "mini-pushes."

In the following example, Chris has been home from the hospital for 3 months. Although basically nonsymptomatic, he is sleeping over 19 hours a day.

MOTHER: I guess he's still sick. That's the only reason I can think of for that much sleeping.

FATHER: (*Quietly*) Sick or lazy.

CLINICIAN: I can't fully explain the reasons why Chris is sleeping so much. I do know that we see this an awful lot. Many people seem to need an inordinate amount of sleep following an acute episode. We talked about it at the workshop.

MOTHER: I do remember—time for recuperation.

CLINICIAN: Right. But, I also think that Chris has to help in this process.

CHRIS: I'm just tired.

CLINICIAN: I understand. I believe that your energy will gradually return. In the meantime, it will take a big effort on your part to be active.

CHRIS: I don't have it.

CLINICIAN: I believe that it's hard. I don't think you can decrease your sleep at this time, but I do think it *will* gradually decrease. In the meantime, I think we have to make use of the 5 hours you are awake.

CHRIS: I really am tired.

CLINICIAN: Okay, well . . . how about . . . seeing if we can come up with one thing you could do this week—just one—that would let you and your parents know that the potential is there for things to get better.

CHRIS: Well. . . .

MOTHER: Anything. . . .

CLINICIAN: At the beginning of the session when we were chatting, you mentioned putting in your vegetable garden.

FATHER: Right.

CLINICIAN: Chris, I wonder if you could help your father with preparing the garden for, say, 15 minutes, two times this week.

CHRIS: (*Reluctantly*) I don't know.

CLINICIAN: Hm . . . I guess that is a lot. How about one time this week?

CHRIS: Well . . . I guess I could.

CLINICIAN: How about you, Mr. S?

FATHER: I can always use help.

In this situation, the clinician acknowledged the parents' confusion and frustration with Chris's excessive sleep. At the same time, she helped the family to accept this symptom as a stage of the illness, one on which neither she nor they would be able to have an impact at this point. Instead, she negotiated a small task with Chris that would primarily provide his parents with a sense that something was happening and offer the hope of future change.

Exceptions

There are times when the sequences we have described cannot be followed. For instance, all of the therapeutic messages of slow and steady progress and one change at a time go out the window when patients must return to work quickly because they are a family's breadwinner. Fighting this rapid return when both patient and family believe it is an economic necessity just increases stress. In such instances, therefore, the clinician's role is to support patient and family to enable them to cope with a difficult situation, to empathize with the problems encountered, and to help make the best of it. Family sessions must focus on creating a family atmosphere that supports the patient's need to work by minimizing other stresses. For example, the clinician might help a patient's wife to tolerate his minimal energy level and inability to help around the house following his return to work. In the following example, Cliff had no choice but to return to work. He had his wife, Rose, and four children to support.

CLINICIAN: It doesn't seem as though there are any other options available.

CLIFF: Nope, that's the way it is.

CLINICIAN: How do the two of you feel about it?

CLIFF: I'm worried. The last time I went back I didn't last 2 months. I'm lucky to still have my job.

ROSE: I'm frightened too, but we need the money. They've been real good to him, but they won't hold the job much longer.

CLINICIAN: I'm concerned too. I wonder if something can't be done to help ease the stress and make this time successful.

CLIFF: Like what? I've just got to do it.

CLINICIAN: Well, I think two things are really important. First that you get plenty of rest and second that you don't have anything *else* to worry about, at least at first.

CLIFF: That's tough. My house is falling apart. I haven't done anything on it for months. I know my wife is upset.

CLINICIAN: That's just what I'm talking about. If you start worrying and doing everything at once, I'm concerned you'll crash. I wonder if the family can't cover for you for just 1 or 2 more months to let you get on your feet at work.

ROSE: Well . . . I guess 1 or 2 months would be okay. After all, if Cliff goes back to the hospital, nothing gets done anyway. We can let things slide if it will help.

CLINICIAN: Good point. Then it's agreed. Cliff, the only thing you have to worry about is work. Remember: Get your rest, even if you feel like doing more. I would like you to hold back until you've been working at least a month.

Family Boundaries

During the chronic course of a schizophrenic illness, generational and interpersonal boundaries within families often become blurred. When the patient is an adolescent or a young adult, one or both parents may become involved with the patient to the detriment of their relationship with one another or with their other children. Wives or husbands come to treat their ill spouses as children, and children come to perform parental roles to fill in for ill parents. Often, the patient's illness dominates the household, so that all decisions and plans are made on the basis of what the patient needs, wants, or will tolerate. This, in effect, puts the patient in control of the rest of the family. These confused generational boundaries are a problem for everyone, as is the central position the patient occupies within the family. The familial structure becomes skewed in such a way that the normal needs of its members cannot be satisfied or attended to properly.

Similarly, vague interpersonal boundaries tend to become a problem. When the illness is severe and chronic, it becomes easy for everyone else to be upset when the patient is upset. It also becomes easy to develop interactional patterns in which other family members attempt to anticipate and interpret what patients might mean or feel when their communications are unclear or absent. Yet these attempts to understand and to be helpful leave patients vulnerable to overintrusiveness from other family members, and leave family members vulnerable to being affected by every mode of behavior from patients.

While solid generational and interpersonal boundaries must be reinforced, it is often helpful to try to make the boundary between the family and the community more permeable. When patients have been ill for any length of time, they and their families have usually become more isolated. The sheer amount of time and energy it takes to cope with the illness, coupled with the stigma of mental illness and the resultant alienation of friends and relatives, leaves both patient and family feeling disconnected and unsupported. Therefore, in addition to the establishment of appropriate intrafamilial boundaries, another significant goal of treatment is decreasing the isolation of families from their social community.

Reinforcing Generational Boundaries

Generational boundaries are reinforced by supporting a solid marital coalition, with both partners meeting their adult needs within the adult relationship and uniting for the sake of childrearing or patient-care tasks. Sometimes families need help with this process, as in the following example.

CLINICIAN: I'd like the two of you to come to some agreement about what the rules are for Joe to keep living in your house.

FATHER: I'd like to have some rules.

MOTHER: But Joes sick. How can we ask him to follow rules?

FATHER: See what I mean? (*To clinician*) She just won't do anything she thinks he might not like.

MOTHER: That's not true. I just can't. I'm the one who suffers. You're never there.

CLINICIAN: I don't want to get into an argument here. But, it's really important that the two of you agree on some basic issues for Joe's sake and your own. He needs structure. You don't have to like the rules, or even each other. (*Parents laugh*) But we need things to be more predictable. What's the least controversial issue we can start with, just for practice?

In discussions like these, the clinician can reinforce generational boundaries by building a parental coalition, first over minor, non-controversial issues, later over more difficult ones. When the patient is the parent, reinforcement of solid generational boundaries sometimes involves gradually moving a child out of a parental role. In the following example, the clinician and family discuss arranging some age-appropriate freedoms for a teenage son of a single-parent mother who has schizophrenia.

MOTHER: I need Willy at home to help with the younger kids. They get on my nerves.

WILLY: I don't mind.

PATTI: I like it better when Willy is there, too.

CLINICIAN: I think it's terrific that Willy helps out so much, but I also think Willy needs a chance to do the things other boys his age do.

MOTHER: I guess that's true, but. . . .

WILLY: If I'm not there, I'm afraid something might happen. I try to get home right after school.

CLINICIAN: Is there anyone else who you could ask to help out occasionally so Willy could get a break?

MOTHER: I guess my sister could come in once in a while. She helped out once before when I was in the hospital.

Thus, the mother is helped to assume responsibility for finding a replacement for Willy. Even though she could not yet completely and consistently function as a parent herself, she could remain in charge of who "parents." Simultaneously, Willy is given a little time off from the task of holding the family together.

Family sessions must also focus on discouraging excessive mutual involvement between some family members and encouraging the development of other family relationships. For instance, to reinforce generational boundaries and firm up a marital coalition, parents may be given tasks that engage them in a social activity as a couple, without the patient or other children. Considering the years these parents have focused on the patient, such activities may be new and uncomfortable. For this reason, a clear rationale must be given, along with a great deal of support for following through. In the following example, the clinician begins to encourage Sandy's parents to go out without her for the first time in many years.

CLINICIAN: I'd like to see the two of you go out alone as a couple sometime over the next few weeks. Sandy is doing well now and needs an opportunity to see how it feels to be on her own for a few hours. Besides, it's time the two of you got a chance to get some relief from your full time job as caretakers. If you don't, you won't be able to be helpful to her during the times she really does need you.

MOTHER: I don't think I could leave her.

CLINICIAN: What would be in the way?

FATHER: She'd worry from the moment we left the house.

CLINICIAN: Is there anything you could do to help her worry less?

FATHER: Maybe we could have someone look in on Sandy?

CLINICIAN: That's a start, sounds good.

MOTHER: I'd still worry.

CLINICIAN: That's okay. This is a new experience, and you'll worry until you get reassured. It's okay if you don't enjoy it, as long as you go. That's enough for a start.

If couples have not spent time together in several years, it's important to begin with activities that do not require a great deal of interaction or intimacy (e.g., a movie, bowling). Later, activities that involve more talk can be suggested (e.g., dinner at a restaurant). This reinforcement of generational boundaries and the parental or marital coalition serves a number of functions. Most simply, it builds in pleasant activities for overstressed family members, helping to recharge their depleted energy in order to cope in the future. It also helps to strengthen other family relationships and to decrease the focus on the patient. This in turn decreases the stress patients sometimes experience when they feel responsible for the worry and pain of other family members. The reinforcement of generational boundaries also eases the burden that cross-generational alliances put on the younger generation to meet parental needs at the expense of their own needs to grow and differentiate. Children of patients can be at least partially freed from roles in which they must overfunction. Finally, the stage can be set for enhancing both the patient's and family's social network (to be discussed further in Chapter 5).

The next example came from the session after Sandy's parents did their task and went out for coffee.

CLINICIAN: Sandy, your parents were concerned about how you'd do when they went out. How did it go?

SANDY: Great! I felt so good seeing them go out . . . I can't remember the last time they did. You know, I've always felt terrible—like I was stealing their fun. They just gave me a gift.

MOTHER: Then how come you waited up for us and asked us where we'd been? You seemed angry.

SANDY: Well, I was a little nervous being alone, but I was okay.

Interpersonal Boundaries

Respect for interpersonal boundaries often increases spontaneously following the educational workshop, perhaps as a result of decreased anxiety and guilt, or perhaps because it becomes clear that interpersonal intensity is not helpful to a patient vulnerable to stimulation. Nonetheless, the need often exists for ongoing help and suggestions in establishing appropriate interpersonal boundaries when one family member has been dysfunctional over a long period of time.

Within the family sessions, it is possible to create rules and processes that make clear the importance of interpersonal boundaries. For instance, simply requiring that each family member speak for him or herself helps to stress this point. Thus, each time any family member makes assumptions about what others think or feel, they are asked to check it out and to respect the answer they receive. In the following example, a mother is helped to accept her son's overt messages rather than responding to her perception of his internal pain.

MOTHER: I can't leave Joe alone to go shopping. I know how terribly lonely he is. I just can't bear going out without him.

CLINICIAN: I think you should check that out with Joe.

MOTHER: You don't want me to leave you alone, do you?

JOE: I don't mind. You can go shopping.

MOTHER: You don't mean that.

JOE: (*Says nothing*)

CLINICIAN: Joe, your mother isn't convinced you mean what you said.

JOE: I *do* mean it, but I don't know what else to say.

CLINICIAN: (*To mother*) I think we have to believe Joe. If he changes his mind, he can let us know, but right now he says it's okay. We need to respect what he says.

MOTHER: I guess I believe him . . . it's just that it bothers *me* so to see him alone.

CLINICIAN: That's another issue. Let's talk about it.

In this example, the clinician begins to help Joe's mother to recognize that her own feelings of sadness about Joe interfere with her ability to accurately hear his messages. Understanding this can help her to respect his messages and her own needs as well.

Interpersonal boundaries are also stressed when clinicians encourage family members to recognize each other's limitations and vulnerabilities as well as to recognize each other's strengths. This is the first step in helping family members to tolerate each other's requests for distance. In the following example, the patient and his parents are helped to see that the need for distance relates to survival and does not constitute rejection. Allowing family members to do things separately is reframed as positive and healthy.

CLINICIAN: It sounds like it's been a rough week for everyone.

FATHER: Yeah, work was rough for me and then coming home didn't help. Tom had a few bad days.

CLINICIAN: Sounds like you need a break.

FATHER: I'd love to have one but it wouldn't be fair to Joan [his wife].

CLINICIAN: What's fair is less important than what each of you need. Joan will get a turn but right now I think it's really important that you get a break. In fact, I think it's the most positive thing you can do for Tom *and* Joan. After all, it's tough enough to tone down stress under the best of circumstances, not to mention when you're really stressed yourself.

FATHER: Well, maybe I could get away if Joan wouldn't mind. I was invited to go fishing Saturday. . . .

MOTHER: I don't mind, not as long as I get *my* chance too.
TOM: What about me? Doesn't anyone care about me?

The clinician helps Tom's parents to recognize that their exhaustion is a normal response to a difficult situation. He then encourages them to be more supportive of one another. In this case, he suggests each allowing the other "time outs" from the recurring stresses in the home. While Tom had a somewhat negative reaction initially, he eventually adjusted to not being the constant center of concern for both his parents.

To avoid the strain of patients and family members having to request space each time they need it, interpersonal boundaries are also stressed by encouraging family routines that build in time outs. This allows the patient or others to retreat to their rooms or to go for a walk when feelings of agitation or overstimulation arise. During times when this routine doesn't work or is disrupted, patient and family are asked to discuss and agree upon signals that indicate the need for psychological space, as well as the need for support. In the following example, a patient and family discuss the patient's response to the stress of dinner guests and try to develop more appropriate methods of distancing for the future.

FATHER: I was so embarrassed. Here we had eight friends over. Jane knew everyone. And what does she do? She lies under the table for half the evening.
CLINICIAN: What was happening, Jane?
JANE: I was really tired.
CLINICIAN: How come you didn't go to your room?
JANE: I knew how much they wanted me there.
CLINICIAN: (*To parents*) Did you want her there?
MOTHER: Well, we would have liked her to be there, but not if she was so uncomfortable and inappropriate.
JANE: Well you *told* me you wanted me to stay.
CLINICIAN: I wonder what can be done to avoid this problem in the future?
FATHER: All she had to do was *say* something.
CLINICIAN: Maybe Jane didn't know that. Sounds like she was trying to stay because she wanted to please you. Jane, do you think you could let the family know more directly when things are too much or when you need time to yourself?
JANE: (*Reluctantly*) I guess so.
CLINICIAN: Do you really think it would be okay with your parents if you left?
JANE: I'm worried they'll be mad or disappointed.

MOTHER: It's okay, really.

FATHER: Much better than doing something like lying under the table.

CLINICIAN: Do you believe them now?

JANE: Yes.

CLINICIAN: Fine, try being more direct next time. Tell your parents when you want to leave. (*To parents*) Now, if for some reason, she can't tell you, it's okay to suggest she go to her room if she starts sending you signals by acting inappropriately.

FATHER: I wanted to tell her this time, but I was afraid of a blow up.

JANE: I wouldn't have blown up. I wanted to leave. I just couldn't.

In this case, the clinician reinforced the need for each family member to give clear signals and attempted to diffuse the fear that honest communication would lead to disappointment or to an explosive confrontation. Most patients and families can identify "signal" behaviors and learn to verbalize their messages or check out how others are really responding. By helping families avoid tendencies to engage in "mind reading," or tendencies to ignore messages in order to avoid confrontations, both the patient's ability to function appropriately and the family's rights to expect reasonable behaviors are reinforced.

Interpersonal boundaries are also strengthened by discouraging family members from ignoring, reinterpreting, or trying to make sense out of unclear messages from patients. Rambling, vague, and nonsensical communications are frustrating to everyone. Since the symptoms of schizophrenia include loose associations and thought blocking, it is not surprising that family members sometimes find themselves involved in bizarre patterns of communication with patients. Tolerating poor communication gives a message that the patient need not learn to be clear in interaction with others. The world outside the family will not take the time to make sense out of the nonsensical, so patients must learn to be clear. Families are encouraged to give responses such as "I don't understand that," or "That's unclear, could you try again?" when patients are having difficulty expressing a thought.

The following example of a father–son interaction came from a session early in the treatment of Jason, who had been ill for several years. His father, who is very supportive, attempts to understand the highly confused messages of his son.

FATHER: I've always tried to treat my children the same. Yet I think Jason has always been jealous of his brother and me spending time together.

JASON: Lifting weights is important.

FATHER: What?

JASON: For muscles and repetitions are in circles.

FATHER: (*Pause*) Oh. I guess I see. His brother has weights down in the basement. He's been working out for football. I guess Jason is jealous of the attention he's getting . . . being an athlete and all.

CLINICIAN: That's incredible. (*Laughing*) You know, I really didn't understand what Jason said at all. Are you sure that's what he meant?

FATHER: (*Smiling*) Not really. I didn't understand him either. I was just guessing.

CLINICIAN: I think we'd both be better off checking it out with Jason. (*To Jason*) Could you explain what you meant? Neither your father nor I understood.

JASON: I don't know what I meant.

CLINICIAN: *Are* you jealous of the time your father spends with your brother?

JASON: Yes.

In this example, the clinician begins to reinforce appropriate communication by preventing Jason's father from mind reading and assuming the burden of decoding Jason's unusual communications. He also attempts to achieve these goals by encouraging Jason to answer questions directly.

Families and patients are also encouraged to develop rules to live by that do not violate any individual's integrity or privacy. During the acute phase of schizophrenia, family members often must monitor patient behaviors in order to protect the patient, family, or home from harm. The development of a sense of reassurance that such behaviors will not recur takes time, and the presence of continuing symptoms can further delay this process. Thus, overmonitoring behaviors are common and difficult to change.

In a discharge planning session which occurred while Wally was still an inpatient at a state hospital, his parents discussed their fears about his return home.

FATHER: I don't know if we can have him come back. No matter whether he was crazy or not, he did set a fire in his bedroom. It's a lucky thing no one was hurt.

MOTHER: I'm worried sick. He looks okay now, but what if he stops taking his medication? We might be back into the same old thing of having to stay up all night to watch him.

CLINICIAN: Well, let's take one thing at a time. You had good reason to worry before because Wally was out of control. He's not now, but before he comes home, we will have a few sessions to make sure you all agree that he's ready. We also need a commitment from Wally that he will agree to some basic rules for living in the house.

MOTHER: Like making him promise to take his medication?

CLINICIAN: That's a start. We'll meet together and you can bring up the concerns you have. I know you'll worry some for a long time, but we'll do everything we can to make things as safe and predictable as possible.

Initially, the clinician tries to insure as structured and predictable a home environment as possible. This includes supporting the family's attempts to guarantee controls on the patient. He acknowledges that some fear is appropriate but gives the message that there are things both the clinician and family can do to enhance the safety of the situation.

At the beginning, family members are asked to set firm but reasonable rules and limits, to be available to patients but not to center their lives around them. Over time, however, support must be given to enable families to take small risks that allow patients to develop the ability to control and maintain themselves. From the earliest sessions, patients are asked to assume some responsibility for letting their families know their needs. Both patients and families are asked to use the clinician whenever they have questions and concerns about these guidelines.

Family–Community Boundaries

The isolation that develops when patients and family members must deal with any chronic illness, be it mental or physical, probably decreases stress tolerance over time. For this reason, family members, and eventually patients, are helped to connect with friends or members of their extended family, both to have someone to turn to for practical help or emotional support, and to have people with whom they can become active, thus temporarily distracting them from the problems associated with the illness. When work or social organizations are available and helpful, these activities are also supported. Essentially, patients and families are simply encouraged to use whatever resources they have for coping with stress.

For direct help and comfort about the illness, however, there is nothing like talking and relating to those who have been through a similar experience. For this reason, it is extremely important to help family members to connect with other families of patients with schizophrenia. In many communities, groups are already in existence. Such organizations as NAMI (National Alliance for the Mentally Ill), PAMI

(Parents of the Adult Mentally Ill), and their equivalents provide support, self-help, and opportunities for political advocacy for patients with these illnesses. In our particular project, we have not only distributed information about those groups which are external to the helping system, but also have provided families with the opportunity to get together every 6 weeks to discuss issues of common concern. In addition to diminishing family isolation, often families are able to help one another in ways professionals cannot.

In the following example from a multiple family group, family members share their reactions to the way others have responded to their concerns.

MRS. A: Like I was saying, you don't really know until you have been through it. People just can't understand.

MRS. M: My sister calls up and she says things like, "You shouldn't worry so much." "Have faith in God" or "Tomorrow will be a better day" . . . and I don't say anything because she just doesn't understand. What good is it to have faith in God when my son is doing another one of his rituals or when he's up all night with the music on.

MR. B: They really don't understand. I've stopped talking, too. When they ask me how she is doing, I just say, "coming along." I figure that covers just about everything. (*Group laughs*)

MRS. A: Maybe that's a good idea. I'm serious. At least I wouldn't be explaining all the time.

MR. B: Feel free to use it. . . But I wanted to get back to Mrs. M because it sounds like she's having some of the troubles we used to have and I know how hard it was.

MRS. M: It's terrible, just terrible.

MRS. J: Well, you're new here, but you should know we've all been through some of this. One of the things I learned was to say "No" to him—like that he can't have the music on at night, I need my sleep. It was hard, but after a while, things really settled down.

In terms of advice, Mrs. J and Mr. B clearly have much more credibility than a professional could have in this context. They have been through similar experiences with someone they love. They have developed coping mechanisms out of the painful crucible of trial and error. The process of sharing experiences and solutions helps people to feel less alone and less stigmatized.

Coping with Dangerous Behavior

The most frightening problem encountered by clinicians and families is the potential for or presence of dangerous behaviors. Families are particularly sensitive to this issue in part because of the attention the media has given to the behavior of those few patients with schizophrenia who commit violent crimes or behave in dramatic ways. The first step, therefore, is to reassure families that most patients with this illness are not violent to others or to themselves. If patients have not been violent in the past, it is unlikely that they will be in the future. This simple reassurance can do much to decrease emotional intensity of those families in which violence is not an issue. However, for those families whose patient members have been or seem now to be prone to violence, it is possible to be helpful in a number of additional ways.

The best time to cope with violence is before it occurs. Clinicians must ask patients and families to review the kind of situations that have resulted in violence in the past. It is important to encourage them to be as specific as possible so that common themes can be discerned. Who tends to be present? Are there particular topics that set things off? Are there particular times of the day that are stressful? Have particular medications helped in the past? If a situation can be defined in sufficient detail, the clinician then can proceed to help the family and patient to establish rules for interaction at home that will serve to diminish the likelihood that these situations will occur.

In certain situations, it can also be suggested in advance that if violence seems to be brewing, either the patient or family members agree to leave the room or the house until things have settled down. For those patients or family members who know in advance that they are about to be upset, this sometimes allows the time and space for each to regain control. If patients are paranoid, confrontations about paranoid ideations can become the precipitants of violence. This type of violence sometimes can be avoided by simply helping families to avoid direct confrontations with the patient's paranoid ideas. Instead of saying, "That's not true," to patients who think they are being poisoned, it is suggested to family members that they respond, "I understand that you must feel upset and frightened if you think that."

As is done for all problems of an emergency nature, families and patients are given the message that a member of the treatment team is always available to them for support and suggestions, and that they should freely use the team when they have any concern, rather than waiting for things to develop into a crisis. They can also be instructed on how to proceed with an emergency commitment or how to receive emergency help from police who are reluctant to respond to calls about mental patients.

Dangerous behavior, however, is not just violence. It also takes the form of lack of concern about self and others, or lack of good judgment about a situation. Families sometimes complain that patients

smoke in bed or do not watch where they flick their cigarette ashes.
Parents worry about patients wandering the streets at night, fearing
they will be mugged or raped. Clinicians must approach these problems
by acknowledging the validity of familial concern and attempting to
negotiate an appropriate resolution to the problem, as in the following
example.

MOTHER: I have to follow her around. She flicks her ashes all
over the place. You should see our couch and rug. It's a miracle there
hasn't been a fire!

CLINICIAN: That *is* a problem. But I'm curious. Janet doesn't leave
the house at all and nobody else smokes. Where does she get her
cigarettes?

FATHER: I buy them. I mean she has nothing else. . . .

CLINICIAN: I understand . . . well, I see two paths we can take.
First, you could stop buying the cigarettes. If she needs them, then
she'll have to go buy them. Or, since you are good enough to get
cigarettes for her, I think in response, she can be more careful and
use an ashtray. If she can't, then I think it really is important that
you not buy them for her.

FATHER: That will be hard.

CLINICIAN: Are you willing to try?

MOTHER: Do we have a choice?

CLINICIAN: How good is your fire insurance?

FATHER: We don't have a choice.

Another type of dangerous behavior frequently encountered involves suicidal threats. This is a particular risk after the acute illness
has subsided since many patients become depressed during this time.
It is difficult to manage such problems since constant monitoring of
patients is a stress to both patients and families, yet families feel they
must monitor patients who are talking about killing themselves. The
clinician must carefully assess the level of risk. If it is significant, then
frequent monitoring or even a short hospitalization may be necessary.
If clinicians feel they have a good relationship with patients, they can
attempt to extract promises to call any time they are feeling suicidal.
While clinicians should be conservative in these situations, they must
help patients and families to get on with their lives as soon as possible.
For families, this often means accepting the inevitability of some risk.
Even overmonitoring does not guarantee the patient's safety. Therefore,
family members and patients should be helped to continue on the
road toward normalization of the family routine.

In the following example, a crisis session was called following Diane's attempt to cut her wrists. While she did not actually hurt herself, she frightened her parents.

CLINICIAN: What's happened?
DIANE: I couldn't take it anymore. What's the use of living? There isn't any. I'll never be well.
MOTHER: (*Tearfully*) Oh, my God.
CLINICIAN: I can understand why everyone is upset right now. So you've been feeling pretty hopeless?
DIANE: Yes.

There continues a discussion about the frustration involved in the slowness of change and Diane's anger at her parents for watching her every move. Finally:

CLINICIAN: What can we do to prevent this from happening again? Do you have any ideas how we could handle this?
FATHER: We should have called you. We knew she was really upset. It's our fault.
CLINICIAN: (*To parents*) I don't think you could have predicted this or even prevented it from happening. But what got in the way of your calling?
MOTHER: We didn't want to bother you.
CLINICIAN: I wish you would bother me anytime you're worried. Most of all, I wish you, Diane, would call me anytime you're that down. Could you do that?
DIANE: I guess so. I almost did this time.
CLINICIAN: I'd really appreciate that. I care what happens. For right now, maybe we should consider your coming into the hospital for a couple of days so that you can feel better and more in control.
DIANE: I don't think I need it. I promise to call if I feel that way again.
CLINICIAN: How do the two of you feel about this? Do you feel you can trust her word?
MOTHER: As long as I'm home . . . and I'll be there over the weekend.
FATHER: I think so, but I know we'll still worry.
· MOTHER: Oh, yes, we'll worry.
DIANE: But *that's* what drives me crazy. It's like they're my shadows.
CLINICIAN: Okay, let's look at some ways that you can feel you have a little more freedom without making them more nervous.

In this example, the clinician first attempts to deal with the immediate issue of suicide and what can be done to prevent this from being an issue in the future. She then moves to dealing with the interactional issues that provoke such behaviors on the patient's part when it becomes clear that the family's current solution actually increases the patient's distress.

Other Family Problems

Families with chronically ill patients are not immune to problems that create stress and conflict in all families. In some ways, because of the levels of stress they have experienced for long periods of time, and the magnitude of problems with which they have had to cope, these families may have learned to ignore all but the most blatant and urgent of problems not related to the illness. Nevertheless, marital conflict, problems with other children and depression are common. To attempt to deal with all these problems at one time is an overwhelming, frustrating, and probably antitherapeutic task.

It is important to remember that the initial therapeutic contract is to help the patient with schizophrenia recuperate and to help the family cope with the illness. During the course of treatment, this must remain the primary focus. Other problems should be addressed only when they impede the progress of the patient or family toward the primary goal, or when the patient or family specifically gives the clinician permission to do so. When it is necessary to deal with one of these other problems directly, the clinician should explicitly recontract with the family, gaining their agreement to work on the new issue. If this is not directly related to the patient, patients can be asked to leave during this process so as to concretely control the level of stress they experience, reinforce the generational boundary, and insure the privacy of other family members. For instance, this might be the case if parents begin to work on marital or sexual issues.

MOTHER: I know our going out is supposed to help Peter [their son], but, to be honest . . . well, I don't really like going out together.

FATHER: Yeah, well, I guess since you're our therapist, you should know my wife and I have been having problems for quite a while.

CLINICIAN: I appreciate your honesty; since you both seem uncomfortable talking about it. I apologize for putting you both in an uncomfortable situation with the last task. . . .

MOTHER: Excuse me. We talked about it before we came today, and we'd like to discuss our problem with you if it's okay.

CLINICIAN: Well, Peter seems to be doing all right at this point. Peter, your parents want to talk to me about some problems they've been having. Is that okay with you?

PETER: Yeah, sure.

CLINICIAN: Okay. Since it sounds like it's just between them, I'd feel more comfortable if you could wait in the waiting room for right now.

PETER: Sure, but I know they've got problems.

CLINICIAN: I know you do, but they should work them out with each other . . . just like there are some problems I've seen you about by yourself.

PETER: Okay.

Patients need not always be asked to leave during such discussions. Sometimes hearing parents work out disagreements, and learning to stay out of the conflict is a good experience. At other times, however, the message-value of removing the patient is a more appropriate therapeutic intervention. It can reinforce the message that parental issues belong to the parents.

Whatever choice the clinician makes regarding the inclusion of patients, family problems are labeled as understandable and predictable based on what these families have experienced. Normalization of these issues reduces stress. Even under these circumstances, the clinician avoids stimulating an emotionally charged atmosphere and attempts to be helpful in concrete ways.

The guidelines for managing other family issues are based on avoiding the assumption that clinicians have a right to move into all areas of a family's life simply because they have become a captive audience of the patient's illness. Each additional issue placed on the agenda must be negotiated with respect.

Many times, however, it is not necessary to focus directly on other family issues. Often other family problems seem to dissipate by themselves as the patient-related stress eases and families reorganize themselves to be less focused on patients. Sometimes getting two parents to agree on management rules for their problematic son or daughter has the indirect effect of helping their marriage. Other times, decreasing patient symptoms and setting limits on behaviors in the house allows siblings to be less stressed and to move toward a more normal life-style. A few months after Mark got his first job in several years, the relationship between his parents showed a dramatic improvement, although it had never been a focus in therapy sessions. In a session with the patient, they reported their plans to go away together.

MOTHER: I'm so excited, Josh [her husband] and I are going to New York for the weekend.

CLINICIAN: Great! You folks could use a trip like that. In fact, I could use a trip like that myself.

FATHER: You know this is the first time we've gone away together since Mark got sick 7 years ago.

MOTHER: And I'm only a little worried. Not enough to stop me from going. (*Laughs*) You know, we haven't gotten along so well in years.

Unremitting Symptoms

While unusual, a small percentage of patients have symptoms that remain, regardless of the dosage of medications, type of treatment intervention, or length of illness. Many families and patients naturally respond with anger and a sense of hopelessness. Clinicians must help such patients and families to accept the inevitability of the symptoms but, if possible, to learn to cope with them more effectively. The presence of symptoms does not mean that patients cannot learn to function in some areas and to be more considerate of their families.

George had been ill for over 10 years when he and his family entered the program. During that entire time, he had never been symptom free and had never remained outside a hospital for more than a few months. After a year's treatment, he still heard voices. Nevertheless, he was able to enter a vocational training program, make a few tentative friendships, and to live away from home in a structured environment. Even with these positive changes, both he and his family continued to focus on the hopelessness of his illness and the persistence of his symptoms. In such situations, the clinician must help everyone to appreciate small gains, to tolerate the slowness of change, and to stress the importance of only one change at a time.

FATHER: You know George still hears voices. Do you think we should try another medication?

MOTHER: It breaks my heart to see him suffer.

CLINICIAN: What do you have to say, George?

GEORGE: Well, I do hear voices. I entered a science fiction novel 10 years ago, and I never came out.

CLINICIAN: I know you've said that before. (*Pause*) By the way, how's work going?

GEORGE: (*Brightening*) Pretty good. I'm earning minimum wage.

CLINICIAN: (*To parents*) I know George still has symptoms, but I would really hate to see us change anything. He's doing better than he's done in a long time.

FATHER: Well, that's true. At least he doesn't go to the hospital constantly these days.

MOTHER: But, he's so *lonely*.

CLINICIAN: We'll try to get to that, but one thing at a time. He's really doing very well compared to last year. When we don't have any other crisis, we'll work on helping George to find friends, that is if George wants to.

GEORGE: My voices are good company.

FATHER: We're glad he's in the training program, but I still think we should try some other medication. It's not fair that he's still so sick.

CLINICIAN: I agreed it's not fair. I wish we could make the symptoms go away, too. But I have to say I'm really impressed with how well George has done under the circumstances, and I think it will continue. I think you all should feel proud.

GEORGE: I do!

Resistances

The strong emphasis on the initial process of connecting with both patients and family members, the genuine collaborative nature of the treatment, and the methodical nature of the clinician's approach, helps to diminish resistance. Resistance to treatment is less of an issue than resistance to change. Resistance to change tends to occur when long-standing patterns of coping are challenged or when the changes required cannot be made without temporarily increasing anxiety or pain. In the following example, both of Rick's parents were uncomfortable leaving their son alone, even for a few hours.

MOTHER: Do you know that we have never gotten a babysitter for our kids? Even before Ricky was sick we didn't go out by ourselves. Why have children if you're not going to be a family.

CLINICIAN: I understand and I think the two of you have been good parents. I also know that what I'm asking you to do is very painful and difficult, but you and I know that our hope as parents is to one day see our children establish a life of their own.

MOTHER: (*Tearfully*) Yes, but it will never happen.

CLINICIAN: I think it can, but the first step is to let Rick try to be on his own for just a little while. Since he won't go out, I feel the only way to do it will be for the two of you to go out without him, even if only for a few hours. I don't underestimate how difficult it will be, but it is another way of showing your caring for Rick.

FATHER: Well, I'll try it, but 2 hours is too long. How about one?

CLINICIAN: Fine with me. It's a start. How about you two?

RICK: (*Uncomfortably*) Okay.
MOTHER: (*Uncomfortably*) Okay, but I won't have a good time.
CLINICIAN: I know. I'm only asking you to do it for Rick's sake.

Resistance is lessened by acknowledging the pain and difficulty of these changes. This imparts an empathic understanding by the clinician yet continues to underline the importance of changing certain behaviors. The clinician must show a willingness to negotiate for a small change if the task presented seems overwhelming. One of the most difficult tasks for parents is that of beginning to set limits on a son or daughter who they feel is too sick to respond. In the following example, this problem led to an impasse in treatment.

CLINICIAN: I think we've hit a roadblock, and I don't know how to get around it. Things are not getting better.
MOTHER: That's for sure. Katie just lies around making nasty comments. I'm constantly nagging at her to get up.
CLINICIAN: I understand how frustrating that must be and how difficult it is for the two of you to set some rules and then back off.
FATHER: You should try living in our house for one day—then you'd see.
CLINICIAN: I'm sure it'd be really difficult for me, too. I don't underestimate that. I realize I'm asking for a lot. You've been super-caring parents and now I'm asking you to show your caring in a different way. If you could set a few rules on some of Katie's behaviors for just 1 month, I think we'd be on our way.
MOTHER: I just get so angry. There's no point in rules, she doesn't listen.
CLINICIAN: I understand that it will be rough for everyone to take this first step. But you've tried it your way for 8 years, please give our way a try for 1 month.
FATHER: Can we have an appointment next week?
CLINICIAN: I think that would be a good idea.
FATHER: Allright. We'll try it your way for 1 week and let you know next week what happens.

Without blaming, the clinician states the fact that the family's approach had not been effective, and asks the family to agree to try something new. While little change can be expected in 1 week's time, in areas that are difficult to change, clinicians must sometimes settle for very small commitments to get a foot in the door. In this case, 1 week was gradually extended to 2, and rules developed in one area were gradually extended to the development of rules in another.

Techniques of reframing and relabeling also can help overcome resistance to change, particularly in the area of overinvolvement and overprotection of patients. Parents who cannot allow the patient space and distance often cannot do so because of their own conception of good parenting. For example, parents may believe that a "good parent" would never leave a sick child to manage alone. Clinicians then can help by redefining what is good parenting for patients with this illness.

CLINICIAN: I know you've made lots of sacrifices for your son, and now I'm asking you to make another one, the ultimate one. I'm asking you to live with the anxiety of letting him make some mistakes on his own. The hardest part of being a good parent is to let go.
MOTHER: I never thought of it that way, but you're right. It hurts to let go when you think something might happen.
FATHER: You want to protect them, you know.
CLINICIAN: I know.
FATHER: But you're saying we can't forever. He has to be on his own.
CLINICIAN: Only a little . . . he'll always need you, but he also needs a little freedom.

The most difficult resistances by far are those raised by schizophrenic patients who do not believe they are ill. In such cases, it is particularly important that clinicians form and maintain an alliance with the patient and the family around issues that the patient can accept. Clinicians should present patients with alternative reasons for therapy, such as helping patients to begin to get ready for work or independent living. Such goals acknowledge that problems exist, but bypass the inevitable power struggle caused by insisting upon focusing on the patient's illness.
As discussed before, separate sessions with resistant patients sometimes help to increase the therapeutic alliance. If resistance remains, open discussion about the issue between the patient, family, and clinician allows for the negotiation of a contract that offers all parties the chance of gaining something from the sessions. In the following case, Joel continually refused to accept that he had an illness and was on the verge of pulling out of treatment.

CLINICIAN: Even though I strongly believe we can help you, I understand that you believe there's no need for you to be here [in treatment].
JOEL: I don't see how.

CLINICIAN: Well, forgetting about whether you have an illness, I think we can help you regarding school [Joel wants to go to a local college].

JOEL: I don't need your help.

FATHER: But you need ours. You don't have money or a place to stay.

CLINICIAN: Perhaps we can negotiate a compromise. How about if Joel continues to take his medication and comes to sessions. In return, the family will agree to support him while he goes to school.

MOTHER: That's fine with us.

JOEL: Well, if you put it that way, I have no choice.

This resolution is not the most desirable one, since Joel is clearly cooperating only under duress. Nevertheless, it is better than the alternative, that is, his leaving treatment completely. As one of our colleagues is fond of saying, "It's hard to do any kind of therapy when the patient is running down the street." At least with this contract, clinicians can buy time to form an alliance and prove their usefulness.

Some specific problems occasionally arise when patients have had their first break, and their family is not familiar with the illness. Patients who are ill for the first time, and their families as well, often hope and believe that the episode was a once in a lifetime event. It is an understandable hope and 20% of the time, it is true. It is the job of the clinician to allow that hope to continue while at the same time setting up a management program that gives patients their best chance of survival. The question, "Why do we need anything?" has to be anticipated and answered in a way that does not frighten patients and families away, yet spells out the realities of the illness. In the following example, the clinician is dealing with that exact question.

MIKE: I don't know why we're coming here anymore. I'm feeling a lot better.

FATHER: I've been asking myself the same thing. He's doing a lot better.

CLINICIAN: You really are doing well, and you may not need to come much longer. But remember when we talked about making a contract for a year? I'd like to make sure we get through that year. It's the highest risk time. Maybe if you'd like, we could meet a little less frequently?

MIKE: (*Laughs*) How about once a year?

FATHER: Seriously, how about once a month. It is a 3-hour drive to get here, and he's doing okay.

CLINICIAN: I think I can live with that, if you promise to call if anything comes up.

MOTHER: Oh, we'll call. We don't want it to ever happen again. I just don't think it will though.

On the other hand, patients with a chronic history of schizophrenia and their families are likely to be resistant for other reasons. Rather than being overly optimistic, they have a sense of hopelessness, having been the medication and therapy routes before with no appreciable success. They also ask the question, "Why do we need this?"; but this time, the question emanates from a feeling of futility. Usually, even in the most discouraging situations, there remains a core element of hope that this time might be different. It is to this core of hope that clinicians must appeal. They do this by expressing an understanding of what these patients and families have gone through in the past, while asking for one more try.

SUMMARY

This chapter has described the ongoing phase of family treatment that extends from patient discharge from a hospital until they are ready for a more intense focus on returning to social and work functioning in the community. Small tasks are used to accomplish the goals of gradual reintegration of patients into the family and the community. Contacts include regularly scheduled family sessions, crisis sessions and telephone consultations. Each session is conducted in a carefully controlled manner with phases that emphasize social contact, review of assigned tasks and new problems, problem resolution, and the assignment of new tasks. The content of the sessions during this period tends to include such topics as the importance of early warning signs, strategies for living together, medication compliance, and gradually increased responsibility for the patient. During all sessions, appropriate interpersonal, generational, and family community boundaries are emphasized. This phase may last a few months or a few years.

SOCIAL AND VOCATIONAL REHABILITATION

That the mental health system has been generally unsuccessful in devising methods capable of rehabilitating its psychiatric patients would seem to be a gross understatement.—*William A. Anthony (1977, p. 658)*

If and when patients are able to demonstrate that they can maintain themselves outside a hospital without major crises, and after they are able to gradually resume some responsibility within their families, it is possible to begin to focus on their reintegration into a larger social and work world. The time it takes to reach this stage differs from patient to patient. Some are able to return to work relatively quickly and/or are able to establish meaningful social contacts. Others, however, go through a prolonged period of amotivation, apathy, and depression. Such patients frequently complain of loneliness and hopelessness while their families complain of the patient's lack of interest in life and the frustration of trying to find ways to help. Over time, these patients and families become increasingly aware that the patient's quality of life is poor. Thus, it is imperative to help them to improve their social relationships and to increase their positive involvement with social, community, and vocational activities.

This chapter will focus on the difficult task of moving patients from relatively low-level, stable functioning within the home to becoming involved in community activity, including work and a social network. While the areas of work and social functioning will be discussed separately for purposes of clarity, in actuality the focus of treatment may alternate between the two. In all cases, the decision of which area to emphasize at which point is made in conjunction with the patient and the family.

The basic overall theme that guides a psychoeducational model of intervention continues to apply: Only one change should be made at a time. Thus, when therapy focuses on engaging patients in a larger social network, vocational efforts are held in abeyance. When attempts are being made to move patients into work or training programs, no focus is placed on improving the social aspects of their lives. Priorities should be set for specific patients and their families depending on which tasks come more easily or which need the most attention. Some patients find the relatively structured tasks of a work environment easier to handle than negotiating informal social relationships. If this is so, the clinician may suggest establishing goals in the vocational area as the first step outside the home. Other patients feel less threatened by social interaction than by the demands for performance inherent in even low-level employment or vocational training. Thus, for these patients, the first steps outside the home may best be social ones. It is important to understand, however, that it is not only the abilities of the patient that must be taken into consideration in making this decision, but the needs and abilities of families as well. For instance, some patients must contribute to the financial support of their families. When a family's economic survival is even partially dependent on the patient's ability to work, every effort must be made to return the patient to his or her employment as soon as it is feasible.

RATIONALE FOR SOCIAL REHABILITATION

Schizophrenia has an inevitable impact on the social life of patients as well as on the social networks of their families. Over time, some of the symptoms of schizophrenia, such as attention problems, delusions, or paranoia may have caused patients to question or misperceive the intent and meaning of communications from others in their social world, particularly communications from friends and family. When patients interpret the casual or even well-meaning comments of others negatively, it is not surprising that they come to avoid social contact. Even those patients who are not suspicious tend to have a heightened sensitivity to environmental stimulation that often leads them to withdraw from social interaction in order to gain some perception of control over the context in which they live.

The isolation brought about by purposeful withdrawal can be further intensified by the negative symptoms of schizophrenia. It is very difficult for patients to engage in social interaction outside their immediate family when their functioning is impaired by apathy, amotivation, and decreased energy. Frequently, patients complain that going out is "too much of an effort" or that they have "no desire" to do so, despite their complaints of loneliness. Even activities that were pleasurable for patients in the past hold little, if any, interest for months and even years after an acute psychotic episode. Thus, most patients, especially those who have been ill for a number of years, are relatively isolated with no support system beyond that of their families. Patients who have developed bizarre behaviors or socially unacceptable mannerisms are usually even more isolated. Ultimately, when their desire for social contact returns, they lack the ability to relate in ways that will allow them to be accepted by the rest of the world.

The longer social isolation is allowed to continue, the more social skills tend to decrease, with odd behaviors becoming entrenched over time. Repetitive negative responses from the environment further reinforce dysfunctional patterns and the need to withdraw. Even those friends who attempt to maintain a relationship by repeatedly initiating contacts over the years, sooner or later run out of patience in dealing with the intensity of the patient's social problems or the lack of response to their overtures.

Thus, despite the extreme difficulty inherent in beginning to connect relatively unmotivated patients with a wider variety of social contacts, efforts must be made to begin this process as soon as some stability has been achieved. It is helpful if clinicians take the lead in beginning this process since friends, acquaintances, and family members are often unsure on the one hand of how much to push the patient, perhaps leading to or causing the resurgence of positive symptoms, or on the other, of how much to tolerate the patient's lack of initiative or reciprocity, perhaps reinforcing a deficit state and settling for far less than the patient is capable of achieving (Breier & Strauss, 1984).

Family members of patients coping with this phase of the illness often describe their own social isolation. Caring for someone who has a debilitating chronic illness takes a great deal of energy. Out of necessity, patients become the focus of all family and household activities, with most decisions based on what patients need or can tolerate, rather than being based on the needs of other family members. The effort required to cope with the issues inherent in living with this illness leaves everyone in the family without enthusiasm, interest, or even the ability to manage much social activity outside the home.

The sheer emotional and physical exhaustion families experience in coping with patients tends to be further complicated by fears of leaving patients alone out of concern about what they may do to themselves, others, or the family home. As one parent stated, "It's difficult to go to a party and enjoy yourself when you're afraid of what you might find when you get home." The isolation of family members also can be exacerbated by the stigma associated with mental illness and by the negative attitudes they may have encountered in both friends and strangers. Their embarrassment over patient behaviors may also lead to isolation. For instance, one family described their son's intense questioning of everyone who came to their home. He demanded to know whether or not each visitor was a secret agent of the CIA. It is understandable that, as time went on, family members invited fewer and fewer friends to the house, becoming more isolated themselves as a result.

Finally, family members become more isolated because so few of their friends and extended family truly understand what it means to live with a chronic mental illness. Some people they would like to turn to for help and comfort are unavailable or unsupportive. For instance, one mother of a patient complained that, "My sister says she doesn't want to hear about it; she's got problems of her own." While the isolation that occurs when friends and family are this unavailable is obvious, family members also can become uncomfortable and upset by uninformed attempts to help. For instance, many families come to avoid discussing the issue because other people just don't understand. One wife of a patient stated, "People tell me just to ignore it when he acts up. Well, that advice doesn't help when Henry's doing something crazy and you're at your wit's end."

To combat the isolation of both patients and families, specific attempts must be made to facilitate their use of existing support systems and to facilitate the establishment of new ones. This chapter will begin with a discussion of tasks that will diminish the patient's social isolation, followed by some suggestions about how to help family members in this regard.

CONTENT, TIMING, AND STRUCTURE OF SOCIAL TASKS

The Initial Step: Moves with Other Family Members

The goal of increased socialization for patients cannot become a focus until their symptoms have been stabilized and they have begun to assume some responsibility for their behavior within their families. In fact, the gradual reinvolvement within the family that was described in Chapter 4 is the first step in the resocialization of patients. Social failure and rejection within the family unit is less devastating than failure in the broader social environment. Progress in the area of functioning within the family can also be used to determine when patients might be ready to move toward the more ambitious goal of beginning social contact outside the family. When "in-home functioning" has been sustained and/or steadily improving for a number of months without crises, the clinician can begin to attempt to help the patient move to the next level. In fact, if things have gone moderately well within the family, family members can be effectively used in helping the patient to make the first moves outside the home. For instance, tasks given to patients have a greater chance of success if they are grounded in tasks already given within the family, and if the initial tasks assigned to the patient outside the family are assigned with the cooperation and participation of another family member.

The following example came from a family session 8 months after the patient's discharge from the hospital. Roger no longer experienced overt psychotic symptoms and had successfully completed most of the small tasks assigned to him with only minimal difficulties. However, he rarely initiated activities within the home and never left the house unless it was absolutely necessary. During this session, the clinician began to ask for family input in creating a task that would help Roger to begin to become more socially active.

CLINICIAN: It seems that Roger is doing really well. He's made a lot of progress. I think it's taken effort on everyone's part and you really should be pleased.

MOTHER: We certainly are. Roger's so much better.

CLINICIAN: Yes he is, and because things have gone so well, I think now's the time to begin to focus on doing more outside the house. Maybe moving toward having some friends.

FATHER: Good idea. He's always alone. He never calls anyone.

ROGER: I don't have anybody to call.

CLINICIAN: If you did, would you call?

ROGER: (*Hesitantly*) I guess so.

MOTHER: We've asked him to call some of his old friends but he just won't.

ROGER: They're busy. I don't even know them anymore.

CLINICIAN: We've talked before about some of the problems with just picking up where you left off before this illness and I'm sure there are problems picking up on old friendships, too.

FATHER: I think he's embarrassed, you know, about being in a hospital and not doing as much as they might be. . . .

ROGER: We're just different, that's all.

The clinician then discussed some of the social difficulties that arise for patients during the course of this chronic illness. He particularly focused on the fact that many of Roger's old friends, friends with whom he had had only minimal contact in the several years since he had become ill, were unavailable, having moved on in their lives. Although Roger readily acknowledged that his old social network was neither available nor of interest, it was difficult for Roger even to consider the idea of mobilizing himself to find a new set of friends. Despite these major problems, the clinician started to emphasize the importance of friendships and social activities. He began to focus on creating a task that would help provide a structure within which Roger could begin to develop positive social contacts without causing too much stress. In this case, a family member was used as the initial conduit to the outside world.

> CLINICIAN: Well, we need a first step. Any thoughts?
> ROGER: No.
> FATHER: I can see the first step's a problem. He doesn't have anyone to start with.
> CLINICIAN: That's not entirely true. He does have the family.
> FATHER: I thought we were talking about going *beyond* the family.
> CLINICIAN: We are, but maybe going beyond the family *with* one of you would be a first step.
> MOTHER: I'd be happy to do something with him. (*To Roger*) How about you going to my bingo game with me?
> ROGER: (*Looks down silently*)
> CLINICIAN: (*To mother*) Well, I think that's a good suggestion. But, you need that time away from the family. You've said how important that is to you.
> MOTHER: Well, yes, but . . . if it would help Roger. . . .
> FATHER: How about if Roger and I go to a *Pirates* game. I've wanted to go anyway.
> CLINICIAN: Roger, how about it. Would you go to a ballgame with your Dad?
> ROGER: Well, okay.

In this part of the session, the clinician moved toward developing a task that was primarily social and out of the home. Rather than accepting the offer of Roger's mother (since she was already more involved with Roger than his father and also needed her own separate social contacts), he accepted the father's offer of taking Roger to a ball game. Roger's father had always been concerned, but somewhat distant. Thus, while this task did not directly establish new social contacts for Roger, it served several functions: It began to get him out of the house, to desensitize him to crowds, and to facilitate an experience more related to the interests and activities of other young men his age.

As in earlier phases of treatment, whenever a social task is assigned, task performance is discussed during the subsequent family session. If positive social interaction has occurred, its importance is emphasized and reinforced. This is particularly important since too often small social contacts are taken for granted as a natural part of life when they are not natural at all for these patients. In the session that followed Roger's excursion with his father, the clinician asked Roger and his family for feedback.

CLINICIAN: If I remember correctly, last time we talked about you and your dad going to a ballgame. . . .

ROGER: Yeah, the *Pirates'* last game.

CLINICIAN: How did it go for you?

ROGER: Pretty good, except Dad and I had an argument about me having another beer.

FATHER: Well, he already had had one, and I remember our discussions about drinking. . . .

CLINICIAN: Okay, we'll get into that in just a few minutes, but first, (*To father*) how did it go for you?

FATHER: Much better than I thought. I was a little worried before we went . . . you know, that Roger would have problems. But, he did fine, really seemed to enjoy himself. To be honest, I think that it was the closest we've been for a long time.

CLINICIAN: Sounds good. Do you agree with your dad, Roger?

ROGER: Yeah. I really liked being with him . . . I didn't mind the crowds.

CLINICIAN: I'm glad to hear you both enjoyed yourselves, except that the *Pirates* lost. I'm really pleased to hear both of you say you enjoyed each other's company, and also pleased that you didn't mind the crowds. That opens up a lot of possibilities for future activities. Now, it did seem as though there was one problem, and that was the drinking. Let's discuss it a bit and see what can be done to resolve it, and then we can plan the next task.

ROGER: Fine, except not another game where the *Pirates* lose.

The clinician focused on the positive aspects of task performance, reinforcing the enjoyment that both Roger and his father gained from doing it. He then turned to the problems that had arisen during the performance of the task, helping the family to achieve a solution before attempting to focus on developing a new task.

Sometimes the development or redevelopment of conversational skills and increased awareness of the needs of others is essential before the patient can begin to engage in appropriate social activities. Many patients lose their ability to make small talk, or the sensitivity necessary to understand the impact of their words and behaviors on others. Within the sessions themselves, social conversation and problem solving between family members or with the clinician can provide a practice ground in which patients are encouraged to communicate in a clear, simple and direct manner. This not only allows the clinician to give feedback about appropriate communication skills, but gives impetus to patients to continue to have conversations at home with their family members. For instance, Sharon who had been hospitalized intermittently for 6 years, had been largely uninterested in conversation even within the family. While she once fled to her room when she encountered family members, over the months she had participated in the program she had begun to have an interest in being around the family, and even in being present when her mother had guests. Unfortunately, she continually initiated conversations with her mother by calling her fat and suggesting she diet, often in front of others. The mother's response was first one of tolerance, then of irritation, and eventually of anger. This problem was discussed during a family session.

MOTHER: I could have killed her. I don't mind when she says these things to me by myself, but in front of my friends. . . .

CLINICIAN: I can imagine how embarrassing that must have been. Why are you saying these things to your mother, Sharon?

SHARON: She's too fat and it's not good.

CLINICIAN: I'm sorry, I don't understand. . . .

SHARON: She has to be more careful. . . .

CLINICIAN: Go on.

SHARON: Fat isn't healthy.

CLINICIAN: All right, if you're concerned about your mother's health, let's look at how you might let her know that without embarrassing her. When you start going out with friends, you'll need to be able to let your friends know how you feel in a positive way, too. So, let's practice.

SHARON: Okay.

In this discussion, Sharon was finally able to state that she was concerned about her mother's health. While she may have had other reasons for making such statements, the clinician chose to focus on the caring element of the message, and to help Sharon to develop a more socially acceptable way of expressing it. This allowed the clinician to discuss better ways of communicating messages within the family, a skill that eventually could be generalized to interactions outside the home. After Sharon agreed to limit her comments about her mother's weight to private times and Sharon's mother was less upset, the clinician focused on the issue of preparing Sharon to be understood by the outside world.

CLINICIAN: I'm glad we've straightened this out. However, I get the sense that it often isn't clear what Sharon is saying.

FATHER: True. We spend a lot of time trying to figure out what she means.

CLINICIAN: I'm sure that gets to be hard work. I'd like to work on making it easier for everyone to have a conversation. What about

just telling Sharon when her messages don't make sense or are upsetting? She needs to know or she will have a lot of difficulty in making
friends outside the family.

MOTHER: Do you think she can handle it? She used to get really
belligerent when we confronted her.

CLINICIAN: I think she's ready now, but let's check it out. Sharon?

SHARON: You can tell me.

The clinician then initiated a conversation within the session,
encouraging family members to discuss a noncontroversial topic. During
this discussion, the clinician gave everyone suggestions on how to
keep their communications clear and simple. The session ended when
the clinician assigned a task requiring Sharon to strike up a conversation
with a family member about a neutral issue such as a television program
or a current event. During the next session, everyone's reaction to
this assigned task was discussed, and a new, somewhat more ambitious
task was given. This task involved talking to someone outside the
nuclear family. Sharon successfully responded to the second task by
initiating a conversation with an aunt who was visiting. While the
conversation was brief, it was socially appropriate.

The use of the family as an initial testing ground for the patient's
moves towards social interaction outside the home has several advantages. It allows trial and error within a reasonably safe environment,
provides the clinician with direct feedback about the patient's abilities,
and can indirectly improve family relationships. For example, it is
often suggested to families that they stop at a restaurant following a
family session. There, the patient can be exposed to the "outside
world," and be required to minimally interact with strangers (at least
with the waiter or waitress in order to eat). This type of task has the
added benefit of encouraging the whole family to get out socially,
laying the groundwork for later tasks that will encourage both patient
and family members to go out on their own. Finally, discussing the
success or problems encountered in this type of brief outing allows
the clinician to design future tasks that are appropriate and that will
be likely to give everyone a chance to experience success rather than
failure.

Occasionally, out of a desire to have things return to the way
they were before the patient's illness, family members will make too
many suggestions for social interaction, usually focusing on things
that once were of interest to the patient. When patients fail to respond
to these suggestions, family frustration can increase, and, paradoxically,
their search to find a magic technique that will stimulate the patient
may intensify. Since most patients with this illness do not respond
well to pressure, even in this later stage of treatment, continual attention

must be given to helping family members to maintain realistic expectations, to tolerate the slowness of change, and to use their energies to work toward feasible, not ideal, goals. For instance, the parents of one patient in the early postpsychotic phase of recovery became involved in trying to find ways to stimulate the return of some signs of life to their apathetic, disinterested son. Since the patient, Adam, had once been an avid tennis player, the family, out of desperation, decided to take him with them to a week-long clinic at a tennis ranch, involving a number of families with young people his age. Although the likelihood of problems with this plan was discussed during several sessions, they were deeply disappointed when he spent the entire week sitting in his room at the ranch. During the next family session, the vacation was discussed with the primary goal of defusing everyone's anger and disappointment.

FATHER: I was sure that this would do it. He used to love to play tennis and all he did was stay in his damn bed. It made me furious. I wouldn't have minded so much if he only would have tried, at least a little.

ADAM: (*Blandly*) I was tired.

DAVID: [brother] (*Disgusted*) You always say that!

CLINICIAN: Whoa, let's slow down for a second. I haven't even heard how the trip was for the rest of you yet.

MOTHER: It was great. We had wonderful weather, great instruction, and all the court time we wanted.

This led into 10 minutes of enthusiastic conversation about the positive aspects of the trip for other family members. The whole family with the exception of Adam, participated in the discussion, and everyone seemed to have found a way to get something out of the trip. The clinician then returned to Adam's lack of participation in the activities of the vacation.

CLINICIAN: Boy, it sounds like just the vacation I could use. It's too bad you weren't able to enjoy yourself, Adam.

ADAM: I was tired.

CLINICIAN: Yeah, I know. Maybe in the future you'll enjoy yourself more.

ADAM: Maybe.

CLINICIAN: (*To family*) You know, I think it's real easy to keep looking for the magic answer and then to get upset and frustrated when it doesn't work the way you hoped it would—like the tennis trip for Adam.

FATHER: We keep hoping that if we only find something he likes, then he'll show some enthusiasm. It's really frustrating to see him like this.

CLINICIAN: I know, but remember, we did talk about it being pretty early to expect much from Adam in a situation like that.

MOTHER: That's true, but we still hoped—

FATHER: I for one can't sit by and watch him just vegetate.

CLINICIAN: But the point is, he did *go* with you, and if I understood it, he at least went out to eat with you in the evenings.

FATHER: Sure, but there was no other way for him to eat.

CLINICIAN: Nevertheless, he did it, and he did it without getting symptoms.

MOTHER: That's true, 6 months ago, he would hear voices if we even had company for dinner.

CLINICIAN: I'm not saying you should be satisfied with the way things are, but only that we should try to appreciate small gains. I agree that the pushes have to continue.

MOTHER: Pushes?

CLINICIAN: Pushes. The tennis clinic was a push. "Come out and try it" is a push. We'll all keep pushing but just a little at a time. I think we have to give up on "what once was" and slowly move toward "what can be."

In this example, the clinician elicited the reactions of all family members to the vacation in order to stress that everyone else's needs were also important, and to emphasize the fact that it was not necessary for everyone to center all of their energies on Adam, particularly during this phase of slow progress. She then moved to a discussion of the family's frustration about the slowness of change, but emphasized that some change had occurred. She encouraged the family to "hang in there" and continue trying to help, while keeping expectations low. The session ended with the following discussion in which Adam, his family and the clinician worked to develop a task that was more in line with Adam's present capabilities.

CLINICIAN: Overall, it sounds like it was an enjoyable vacation for everyone and even Adam got out a little more than usual.

MOTHER: That pretty well sums it up.

CLINICIAN: I was wondering what task we should assign for next time. Something that could keep some of the positive momentum going, but not as adventurous as a ski trip to the Himalayas.

FATHER: (*Laughing*) Well, not until next year at least.

DAVID: You know, I've asked Adam if he wants to go out with me and my friends.

CLINICIAN: Oh? And. . . .

DAVID: He's always "too tired."

ADAM: You always want to go out too late.

DAVID: Well, would you go anyway if I went out earlier?

ADAM: (*Pause*) I guess so.

CLINICIAN: David, I think it's great that you've kept asking. I don't think you always have to try to include Adam, but once in a while might be nice. Maybe the two of you can make some plans while you're here.

The session thus ended with the initial frustration of the family being replaced with an increased awareness of the improvement that had occurred, and somewhat more hope that it would continue. Adam's planning of a social activity with his brother was viewed as an appropriate and positive step in the resocialization process. However, since all too often siblings, as well as parents, sacrifice too much for patients, care was taken to insure that Adam's brother not be led to believe that he should always be available. He, too, needed a life of his own, and occasional freedom from being his brother's keeper.

More Independent Social Excursions

Properly planned social activities with the family are used as springboards for the development of more independent social excursions in the next phase of treatment. Patients still may not have much internal motivation or desire to participate in outings. However, family related activities may be sufficiently reinforcing to make them less resistant to the idea of doing something on their own, if not actually willing to initiate activities in the future. During the week following the session just discussed, Adam went out with David and three of his friends for a movie and pizza. This example comes from the session following their outing together.

CLINICIAN: Well, how did it go?

ADAM: Pretty good.

DAVID: Not as bad as I thought. He talked to my friends about the movie and seemed to have a pretty good time. Except at the end. He wanted to leave before we were ready to.

ADAM: I was tired.

DAVID: (*Sarcastically*) Again, he's "tired."

CLINICIAN: This time, it's to be expected. Overall, it sounds like you both had a reasonable time. I'd like to hear about it. What did you see?

The clinician spent the next 10 minutes discussing the outing. This served to reinforce its importance, to enhance the positive aspects of the evening, as well as to gain an understanding of how Adam reacted to social interaction with peers. Following that, she focused on developing a new task that would build on the success that had been achieved.

CLINICIAN: What I'm hearing is that both of you had a nice time— better than either of you anticipated?

FATHER: I haven't seen Adam show that much feeling in a long time. His mother and I were both pleased, and thanked David.

DAVID: I keep saying it was no big thing.

CLINICIAN: Okay, but for Adam it was a good start. I think your fatigue, Adam, was natural. After all, it's been a while since you've been up that long. Would you be willing to go out again?

ADAM: Yeah, I'd like to. I already asked David if he'd like to go out again with me.

CLINICIAN: And?

ADAM: He said fine. So, we're going bowling with Don and Hank on Thursday night. Every other night, there's a league.

CLINICIAN: You checked it out?

ADAM: Yeah, I called the bowling alley.

CLINICIAN: Are these plans all right with you, David?

DAVID: They're fine. As I said, I had a good time the last time. Maybe this time, Adam won't say he's tired.

CLINICIAN: Maybe. But even if he does, I think it's positive that he initiated something and made the arrangements. That's better than any task I could have come up with. By the way David, I do want to make sure you still are doing things on your own. Adam doesn't have to go every time.

The clinician reinforced David's cooperation and the family's acknowledgment of it. Again she checked with David about his comfort in being Adam's initial but temporary link to a social life, and stressed his right to a private life without his brother. Finally, she reinforced, without overemphasizing, the fact that Adam had initiated a new social activity.

An Alternative Beginning: Assigning Tasks to Other Family Members

Sometimes, especially when the patient is very resistant, it helps to begin with a focus on enhancing the social life of other family members. For instance, Julian spent the better part of a year resisting all suggestions from family members and professionals regarding social activities. If tasks were assigned, Julian would either ignore or sabotage them. Since progress was at least temporarily at a standstill with Julian, the clinician switched the focus to Julian's parents. Their social life had become practically nonexistent over the years of coping with Julian's illness, but they were able to talk with pleasure about once having belonged to a bowling league "before Julian's problem." Based on the rationale that Julian needed good role models, and that they needed a respite which would help to renew their energies, a task was given to the parents to find out about bowling leagues in their area. At the next session several weeks later, they reported that they had not only found out about a league for couples, but had joined it and had already gone once. Interestingly, as soon as everyone stopped pushing Julian, he became less negative and soon expressed interest in going bowling with his parents. Not wanting to allow Julian to interfere with his parents' only night out, the clinician suggested they go bowling as a family on another night. By the next session, Julian and his parents had gone bowling together. Julian spontaneously talked about having a good time and expressed a desire to continue bowling regularly. He had already made inquiries at the alley and had found out that there was a family league they could join. Thus, the technique of beginning with a task for Julian's parents served several functions: It ended a power struggle between the clinician and the patient; it removed Julian from the powerful position of being the center of everything his parents did; it gave Julian's parents a positive social outlet; and it eventually provided a way for Julian to begin to be involved in activities outside the home.

Some patients do not require this level of effort or involvement to get them reinvolved with a social or work life outside their families. In such cases, much of this phase of treatment can be passed over lightly. With those patients who have difficulty with social contacts, however, the move to socializing outside the family must be a slow and careful one.

Moving Outside the Family

The family neither can remain the exclusive social outlet for the patient, nor continue to be available on every foray he makes into the outside world. Sooner or later, the patient must make a transition into a peer-oriented social life. Nevertheless, this transition tends to be a major one, accompanied by a good deal of stress. Therefore, it is often important that the clinician provide increased support and structure for the patient during this time to insure that the transition is a gradual, controlled, and safe one. Although this may seem to be an excessively conservative or protective stance, care is required to help most patients to avoid embarrassing as well as dangerous situations that can arise out of even seemingly simple tasks. For example, early in the application of this model, Paul was given the rather vague task of striking up a conversation with a stranger. Being compliant, he approached a stranger on a corner and asked how to get to a certain area of the city. When the stranger responded by telling him that he was already there, Paul became embarrassed and withdrew to his room for several days. Ben, who had more difficulty knowing what was socially appropriate, was given a similarly vague task. In his enthusiasm, Ben got on a public bus and proceeded to ask every person, one at a time, if they were Jewish. A number of people took offense and one person hit Ben. These tasks were clearly too vague, left too much room for error and thus failed to give either patient a much needed "success" experience.

These examples should make it clear that the assignment of tasks designed to help patients to begin to function outside the home without the help of their families requires considerable thought. Although it may seem insulting to assign small, highly structured tasks to intelligent individuals who once functioned in complicated employment situations, these small, specific tasks are absolutely essential. Not only are these patients functioning at less than their optimal capacity during this phase of the illness, but they badly need opportunities to gain increased confidence by experiencing small successes, however insignificant they may seem to those not struggling with the symptoms of schizo-phrenia.

When the patient, family, and clinician begin to focus on the move outside the family, the first major decision involves where to start. If the patient has been ill for any length of time, his old social network has dissolved, leaving him limited access to peer related social interaction. Therefore, the initial social contacts outside of the family tend to be dictated by the availability of resources. The presence or absence of extended family (cousins, uncles, etc.), neighborhood acquaintances, church groups, social organizations (e.g., YMCA), social clubs, or volunteer and self-help organizations will have an impact on the choice of tasks. Decisions about which resource to pursue are based not only on availability, but also on each patient's particular skills and interests, the level of stress and personal involvement inherent in the contact, and the amount of initiative it requires of the patient.

In the following example, Marty is discussing an outing he had at the movies. In Marty's case, there was a large extended family, many of whom were willing to spend time with him. After considerable discussion, Marty had expressed some interest in a particular cousin, Pete, who was a film buff. When Pete's family had visited several weeks earlier, Pete had invited Marty to go along to a movie "sometime." Marty had been extremely reluctant to make a call to Pete to take him up on his offer, but had finally agreed when the task was presented as one step towards permission to join a vocational training program.

MARTY: (*Blandly*) I gotta say, for most of it, I had a good time. It was a good movie—really funny.

CLINICIAN: It sounds like it . . . sounds like you are happy you went.

MARTY: Yeah. Pete was cool. He even introduced me to a couple of girls. One of them was *really* good looking.

MOTHER: You didn't tell me that. What was her name?

MARTY: Well. . . . (*Long pause*)

CLINICIAN: Sounds like Marty may want to keep that information to himself for right now.

MARTY: Yeah, I don't want to talk about it.

MOTHER: But, why?

MARTY: (*Pause*)

CLINICIAN: Well, remember we've agreed that there would be no secrets about the illness because we needed to share as much information as possible to work together. This is different, though. Most guys don't want to talk to their parents about what they do with girls.

MOTHER: (*Reluctantly*) Well, okay.

CLINICIAN: Did you have any problems with the task that you want to talk about?

MARTY: Well . . . at the beginning of the movie I was a little uncomfortable. I thought . . . well . . . I thought the people knew what I was thinking.

CLINICIAN: Oh?

MARTY: Yeah, but . . . after a while it went away. That's the first time that happened in a long time. Usually once that feeling starts. . . .

CLINICIAN: I'm glad to hear it. It sounds like you felt more in control, and that let you push past the feeling and still have a good time.

FATHER: He didn't even tell us about it. He always used to tell us when he had a symptom.

MARTY: I didn't want to worry you. I really felt I handled it.

CLINICIAN: Sounds like it—and had a good time on top of it. Would you like to go out again?

MARTY: (*Smiling*) He already asked me for next weekend.

In this example, the clinician reinforces Marty's ability to have made an initial social excursion outside the home with a member of his extended family. He tied the assignment of a social outing to

Marty's interest in getting into a vocational program to increase his motivation to handle the task. At the same time, he dealt with two other issues that related to increasing Marty's ability to function independently. First, he reinforced the appropriateness of Marty keeping some issues (unrelated to the illness) private from his parents. Second, he reaffirmed Marty's beginning sense of awareness that he was developing greater control over his symptomatology and that occasional symptoms need not impede his ability to have a good time socially.

Initial excursions to social organizations or clubs should be discussed thoroughly before they occur in terms of anticipated goals, gains, and problems. Often, patients have distorted perceptions of what will be expected of them, as well as distorted ideas of how they will be viewed by others. Years of social isolation, and fears about the stigma of mental illness often lead patients to become easily embarrassed and intimidated, feeling as though they have nothing to contribute to relationships. Thus, some patients have problems initiating social contacts, not for lack of interest or initiative, but for fear of encountering social rejection as a result of having had a mental illness. In the following example, the clinician focuses on helping Kate, despite her fear, develop some social acquaintances in addition to her husband, Rich.

RICH: You know I can't always be there. I'm working 60 hours a week just to make ends meet. I don't have the energy to be her only friend, too. I mean, I love her, but. . . .

CLINICIAN: I understand, and I know you care for her and she for you. I'd like to see Kate develop some of her own friends, too.

RICH: She used to have friends. She belonged to a woman's group at our church and really liked it. I told her a hundred times to get back into it.

CLINICIAN: Kate?

KATE: I couldn't go there again. They all know about me being in the hospital. I'd be so embarrassed. What would I say?

CLINICIAN: There's no simple answer about how to cope with people who know you've been ill. Some people will be uncomfortable with you, because they don't understand. Some will be curious about what it's like. But my guess is, most of the women will be really glad to see you.

KATE: You think so?

CLINICIAN: I do. It may be a little difficult at first, but I think most people will be.

KATE: Well, it's nice to think that most people will accept me, but what about the others? I don't want to deal with them.

CLINICIAN: That's your decision. I don't know if it will help but I can tell you that most patients who return to clubs or work after a hospitalization are surprised by how nice everyone is. It sounds like you really liked the club before. I'd hate to see you give it up.

KATE: I guess I might enjoy going. I'm so bored, and I know I pester Rich all the time. He's all I have.

CLINICIAN: Maybe you can give the women's club a try one time. If it's really uncomfortable, we can come up with another idea. My guess is it won't be.

KATE: Well . . . I'll try. Maybe on a day that I feel good.

In this case, the issue of embarrassment and stigma was raised by Kate. Stigma is, unfortunately, a common and realistic problem. Some people will be intolerant, and others will be obnoxious or intrusive. Discussing the issue of stigma and some possible ways of dealing with this problem can help the patient and the family to be better prepared to deal with it if and when it occurs.

CLINICIAN: What will you say if someone asks about being in the hospital?

KATE: I don't know . . . that's what I'm afraid of.

RICH: You should tell them it was great. Too bad they couldn't be there with you.

KATE: (*Laughing*) I couldn't.

CLINICIAN: It'd be nice if you could sometimes. A little humor might make everyone more comfortable. Maybe you could also just say that you're feeling much better now and thank them for their concern.

KATE: I could try.

CLINICIAN: How about if we practice right now? I'll be an old friend.

The clinician then proceeded to role play with Kate a number of possible situations. Her reactions and responses were discussed and concrete suggestions were offered to help to give her a sense of control and help to decrease her anxiety. At no time did the clinician negate the reality of her concern.

After initial social excursions, it is important to have a session to reinforce their positive aspects and to deal with any problems that may have arisen. Often, the "slights" and negative comments made in any social gathering are overinterpreted by patients sensitive to signs of rejection. The following incident comes from a session two days after Rita had gone to an arts and crafts class for the first time.

CLINICIAN: I'm confused. I'm not sure whether you had a good time or not.

RITA: Well, as I said, I liked making the picture. That was a lot of fun. But, everybody seemed to be cold to me. They knew I was different.

CLINICIAN: Hm . . . do you think you acted differently?

RITA: No . . . I don't think so. But they must know I am, otherwise they would have been nice.

MOTHER: Oh, honey, they don't know.

CLINICIAN: I agree with your mother, Rita. I doubt that anyone could know unless you told them. You certainly don't act differently than anyone else.

RITA: Then why were they so cold?

CLINICIAN: Well, I'd guess it was a pretty normal situation. You know . . . it was a new class with people who didn't know each other. It takes a while for people in a new group to warm up to each other. I doubt if anyone was super warm to any of the other people either.

RITA: Well, I guess no one talked very much. But, I'd really like to make friends there.

CLINICIAN: Give it a little time and it might happen. Meanwhile, are you enjoying the class itself?

RITA: Yes.

CLINICIAN: Good. Maybe we can talk about some ways you can initiate conversations with your classmates so they know you're interested in them.

RITA: That would be good.

The clinician stressed that Rita's perception of "coldness" was real, but normal, for strangers and not related to Rita being "different." She then discussed ways of approaching classmates based on mutual interests. To help Rita develop a sense of control and comfort, she discussed strategies for bridging the social gap. She intentionally did not go into detail about either the makeup of the group or Rita's behavior since this would potentially contradict the "normal" message. If the "coldness" problem continued, then these issues could be more thoroughly addressed in future sessions.

At times, the clinician must become creative in devising ways of helping the patient to initiate social contacts. For instance, clinicians may be able to focus on a patient's interest or hobby as a way of overcoming social isolation. Rob, a patient who had been ill for over 10 years, liked building electronic kits and was quite good at it. Socially, he was extremely isolated, having no contact outside his family and the clinical team that provided his treatment. Recognizing the severity of his social problem, Rob's clinician looked for a way to tie Rob's hobby with social contact. The following dialogue occurred in a session after a detailed discussion of Rob's latest electronic project.

CLINICIAN: Rob, did you ever build a, what do you call it? A . . . ham radio?

ROB: No, but I've seen the kit.

CLINICIAN: You have? Good. I was wondering, since you didn't get out of the house much, it might be interesting to build one. You could have contact with people all over the world on it.

ROB: Hm. . . .

CLINICIAN: Would it be hard to do?

ROB: No . . . the kit looked easy. I'm not sure about talking to people though.

MOTHER: He can build anything, really.

CLINICIAN: Are you willing to at least build the radio?

ROB: (*Pause*) I'll check it out. It's better than the idea of joining a club like you talked about the last time.

In this case, the clinician gives an initial task (building the radio) that does not require social contact, but which offers the opportunity for at least indirectly increasing contact with others in the future. Although this particular task takes a very indirect path to social interaction, more direct approaches had been ineffective with Rob. In fact, with most seriously isolated patients, direct ambitious social tasks often lead to increased stress and major compliance problems. Thus, a particularly low-key approach is often indicated with such individuals.

Another way of reintroducing patients into peer relationships is to provide a group for them. The use of such patient groups as an adjunct to family treatment has a number of benefits. First, it provides an experience with other people who are likely to tolerate the patient's current level of functioning. As has been stated, many patients complain that, even if they wanted to, they would have difficulty in finding someone who would like to be with them, and who would not make them feel socially inept. Secondly, a group of patients with similar problems tends to facilitate the development of connections and supports for all members. The recognition of not being alone in having had unusual thoughts and experiences often decreases feelings of embarrassment and loneliness. It also can give a sense of increased confidence and stimulate increased willingness to try tasks that once seemed too difficult or too unrewarding. Rather than maintaining a traditional process orientation, such patient groups often do better with more structure, perhaps involving a task or social orientation. Having clinicians intervene frequently to maintain the focus on concrete issues and skills helps to create a predictable and safe environment.

A focus on insight, self-exploration, or confrontation tends to heighten intensity and thus stimulate feelings of stress and anxiety. Thus, in general, if groups are to be used to help psychotic patients to begin to develop social contacts, it is more helpful if they are carefully structured.

In contrast to rules that prohibit interaction between patients outside traditional process oriented groups, such between-session interaction can be encouraged and even prescribed as a way of increasing the networks of poorly functioning and isolated patients. The social aspects of the group can become self-reinforcing since they provide patients with the potential to form satisfying relationships with realistic expectations for the first time in years. Furthermore, tasks given to a group of patients to plan a social outing for themselves are usually met with considerably more enthusiasm than those tasks given to single patients. The patient group in the following example had been meeting for 5 months. Consisting of nine members, the group was homogeneous in terms of their primary diagnoses (schizophrenia) and the presence of social difficulties, but varied in terms of age, length of illness, and socio-economic status. In the following interaction, the clinician attempted to encourage group activities.

CLINICIAN: I'm a little confused. The last time you planned going to a baseball game. You went, right? And everyone says it was a great time?

JOHN: Yeah.

LISA: Even *I* liked it.

CLINICIAN: But since that time, it doesn't sound like anybody did much of anything. How come?

JOHN: Well . . . I don't know.

CLINICIAN: Anybody have any thoughts?

TIM: It just seems easier when we're here. I figured we'd plan something when we came here.

BILL: You know . . . once it's planned, then you sort of feel you have to show up. Otherwise, I just never get around to calling anyone.

CLINICIAN: Yeah . . . but am I right, everyone did have a good time at the ball game?

BILL: It seemed that way. (*Several nods*)

CLINICIAN: Well, it sounds like a good idea to plan another activity. But I wonder how we can get you guys to pick up the ball more?

JULIE: Maybe we should plan two things?

JOHN: I'd be up for that.

The group continued to plan two activities with the clinician becoming less involved as they talked more freely. The clinician's goal of having group members become more involved in the planning was partially achieved, but the issue of the development of initiative and internal motivation in these patients was one that would clearly take more time and work over many months.

Most groups form cohesive bonds that offer support to the individual members and give them a relatively safe way of entering the social world. Care must be taken, however, to help keep relationships on a nonthreatening friendship level. Many patients will not be ready or able to deal with issues of intimacy beyond that of good social friendships. Pressure for closer, more intimate relationships can increase stress and anxiety and make the group seem unsafe. A rule against dating among group members helps to offer a sense of control and safety.

Family Social Activity

As the patient begins to become active outside of the family, the time and energy of other family members is freed up to allow a greater focus on meeting their own needs. Families have varying levels of interest in this area. Some family members never let go of their friendship groups and continue to use them effectively for support and distraction throughout the course of the patient's illness. As mentioned earlier, however, other families have few or no friends to support them or to help alleviate the pain of coping over the long haul. As one father in a group of other family members stated:

> I think the trouble is that you feel you are isolated. The patients must feel like they're isolated. Certainly the parents and the family members do . . . the experiences that we are all having in common . . . from suicide, sleepiness, or whatever, it's all a part of a pattern and we think we're the only ones this is happening to.

To increase the quality of life for family members, as well as to reinforce generational boundaries and decrease the likelihood of overinvolvement with the patient, it may be important for the clinician to help these family members to make individual social connections outside the home.

Some families are as unwilling as patients to become more active socially. Explanations such as "not enough time or energy" or "not knowing what to do" or "the need to be there for the patient" are common. While these are very *real* issues, it is important to continue to push for outside activities since, minimally, they can increase the family's ability to cope. A number of possible explanations can be given. It often helps to frame the request for family contact outside the home as beneficial to the patient (see example on p. 175). For instance, it can be emphasized that it is important for all family members to nurture themselves in order to be able to help the patient. It also can be stressed that the patient must have some time alone, or at least without family members, in order to begin to move toward more normal functioning.

Whatever the situation, the family's social connectedness should be explored, and where necessary and possible, help should be given to enhance it. Again, there are social options that are available within the community in the form of church or civic groups and activity organizations. Acquaintances developed at work can also become friendships.

It should be noted that some families prefer to maintain a relatively isolated existence. Other families dislike structured groups and would prefer to develop more informal social contacts. The family's life style and values must be respected, as long as their isolation does not impede the patient's progress or impose too much stress on the family as a whole. The decision of whether and how much to focus on the social lives of family members is best made in conjunction with family members. In the following example, the clinician and two parents are discussing the social isolation that has come to dominate their lives.

MOTHER: I'm just exhausted at the end of the day. And Jack [her husband] is no better. We just want to watch television and sleep.

FATHER: That's our life.

CLINICIAN: I know I'm not dealing with half of what you two are, but I can relate to that. Sometimes I don't even want to get ready for bed. I just want to sleep. But, you know when I get pushed to go out, I wind up having a good time.

FATHER: I just don't have the energy. Plus Jay [the patient] needs us for company. He has no friends.

MOTHER: I couldn't go out and have a good time, knowing he's alone.

CLINICIAN: But he also needs time to be alone and he must learn how to handle it. That's important as a step toward having friends. He'll never reach out to others if he isn't alone enough to experience the need.

MOTHER: You mean he has to practice being alone? It seems like he's been alone all his life.

CLINICIAN: Believe it or not, he needs to be alone a little. Now that he's feeling better, I think it would be good if you could leave him on his own, just once in a while.

FATHER: Hm . . . well, I don't know about the evenings.

CLINICIAN: Well, how about a weekend? Maybe the two of you can go shopping together. At least away from the house for a few hours.

MOTHER: I could use some help with the groceries.
FATHER: *Some* social activity! *(Laughs)*

When the clinician saw that his initial attempt to encourage these parents to go out for their own sake was not working, he switched to encouraging a parental outing as an altruistic gesture in Jay's best interests. He did not push for a task that required interaction with others, or even with each other, feeling that it would be asking too much as a first step when they had not done so in years. Rather, he tried to fit the task into the current needs and interests of the family. Since Jay was still their primary concern, they were more likely to do a task they believed would be of help to him.

As is true for patients, another way of helping families to reenter social groups is to provide one for them. Multiple family groups and self-help groups serve many purposes, some of them social. For families in a psychoeducational program such as this, the educational workshop conducted in a multiple family format serves as a first step in the process of making families feel less isolated about the illness. In our program, an ongoing voluntary multiple family group continues to offer a supportive social network. Some self-help groups have the added benefit of providing a base for encouraging social action to gain services for other patients with similar problems. In the following example, several family members share what it has meant to them to meet as a group.

MRS. G: This week, she got on my nerves so, I felt I was about to blow. And then I remembered what you folks said last time about getting away from it, so I went down to the basement and did the laundry. Then I felt a little better and came up and called Gladys [another mother in the group].
MRS. P: I was glad you called. Things have been good for us, but it wasn't so long ago I felt just like you did. *(To clinician)* You know, the four of us have been getting together now and then. It's just so great to talk to other people who understand.
MRS. L: It's like having another family. We're like cousins. *(Laughs)*

Multiple family groups have the added advantage of making it possible to learn a number of coping mechanisms from other families, and even to share resources. For instance, sometimes other families may know of job opportunities that can be explored, or may be even able to help patients to get employment.

MRS. M: You know, that idea John [another member] had last time about Henry looking into his brother-in-law's training program looks like it might work out.

MR. J: I hope it does. Your husband is lucky, he's had some good experience. Our Paul couldn't handle that.

MRS. L: Well, my son went to the vocational rehabilitation center. He really likes it. He had been once before and it didn't work out, but it's changed.

MR. J: That's good to hear. My son had been there before too. How has it changed?

This discussion enabled Mr. J to understand the new vocational program. Armed with facts and information, he was able to encourage his son to give the new program a try.

Again, relationships develop in the context of the group can carry over outside the group and generalize to other situations. The following conversation came from a group that included seven couples, each of whom had a son or daughter with schizophrenia.

MRS. D: I don't know if it's okay or not, but after the last meeting, my husband and I went over to Jon and Marge's house for coffee to continue our discussion. I'd like to bring up a couple of points that we thought of.

CLINICIAN: Before you do, why did you ask if it's okay?

MRS. D: Well, I didn't know if we're supposed to do that, and I didn't want anyone to feel left out. Everyone is welcome. In fact, we were going to go out tonight again.

MR. T: That sounds nice. Especially since we know our daughter's okay right now. If you really mean it, we might take you up on the offer.

MRS. D: We'd love it.

MRS. T: Going out with another couple! I never thought we'd be able to do that again.

In actuality, the idea of providing groups for both patients and family members can be accomplished by using a group format which starts out as a multiple family group for everyone, and then splits into two groups, one for patients and the other for family members. This format gives everyone a chance to discuss common concerns and issues, to see how everyone else is doing, and yet provides a special time to discuss the issues peculiar to being a patient or trying to live with one. In the patient group, topics often include the discussion of symptoms, medication, and the difficulty of getting back into the "swing of things." In the family group, topics include the difficulty of maintaining patience, strategies for encouraging and motivating patients, and the problem of going on with other aspects of their lives.

As mentioned in Chapter 4, other self-help support groups for families, such as NAMI, are becoming more prevalent and offer alternative contacts with others who are likely to understand the problems with which these families are coping. If these groups are available, they offer a valuable resource to family members that cannot easily be found elsewhere.

A FEW COMMON PROBLEMS IN SOCIAL REHABILITATION

Refusal by the Patient to Become Involved in Outside Activities

Years of social isolation take their toll on patients in terms of both their interactional skills and their desire to continue trying to relate to others. Even beginning with small efforts and going very slowly sometimes seems to be too much for patients who remain withdrawn in group or social situations, structured or not. When other attempts to stimulate social contact do not seem to work, it is sometimes possible for clinicians themselves to provide the first step toward a social life. For instance, Frank refused to try all tasks geared to increase his social functioning, and also refused the overtures made by members of his family. Finally, the clinician suggested holding the next session with the patient alone at a local coffee shop that had a number of video games. Frank reluctantly agreed. The two sat at a table for a while having coffee, and then the clinician suggested playing a few video games. Frank again agreed, probably partially to get out of talking to the clinician. Although he confessed he was uncomfortable with the number of people standing around, he played two games. The next few sessions were structured similarly, and slowly Frank displayed less discomfort and a greater receptiveness to the idea of going out with a family member without the support of the clinician. In the meantime, the clinician's experience with Frank in a social situation gave him a better understanding of the problems Frank's family were encountering as they tried to get him moving. Family sessions were reinstituted, with new social tasks as their focus. Although reintegrating Frank into a social world was still a frustrating and slow process, Frank, his family, and the clinician were able to resolve the impasse and begin to develop a more positive attitude.

The Use of Alcohol and/or Drugs

The use of alcohol and/or street drugs can be a significant factor that complicates social rehabilitation. Alcohol and drugs, such as marijuana, are usually problematic for patients with schizophrenia, exploiting their vulnerabilities, and thus increasing the symptoms of the illness. Yet, these drugs are often used in the social situations to which young people are likely to be exposed. The young adult patient is thus often faced with the dilemma of wanting to use alcohol or drugs to feel more a part of a social crowd while increasing the risk of becoming ill again, or refusing to use these substances and experiencing a sense of being even more of an outsider, a feeling that is already a problem. This issue was discussed in the following segment from a session with Barry and his family after Barry had been encouraged to get more socially involved with his peers.

FATHER: Well, he went out all right. Came home dead drunk at 5:00 A.M.

MOTHER: It would have been funny, except we remember what was discussed about alcohol at the workshop, and of course, he was depressed for days afterwards.

CLINICIAN: It's true that there are risks to drinking for people with schizophrenia. What happened, Barry?

BARRY: I went out with Ron, just like we agreed. Had a good time, too. What was I supposed to say, "I can't drink"? There's nothing else to do when you go to a bar, and that's where he wanted to go.

CLINICIAN: That is a dilemma that you'll run into. I certainly don't want you to be a wet blanket—especially since you're just starting to go out. I suppose you will feel the need to drink sometimes. I wonder if there can't be some kind of compromise?

MOTHER: You could go to the movies. . . .

BARRY: And *then* what? Anyway, I like to have a few beers.

FATHER: A few!

CLINICIAN: Is your mother right that you seemed to be affected by it for a few days?

BARRY: (*Pause*) I felt pretty bad this week. A few voices, you know. But I don't know that it was the beer.

CLINICIAN: Maybe it wasn't, but it's a risk. How about cutting down? I'd hate to take away drinking totally. But, to be honest, you have to watch how much you drink more than other people. That's a responsibility you have to yourself.

BARRY: How much can I drink?

CLINICIAN: I don't know for sure—everyone is different. I do know you'll pay a bigger price for overdoing it than others will. It will be your decision, though.

FATHER: I know when I go out, I have a couple of beers and then switch to soda. In my business, I can't afford to wake up with a hangover.

CLINICIAN: I do the exact same thing. How about it, Barry?

BARRY: I guess I can cut down, but I like to be one of the guys.

In this example, the clinician acknowledges the problem of total abstinence for a young man who is trying to reengage with peers who socialize around the activity of drinking. He emphasizes limiting drinking, but does so by underscoring Barry's responsibility to himself and then, along with the father, he suggests one appropriate way of coping with a situation that seems to require social drinking. Later, he will attempt to help Barry develop contacts that don't depend so heavily on the consumption of alcohol.

RATIONALE FOR VOCATIONAL REHABILITATION

Patients who have had schizophrenia for any length of time often have neither the ability to get a job nor the skills to maintain one. The difficulty of accomplishing the tasks of the vocational rehabilitation phase of treatment is magnified by the fact that many patients had their first acute episode in late adolescence before the development of marketable job skills. Thus, many patients, regardless of their current age, have never really worked or have done so only sporadically. Traditional models of vocational rehabilitation have not offered much help to these patients, having reported high rates of failure. In 1978, 287,000 mentally ill clients were seen by vocational rehabilitation services. Only 27% of these clients were actually "rehabilitated" (cited in Brinson, 1980). The long-term picture for these patients is even less optimistic. Follow-up studies suggest that one half to three fourths of "rehabilitated" patients are not functioning vocationally 2 years later (Schlamp & Raymond, 1971). In fact, intense rehabilitation services offered to patients shortly following hospital discharge actually have been shown to precipitate relapse (Goldberg et al., 1977).

Thus, even when patients reach a point where they desire to become involved in school, training, or work activities, there are significant risks associated with negotiating this step without precipitating relapse, and a significant chance that attempts to return to work will end in failure. The nature of work and the inevitable demands it places on any individual act as roadblocks to the vocational rehabilitation of patients with schizophrenia. Any kind of work requires certain skills and abilities that are problematic for schizophrenic patients. These skills include a reasonable attention span, the ability to attend to detail, the ability to understand and incorporate supervisory feedback, the presence of internal motivation, a tolerance of and adherence to routines, the ability to relate to co-workers, and so on. Thus, the issues that must be attended to in order to facilitate vocational rehabilitation go far beyond the development of technical skills. Before patients can become employable, it is necessary for them to gain some mastery in all these work related skills.

These factors make the vocational rehabilitation and employment phase difficult and fraught with potential pitfalls. Nevertheless, if the principles of the psychoeducational model can be applied in a flexible manner to the task of vocational functioning in the same way they have been applied to the areas of family and social functioning, it is possible to have greater success in helping patients move into some sort of employment without stimulating crisis or a relapse.

The Prework Phase: Building Skills for Later Survival

The area of vocational rehabilitation can best be approached after patients have been stable and in reasonable control of psychotic symptoms; have developed the ability to recognize their own early signs of illness; and have increased their participation and responsibility within the family. This point is often at least 10 to 12 months following an acute episode and/or discharge from a hospital. Even then, this topic is only broached by clinicians when patients have been carefully prepared for beginning in a work, school, or training program by discussions and tasks which address the skills they will need to survive in these environments. Before this point, however, it is common for either the patient, the family, or both to begin to push for the patient to get involved in work.

When this push occurs before it seems likely that the patient will be able to handle it, it becomes important to negotiate for more recuperative time by setting smaller goals that will increase the likelihood of success with the major step of starting work (see p. 146). For example, both Mary and her parents were pushing for Mary to get a job 3 months after she had been discharged from a psychiatric hospital where she had spent only 3 weeks, leaving only partially stabilized. Although it was evident to the clinician that she was not yet ready to handle work, both Mary and her family were insistent. The clinician suggested that since it would take a while for Mary to get a job, she should begin to prepare herself mentally and physically to handle the required workload and adherence to routines by getting up at a regular hour and increasing the number of chores she did around the house. Mary and her family agreed to these tasks which were defined in detail. The clinician suggested that whether or not Mary could do these small tasks would be a behavioral message about her readiness to do something as ambitious as working outside the home. At the next session, Mary's family, highly disappointed, reported that Mary had not followed through with the tasks. The following dialogue comes from that session.

CLINICIAN: I hear that everyone is upset.
MARY: (*Looks down in silence*)

FATHER: What's the use. If she couldn't handle the jobs around the house, she'll never be able to handle a job.

MOTHER: I had hopes—I guess it's another failure. You'd think I'd be used to it by now.

MARY: I just can't do anything. I'll never make it.

CLINICIAN: I hate to disagree with everyone, but I don't view this as a failure. All I think that happened is we all learned that Mary's not ready yet to get a job. That's important information. As we mentioned, it really was pretty early. Instead of everyone giving up hope, let's plan some smaller steps that will help in preparing her to get ready to go to work later. After all, work is a giant step.

FATHER: I can remember my first job. Even I was pretty uptight and I hadn't been in a hospital. I guess it is a pretty big step.

While it is usually better to avoid setting up tasks that have a high potential for failure, sometimes ambitious goals deserve a chance if only to help make everyone's expectations more realistic. When a failure occurs, even a small one, it is important to deal with the upset that results. In this case, the clinician defused both Mary's and the family's frustration by suggesting that, rather than failing, Mary was just letting everyone, including herself, know that she was not quite ready to go to work.

As stated, the first step toward work is the assumption of increased independent responsibility at home. Until that occurs, the ability of the patient to assume responsibility in a job or training setting is suspect. Although all tasks assigned relate in some ways to developing patient responsibility, later tasks can increasingly focus on cultivating the skills necessary for vocational readiness. Jobs around the home that involve such things as getting up on a regular schedule, managing an entire project (such as yard work) while limiting breaks, and spending increasing lengths of time on tasks, help to enhance the potential of a successful transition to work or training. The following example came from a session with Bill and his wife in which the discussion centered about the development of a prevocational routine.

CLINICIAN: It sounds like you've got mixed feelings about looking for work.

BILL: Well, I've got to get work. We need the money and I can't see living on Social Security income forever. But I don't know if I can handle it yet.

MILLY: (To clinician) I want you to know I'm not pushing Bill. We've been through so much, I'd hate for us to make a mistake now and have to start from the beginning.

CLINICIAN: I'm glad you feel that way because I'd really like to see us wait a little bit longer before Bill gets a job. Although things have been getting better for you both, I'm still concerned about you handling an 8 hour day.

BILL: Me, too.

CLINICIAN: I'd like to continue working on helping you get ready. I think sometimes we forget about what goes into doing a good job. I think we should focus on some of these things, like sticking to a task and getting up early each day. Even though these tasks may seem silly by themselves, getting into a routine before having to adjust to it *and* a new environment is really important.

BILL: Anything that will help me make a go of it.

CLINICIAN: Good. I know getting up early has been a problem for you. I'd like to see you get up at a regular time each morning, Monday through Friday. Say, 8 o'clock.

BILL: I could do it, but I always feel, "why bother?"

MILLY: There's plenty you can do to help me in the mornings.

BILL: But that doesn't have anything to do with the kind of work I want to do.

CLINICIAN: That's true, but it will help to get you used to doing more—just being on your feet out of bed and in the swing of things for 8 hours.

BILL: If you put it that way, fine.

In this example, the clinician focused on helping Bill to begin to develop a routine that hopefully would carry over into the development of good work habits. Later tasks must elaborate on building this routine. The clinician took care to frame the tasks as important steps toward making the overall plan a successful one to defuse the otherwise likely perception that these small steps and tasks are demeaning.

Patient resistance to beginning work or training is not unusual. At times, this resistance seems related to the patient's accurate sense of not being ready; and waiting longer dissipates the resistance. At other times, the resistance seems less functional and more intractable, and repeated suggestions related to work and training lead nowhere. At these times, families can help patients in the process of developing the motivation necessary to maintain work related behaviors. Often patients develop a comfortable, minimally stressful routine within their families and thus have no strong desire to move towards employment. Families can help by restructuring their rules so as to help push patients toward assuming greater responsibility. In the following example, taken from a session 15 months into treatment, Don's complacency is addressed.

CLINICIAN: I'm not sure what else to do. I can't take Don's hand and make him go to the training program. Yet, I believe he's ready.

FATHER: We know it, too. But, he shows no interest in it. Helen [patient's mother] and I are getting pretty upset.

CLINICIAN: Don?

DON: I already told you. I have an illness and can't work. Besides, why should I? Things are just fine at home.

CLINICIAN: First, your illness does *not* mean you can't work . . . I've said it a number of times. You may have to take it slower, but you certainly can handle the training program. Second—

DON: I *am* taking it slow.

CLINICIAN: Second, I think things are too comfortable at home. I know we've talked about creating a low-key environment, but I think this is going to have to change somewhat.

MOTHER: What do you mean?

CLINICIAN: Don is telling us that he has no incentive to work since all of his needs are being provided for free of charge. That was important when he first came out of the hospital, but now he is feeling and doing better and has to move toward becoming a more productive member of the family and the community.

FATHER: It sounds right. But, he's refusing.

CLINICIAN: Well, when adults live together, as in your family, each has to contribute either through taking on responsibilities or bringing in money. I think Don needs to pay for his keep one way or the other.

DON: I do chores.

CLINICIAN: I know, and that's good. But your responsibilities haven't grown as you've gotten better and that's not good. If you had to go to work or a training program in order to eat or pay for a room, I think you would. What I'd like to suggest is that we set a monetary value on Don's room and board. He can pay for these by doing more chores around the house or by spending a certain amount of time in the training program. If he doesn't want to, then the consequences would be having less to eat.

DON: I don't like this.

FATHER: I'm not totally sure I do either, but if it will help, I'd be willing to try it.

CLINICIAN: I admit it's not the ideal solution, but Don has to recognize that he has to assume more responsibility. This is how I think we should go about it.

The clinician then proceeded to establish, with the family's input, a program that required Don to work for 10 hours a week doing chores around the house, *or* in the training program, to pay for his room and board. Considerable time was spent discussing the specific details of what could constitute 10 hours of work. At the next session, 2 weeks later, Don grudgingly agreed to spend the 10 hours in the vocational training program since "anything would be better than doing chores around the house." After 2 weeks in the program, Don reluctantly admitted that he liked it. Although the solution was not ideal since it set up potential conflict between family members, it effectively helped in supplying the external motivation needed to move Don over the hurdle of complacency.

The Initial Work/School Phase

Getting Used to Routine

The decision that patients are ready to attempt the transition from informal tasks to actual work or training usually is made when everyone agrees the time is right. The exact nature of this next step is dependent upon what is available within the community. If there are no vocational rehabilitation services available, then it is important the clinician choose a time to try employment or schooling when other stresses are at an absolute minimum for patients. It is important that the step of beginning school or work be labeled as "only a trial." If the patient does not succeed, it only means that the timing was not right and more preparation is needed before attempting another similar move in the future. The stress of this step is so significant that it is important that patients be protected as much as possible from any concurrent stresses or strains. It should be recognized that *such* stresses can include not only negative events, but also any change, even positive ones, affecting anyone in the family and their subsequent availability to the patient.

Preparation for this step must include, in addition to prework tasks, a focus on potential stresses. One major stress that is often overlooked is the job interview. A job interview requires that patients present themselves in the best possible light since they are, in effect, selling themselves. Interview questions cover a number of areas but almost always focus on past work experiences and gaps of time in the potential employee's history. This immediately puts patients in the position of having to decide whether and what to say about their illness and hospitalizations. Thus, even before employment can begin, patients usually must face a highly stressful event that requires heightened social awareness and control over anxiety and symptomatology, as well as specific social skills. Needless to say, patients who are poorly prepared for this event are at a significant disadvantage. Such was the case in the next example, which came from the session following Ian's first job interview and subsequent rejection.

FATHER: I feel really bad. The job sounded just right for Ian and. . . .

CLINICIAN: I don't think we have to review the job right now. I agree that it's too bad, but I'd rather see if we can learn from Ian's first interview. Hopefully, that will make the next time go better.

IAN: I don't know if I want a next time.

CLINICIAN: All right. We can talk about that later, too. Right now, if it's okay with you, I'd like to talk about the job interview.

IAN: Well . . . I'm kind of embarrassed . . . I was nervous before I even went. But the guy seemed nice and I started to relax. Then he asked me why a guy who was 25 years old had never worked before. I was so upset, I couldn't think or talk. I just sat there and stared until he asked me to go. Even now, I don't know what I should have said.

MOTHER: Oh, my lord! That must have been terrible.

CLINICIAN: It certainly sounds like you had an uncomfortable experience. You bring up an important question though. What should you have said?

FATHER: I have the same question.

CLINICIAN: Unfortunately, I don't have a pat answer. Some people suggest being honest about your past and others think you should stretch the truth. So, part of the answer is up to you.

IAN: If I told him I had been in a mental ward, I would never have gotten the job anyway. I'd rather lie than tell anyone I was a weirdo.

MOTHER: I think I agree with Ian.

FATHER: I think outright lying can also lead to problems. But, I do believe that you can gloss over some of the rough spots. Like . . . let's see. . . . How about something like this: "For most of the time, I traveled around the country working odd jobs." There is some truth to that answer. You were out of the house traveling for a good part of the last couple of years.

IAN: Yeah, but I was pretty out of it.

FATHER: Well, that's what I meant by glossing over the rough spots.

CLINICIAN: What do you think about your father's idea? He *is* in business.

IAN: Hm . . . I like that, but I don't know if I could do it.

CLINICIAN: Well, how about if we practice a few times. I can pretend to be you and you can pretend to be the interviewer.

Over the next few sessions, the clinician and Ian role-played a number of possible scenarios, reversing the roles of Ian and the interviewer. A refresher role play was held immediately prior to Ian's next job interview. Although the clinician's support of the father's message to "gloss over the rough spots" was less than honest, it took into account the reality that some employers would not understand, accept, or hire a person who had experienced a mental illness.

As previously stated, patients and families often hold onto the hopes and plans for the future that they had before the onset of schizophrenia. Although ideals are sometimes helpful, these goals are often unrealistic and can become an impediment to the patient taking a job commensurate with their *current* skill level. They also interfere with the ability of families to support patients. This problem must be dealt with extensively in family sessions. The underlying therapeutic message should be that the first job the patients take is just the beginning step, not the final one. The first job is important for giving patients a positive sense of self, and for developing dependability, a tolerance for routines, as well as an increased attention span. Accepting a low-level job in no way negates the potential for obtaining a better job in the future. This message helps to buy time to accurately assess vocational potential and gives both patients and the families appropriate feedback. In the following case, Evan had his first "break" during his sophomore year of college when he was studying to be an electrical engineer. Both his father and his brothers were electrical engineers. Eight years following the first episode, during which time Evan had never been able to work or go to school for more than a few weeks, Evan's goal, and that of his family, remained the same—Evan should become an electrical engineer.

CLINICIAN: We've been over the same ground a number of times, but I think it's important to discuss again.

EVAN: There's no discussion. I want to go back to college full time.

FATHER: Evan still wants to be an engineer, and I think that's great. There's nothing wrong with that.

CLINICIAN: No . . . but Evan has returned to college three times. And each time, he had to drop out. Two times because things were so bad, he needed to be hospitalized.

EVAN: This time will be different.

CLINICIAN: I hope so, but I wonder if there isn't some way to lessen the risk.

MOTHER: You know, I've pleaded with them to change their minds. It's no use. When either my husband or my son get their minds made up. . . .

CLINICIAN: Well, I have a lot of concern. You know we believe in minimizing stress and taking one step at a time.

FATHER: We know, but what can we do. There *are* requirements and they're stressful. He can do it.

CLINICIAN: I understand that, for now. Evan is set on becoming an electrical engineer. So I won't argue with that. However, I still can't deny that the treatment team is concerned. We've talked about it quite a bit. What we'd like to discuss is starting part-time rather than full-time. It may take longer, but it is less stressful.

EVAN: No.

FATHER: Well, maybe just to start.

EVAN: *(To father)* You think so?

FATHER: If it would get you back to school. . . .

CLINICIAN: If everything went well, the number of courses could be increased after a few semesters.

In this example, the clinician was aware of the strong alignment between Evan and his father and the stubbornness of their stance despite a lot of evidence that this was a high-risk plan. Rather than entering a power struggle that would probably increase the firmness of their stance, he sought a compromise that would build in less stress and more control.

Dealing with Vocational Demands

Considering the basic principles of the program, the ideal job situation for a recovering schizophrenic patient would incorporate the following factors: First, in keeping with the concept that slow is better, it would be part-time to start. Second, the first day would occur midweek, rather than on Monday, to allow a weekend of recuperation after the first few days on the job (since new situations are most stressful). Third, it would be neither completely isolated nor intensely social, but rather would provide a low level of involvement with coworkers. Fourth, it would involve fairly close supervision from a supportive superior. Fifth, it would be moderately interesting work but not so challenging as to create stress due to complexity. The ideal would be for the patient to concentrate on developing a tolerance for routines, and only then move on to the development of specific occupational goals. Of course, jobs which meet all of these requirements are difficult, if not impossible to find. However, offering these guidelines to patients and families helps them in evaluating the appropriateness of potential jobs, as well as helping them to establish more realistic expectations.

When patients are able to begin work, it is important that neither clinician nor family overemphasize its importance or status, since patients usually are already aware of the meaning attached to reentering the work force in a relatively low-level job. If too much is made of it, they can become more uncomfortable and discouraged. The following example came from a session where Peter reported that he had just gotten, at the age of 28, his first job ever.

PETER: It's nothing much, just working at a gas station.
MOTHER: What do you mean nothing much. It's *great*. We're so proud of you.
PETER: (*Looking down*) Thanks.
FATHER: Yes, it's really terrific.
CLINICIAN: Well, I think it's good. I can understand that it's not your ideal job, Peter, and therefore not "great," but it is a first step.
FATHER: We're proud because Peter did it on his own.
CLINICIAN: Right. Tell me about what you'll be doing.
PETER: The usual. Pumping gas. Doing some oil and tire changing.
CLINICIAN: What hours will you be working?
PETER: Well, I remembered what you said about needing a regular routine. The owner said I can work a steady 3:00 to 11:00 shift. That lets me sleep in and it's not too busy at that time of day. He seems like a nice guy.

The clinician asked Peter more about the specifics of the job, such as who his co-workers would be, how often he could take breaks, and so on. The session concluded:

CLINICIAN: I'm glad you remembered all of our talks. It sounds like a good job. Not perfect, but that's life. We've been meeting monthly, but I'd like to see you folks a little more often as work begins. Just to make sure everyone is feeling good. When do you start?
PETER: Next Thursday.
CLINICIAN: At the end of the week? Good. How about an appointment early the following week?

During the session, the clinician attempted to praise Peter for taking the first step on his own initiative while giving a message to the parents to be realistic in their praise. After checking out the details about the job, the clinician again stated the need to accept the job's advantages and limitations. Finally, he reiterated the fact that starting any job would have some stress and suggested a plan that Peter and his family check in more frequently during this time of adjustment. In fact, to prevent a rapid escalation of stress and the possible emergence of psychotic symptoms in response to the demands of employment, increasing the frequency of therapeutic contacts is usually advisable during the transition to work or training. This can include either in-person contacts, over-the-phone contacts, or both. Monitoring the patient's progress during this time is important in avoiding or minimizing potential problems before they get out of hand. The patient and family must be instructed to call at any time a problem arises or something unusual is noted. In addition, support for the patient must be built in from as many sources as possible. As a part of this effort, family members can be helped to temporarily decrease their demands on the patient in all other areas of functioning during the first few months the patient is in a new work environment (see example on p. 172).

The following example came from an emergency session asked for by Jeff's father. Jeff had been working at an assembly line job for 7 weeks. It was his first work experience in 3 years.

FATHER: I don't know. The first month was great. Jeff was excited and enthusiastic. But these last few weeks, he just seems to have lost his spark. We're concerned. He's staying by himself more and that's what he used to do. We're afraid he's slipping back.

JEFF: I'm not getting sick.

FATHER: I didn't mean . . . well, I guess I did, but. . . .

CLINICIAN: Okay, before we speculate, maybe you [Jeff] can help us understand what's going on. Is your father's description accurate, Jeff?

JEFF: No . . . Yes . . . I don't know. I guess some of it. I mean, like, when I first started at the plant, I was really excited. Everything was new and interesting! Now, it's getting kind of boring.

CLINICIAN: Hm . . . I can understand that. What about the withdrawing.

JEFF: I'm tired when I come home and just need some time to relax. But if I do that, my folks start hanging all over me worrying that I'm slipping. That just makes me want to get away even more.

MOTHER: We didn't know that. I'm sorry. . . .

FATHER: How come you didn't tell us?

JEFF: I never really thought about it until now.

CLINICIAN: Well, thank you for sharing. You know, in listening to you talk, I couldn't help thinking "boy, that sounds like the way I've felt with different jobs."

JEFF: Yeah?

CLINICIAN: Yeah. You were all excited at the beginning and then the routine sets in and it gets kind of humdrum. Then you do your job more for the money, than anything. I'd bet your dad has felt that way, too.

FATHER: Oh, yeah.

JEFF: That's exactly it. I don't really want to quit, but only because I like the money, and . . . I guess I like just having a job.

The next 10 minutes of the session were spent normalizing Jeff's feelings, with the father talking about a similar job he once had. Then:

CLINICIAN: Now that everyone seems to agree that Jeff is having a pretty normal reaction and plans to ride it out, I wonder if we can relax things at home during the evening.

JEFF: I just want some unwinding time.

MOTHER: But, we're interested in your day, and. . . .

FATHER: (*Smiling*) How about if we give you some time to unwind and then you spend just a little time sharing about your day with us.

JEFF: I guess that's fine with me, if you back off. . . .

CLINICIAN: I couldn't have done better. I wish all my problems had such an easy solution.

Monitoring progress without the family, the patient, *or* the clinician becoming overresponsive to every nuance, or feeling the need to take an hourly "pulse" is difficult. The need for patience becomes a theme about which everyone needs frequent reminders. Sometimes, the passage of time is the greatest aid in building skills, decreasing vulnerabilities and convincing everyone that there may be a chance for a more normal lifestyle some day.

School

A number of schizophrenic patients have their first break while away at school. Thus, it makes sense that after a recuperation period, some patients would want to return to school. Being away at school, however, involves coping with a number of tasks simultaneously, that is, the need to live away from home (in a relatively independent fashion) carry academic courses, and negotiate a range of new social relationships. There is a significant risk of the return to school precipitating a relapse, and, therefore, it is important to discuss alternatives with the patient and the family to insure that whatever decision is made is a good one.

For instance, going to a local community college on a part-time basis can be a way for the patients to "get their feet wet" again before returning to a more demanding program. In a local program, all concerned can monitor the patient's progress closely. If the patient does poorly, then the feasibility of going back to school at this time can be reviewed. If the patient does well, then another step can be negotiated, such as increasing the number of courses taken while remaining home, adding more social activities, or returning to a school away from home.

The following example comes from a session with Iris and her family after she had completed her second semester at a local community college.

IRIS: I got a 3.4 G.P.A.
CLINICIAN: Great! You should feel very proud.
IRIS: Do I ever. Especially, after last semester's 2.4.
CLINICIAN: Well, I think last semester involved a lot of adjusting. This time seems a better statement of your ability.
IRIS: Thanks. You know, before I went to the community college, I wanted to go back to Penn State right away. Looking back, I'm glad I waited.
MOTHER: We are, too.
CLINICIAN: That makes it unanimous.
IRIS: I still want to go back. But now I feel more ready.
CLINICIAN: Hm . . . well, I think we should talk about that a bit. Let's discuss the pros and cons. What are the advantages?

The rest of that session and the next two sessions were spent discussing in detail the positives and negatives associated with the decision of going away to school as opposed to staying at the community college. In the end, it was decided that Iris should be allowed to return to school away from home the following fall.

CLINICIAN: I get the feeling that we have looked in every nook and cranny for potential difficulties.
IRIS: *That's* for sure.
MOTHER: I really feel hopeful that Iris can handle it.
FATHER: Me, too. She knows her early warning signs and getting permission to start with a reduced load will help.
IRIS: I feel really excited, and I'm glad you'll continue to see my parents while I'm away.
CLINICIAN: My pleasure. And don't forget your calls to me, at least for the first few months.
IRIS: Once a week, like clockwork.

Vocational Rehabilitation Programs

The availability of a vocational rehabilitation agency offers many benefits to the process of integrating someone with schizophrenia into the work force, but the use of such programs also has certain risks. As was mentioned earlier in this chapter, traditional rehabilitation approaches are often too stimulating, complex, and demanding for the schizophrenic patient to negotiate successfully. Since the requirements of most of these programs are based on experience with the rehabilitation of the physically disabled patient, they sometimes do not take into account the particular cognitive problems and attention deficits of the patient with schizophrenia. In fact, many vocational programs operate using a treatment philosophy that differs radically from the one described in this manual, assuming that clients should have an intrinsic motivation to work and are simply in need of new job-related skills.

This conflict of assumptions and differing views of problems can lead to inconsistencies between psychiatric and rehabilitation systems that should be avoided. The following conversation came from a family session after Larry had dropped out of a vocational program which was to have prepared him to be a carpenter.

CLINICIAN: I can see that you're upset. What happened?
LARRY: (*Slowly*) I didn't know what to do. There were so many people and I couldn't understand.
CLINICIAN: Understand what?
LARRY: Anything. What to do. Anything.
CLINICIAN: Did you ask anybody?
LARRY: No . . . I thought that if I did, they'd think I was stupid and throw me out. I sort of just sat there and hoped they wouldn't say anything to me.

Larry was hesitant to try again. In this case, the problem might have been avoided if Larry had been given a more individualized orientation, and if someone had been available to talk with him daily as he began the program. Another patient did not even get that far. Janet had an initial meeting set up with a vocational counselor in a large office building. She wrote down the room number incorrectly and went to the wrong place. She sat in a hallway waiting room for 7 hours until a janitor noticed her and sent her home. She refused to set up another appointment for almost 6 months.

Because of the likelihood of problems such as these, it is imperative that there be communication between vocational and mental health treatment teams before the patient begins a vocational program and throughout his or her participation in it. Problems are created for patients when they get conflicting messages from two different professionals. It is the task of the mental health clinician to let the vocational counselor know about patients' deficits, problems, and limitations, as well as their strengths. Conversely, it is the task of the vocational counselor to give the clinician ongoing feedback about patient progress, limitations, and vocational abilities. In particular, each must let the other know about changes or increases in demands on patients in either of their respective areas since it is crucial that only one change be introduced at any one time. The following conversation came from a discussion between two members of the treatment team (the family clinician, Paul, and the nurse clinician, Sue), and Carolyn's vocational counselor, Sam. Carolyn had been in the rehabilitation program for 2 weeks and was talking about dropping out.

SAM: I know she's not doing well, but she won't tell me what's wrong.

SUE: I saw Carolyn yesterday and she was upset. She didn't understand why she had to change evaluation areas. She liked the clerical work she was doing and then someone came up to her and said she had to go work in the kitchen.

PAUL: She told me the same thing. Also, she said that someone else had mentioned that her hair was greasy and she'd have to take better care of it to work in the kitchen. That was embarrassing for her.

SAM: Hm . . . I didn't know she was upset by the change. It was a normal one. It's our policy to have a person complete a number of evaluation areas to get a better sense of their abilities.

PAUL: That makes sense. But, I'm wondering if it wouldn't be possible to slow that process down a bit. With Carolyn, it's important to recognize that any change creates a lot of stress. That's pretty common for people with schizophrenia.

SUE: And she has been excited about work for the first time in years. I'd hate to see it fall apart now.

SAM: Me, too. For the first 2 weeks, she did pretty well. What do you suggest?

PAUL: If it's possible, I'd like to see Carolyn remain in the clerical area for a while longer. I think it's helping to build up her confidence and get her into the routine of coming to the center without too much anxiety. Later, we can focus more on assessing her job skills.

SAM: I think I can arrange that.

SUE: Great. I think we should also back off on her personal appearance for a while. As she feels better, I think that her hygiene will improve.

PAUL: I'm not so sure it will improve by itself, but I agree we should focus on one thing at a time. The basic routine should come first.

SAM: No problem.

The establishment of a collaborative relationship between the professionals in these two settings allowed Carolyn's program to be structured in a way which enhanced the likelihood that she could succeed. Without this collaboration, it would have been likely that vocational rehabilitation would have failed. It is easy to underestimate the energy schizophrenic patients must expend at the beginning of a vocational program simply to survive. It is, therefore, easy to give insufficient attention to their increased vulnerability to stimulation and stress. Thus, it is important that patients be able to enter vocational programs at levels commensurate with their present level of functioning and also ones at which they can experience success. It is better to start at vocational levels which might be too low than to overstress patients at these times.

Fred, age 27, had been ill since high school and thus had never worked or participated in any type of training program. After he had been stable for over a year, he was moved into a vocational training program. The following conversation comes from a session held the evening after Fred's first half-day (3½ hours) at the center.

MOTHER: How did it go? We're really anxious to hear.

FRED: Okay.

FATHER: Is that all you're going to say? Okay?

FRED: I took apart a lawn mower engine.

MOTHER: Oh, you like that kind of stuff. (*To therapist*) He's very mechanical.

FRED: I guess so.

FATHER: You don't seem excited.

FRED: I'm real tired.

FATHER: I guess you'll want to sleep a lot this weekend?

FRED: Oh yeah.

MOTHER: Do you want to go back?

FRED: I guess. It wasn't as bad as I thought. I'm glad it's the weekend, though.

CLINICIAN: I'm glad to hear that. I'd also like to know, though, if there was anything that bothered you about the program. I might be able to do something about it if there is.

FRED: (*Hesitantly*) No, nothing about the *program*.

CLINICIAN: Something else then?

FRED: I got lost getting there.

A discussion followed which centered on buses and maps and the cost–benefit ratio of someone driving Fred to the program. After this discussion, Fred decided he would prefer to try to make it on his own, and that he could do so after getting a bus schedule and a map.

With regard to the program itself, it is significant to note that Fred had started in a vocational program where the initial steps were co-operatively planned out by the mental health treatment team and the vocational staff. He was intentionally started at two half-days per week, with his first day being at the end of a week so that he could use the weekend to recover from the stress of his first day. The first training task chosen was based on knowledge of his interests and abilities.

Such a collaborative program is unusual. Nevertheless, there are a number of things that can be done within any vocational program that would enhance the chances of patients gaining the skills necessary to employment. Some of these things relate to issues already discussed, such as the establishment, with patient and family input, of realistic and achievable short-term and long-term goals. Both types of goals are important. They should take into consideration past, present, and potential levels of work functioning. For various reasons, some patients have difficulty in maintaining a focus on goals that are distant and soon lose interest and motivation without some sort of immediate reward. Thus, basic long-term goals should be broken down into multiple short-term ones that enable patients to get more immediate reinforcement as well as allow the counselors to reassess progress frequently. As in other situations, progress usually should be measured along the patient's own "internal yardstick." The following example came from a family session in which Gloria and her husband, John, were discussing her vocational aspirations. Since Gloria had been in a vocational rehabilitation program for 3 months, her vocational counselor, Dave, was asked to join the session.

DAVE: I've got to say that we've been very pleased with how you've been doing with us. I've gotten nothing but positive feedback.

GLORIA: Thank you. I've liked being there so far, but I'm not sure it's leading me toward my goal of being a doctor.

JOHN: Come on. We've been through that before. You haven't even gone to college. How are you ever going to be a doctor?

GLORIA: (*Stubbornly*) I can.

CLINICIAN: I know you're insistent on that as your goal, and you know that I'm not sure it's realistic either. . . .

GLORIA: (*Sulking*) I know.

CLINICIAN: Dave and I have talked about your goal a lot and he's come up with a suggestion that he wanted to discuss with us.

GLORIA: What's that?

DAVE: Well, there are two things. The first is that there are a number of career opportunities in the medical field: licensed practical nurse, radiology technician, and so on. So, perhaps, you can think about some of those as options. Secondly, since you haven't had any experience in this area, we thought that you may want to work in our health clinic with the nurse 1 or 2 hours a week.

GLORIA: Could I?

DAVE: Yes, I've already spoken to her. This would be in addition to your regular assignment. At the same time, I'd like to meet with you to discuss some other career options in the medical field.

GLORIA: I'd like that a lot.

In this example, alternative options are offered to Gloria. The unrealistic nature of her desire to be a doctor is not confronted directly since this had led to unproductive conflict in the past. At the same time, the staff of her vocational program demonstrated enough flexibility to allow her the experience of working with the nurse, and the hope of eventually getting involved in a medical setting in some way.

The development of a program that is flexible, individualized, and considerate of the tolerance levels of patients is crucial. It is important to note that flexibility must allow for movement backwards as well as forwards, dependent upon the patient's response to personal, environmental, and program changes. While attempts should be made to avoid exposing patients to failure, problems with certain tasks are inevitable. Difficulty with or failure to accomplish a task should not lead to termination from the vocational program. Rather, it should be viewed as an indication that the pace of the program was too rapid or the task too complex. The program's response to failures should be to help patients to restabilize at a level at which they were previously functional, and then to attempt to progress again with even smaller incremental steps. The following example came from an emergency session that was scheduled after a phone call from Donald's mother saying that Donald had come home from his training program highly upset and distraught.

DONALD: (Crying) I can't do it. I'm no good.

CLINICIAN: I understand you're upset, Donald, but I need to understand better what happened.

DONALD: It was too much.

CLINICIAN: What was too much, Donald?

DONALD: Today. I worked a full day for the first time.

CLINICIAN: What happened?

DONALD: By lunch time, I was tired and by the end of the day, I was hearing voices.

MOTHER: Oh, no!

CLINICIAN: Okay. It's good that you're telling us this. I'd like you to catch your breath for a minute. I'm sorry you got upset today. I think it was our fault for setting too fast a pace. For right now, you seem to work your best on a half-day schedule. That's important information to have. It isn't all so bad, you know. I've heard good things about your work speed and ability.

DONALD: Yeah?

CLINICIAN: That's right. You know, I think we should go back to your old schedule for right now since you were doing so well at it. Later on, we can discuss a possible increase in time.

DONALD: I'd like that.

Once the situation was clarified, the clinician took responsibility for the difficulty Donald was having with his new work hours. He labeled it as a nonproblem, and then gave Donald positive feedback about his work performance. Finally, he suggested reinstituting the old schedule, holding out the possibility of another move forward in the future.

The need for external structure to eliminate unnecessary confusion and stress is as important in training and work situations as it is at home and in treatment. A structured environment can best be achieved by providing each patient with one vocational counselor who plays a supervisory role. This person can monitor the progress of the patient, and act as a resource to both patient and staff of the training site. Having a specific person available to patients helps to avert potential crises and helps patients to deal with "on the job" conflicts or problems that otherwise could easily have led to patients dropping out of programs. Patients often lack appropriate assertiveness skills that would allow them to address coworker and supervisor conflicts comfortably. Having someone who acts as a mediator helps to tone down conflict while providing a model of someone who engages in successful problem-solving behaviors. Finally, such a person can act as a liaison to the mental health treatment facility. This allows for successful and rapid communication in the establishment of treatment strategies and the avoidance of potential pitfalls.

A FEW COMMON PROBLEMS IN VOCATIONAL REHABILITATION

Patients' Perception of Themselves as Failures

One of the more difficult aspects of training and job searching is walking the fine line between finding something that is interesting to patients but not so complex as to exacerbate their problems and deficits. In other words, job tasks should be challenging but not overwhelming or threatening. Most patients have little self-confidence. If they every had it, they have lost it over the years of illness. Failure at a task is easily interpreted by patients (as well as by the families and often by professionals) as yet another indication of a fundamental lack of worth and brings up the inevitable: "Why try?" Trying, in fact, becomes equated with failure. The following example came from a session with Alan and his wife, Mary. Alan had just been fired from his job as a shoe salesman (one he had gotten himself) for sleeping in the stockroom.

ALAN: Go ahead and say it!

CLINICIAN: What?

ALAN: You know! I told you so! I'm a failure. I can't do anything right.

CLINICIAN: That was the furthest thing from my mind. To be honest with you, I was thinking that it's too bad you feel so lousy since hanging in there as long as you did took a lot of courage.

ALAN: That's crap. All I do is screw up.

CLINICIAN: It's not crap. Look, you've been feeling lousy a long time and yet you got a job on your own and stuck with it for 3 months. In addition, you've still had time for your wife and kids. All I think that happened, is that it was a little of "too much, too soon."

ALAN: I *was* exhausted all the time.

MARY: All he wanted to do was sleep.

CLINICIAN: I'm not surprised. It must have been draining. Well, I certainly haven't given up. I hope you haven't either. Let's talk about the job and what the problems were so we can learn from it. Then we can discuss what our next step should be.

ALAN: I think it was the sales part—talking to all those people. . . .

Alan's failure at the job was framed as a good effort under difficult circumstances. The clinician refused to accept Alan's sense of futility and immediately focused on replacing the sense of failure with a sense of hope, and returning everyone's energies to the task of planning the next step.

Poor Conflict Resolution Skills

Social or vocational rehabilitation programs offer the opportunity to pay attention to other related problem areas that will impede the development of social and work competencies. Issues such as dependability, getting along with co-workers and supervisors, developing an increased attention span and the ability to accept appropriate criticism can all be addressed directly, and indirectly. Cliff's difficulties in accepting criticism were causing him problems in his work situation. He was working for a printing company and quickly began to complain about his supervisor. At the family session, he expressed his fear that he was in danger of getting fired, and his anger at the person he thought would fire him.

CLIFF: I don't care. He doesn't know what he's talking about. I'm doing my job just fine and he's nitpicking.

FATHER: He's your boss.

CLIFF: That don't make him right!

CLINICIAN: That's true. But, we have a problem. You said that you may lose your job if this continues which means we have to come up with some way of handling the problem.

CLIFF: It's a good job, but he's got to get off my back.

MOTHER: He won't find another job as good as this one.

CLINICIAN: Whoa! Let's not give up on this one yet. Cliff, I can't tell your supervisor what to do so the burden is on your shoulders as an adult.

CLIFF: Like what can I do?

CLINICIAN: Well, the fact is he *can* fire you. So, on the one hand, you have to listen to him.

CLIFF: Only if he's right.

CLINICIAN: No, as your boss, you have to listen even if he's not. However, you can also discuss your ideas with him.

CLIFF: I told him. . . .

CLINICIAN: Discuss, not tell. Look, why don't you try this for one week. Do what he tells you to do. If you still disagree with him after that time, maybe you can discuss your ideas with him. Try it for one week and then let's talk about it again in a family session. In fact, maybe we can role-play right now how to handle it. I'll be you and you be your supervisor.

After role-playing a number of possible interactions, Cliff agreed to try going along with his boss for a week. Although there was one small confrontation, he received a lot of positive feedback from his supervisor about his new attitude. He was not fired, and over time he formed better relationships with his supervisor and co-workers. He never admitted that his supervisor was right, but learned to play "by the rules."

Poor Personal Hygiene

Issues that have reached an impasse in family sessions can sometimes be dealt with effectively in the rehabilitation setting. Personal hygiene is a common problem for many patients and a common conflict in many families. For example, Christine took very poor care of herself, coming to sessions looking unkempt and dirty. Neither her family's nagging nor the tasks assigned by the clinician resulted in much improvement in her grooming habits. The clinician and vocational counselor discussed the matter and decided that her appearance was not only unappealing, but that it would be a significant problem in future employment and thus could be addressed legitimately in the training setting. It was decided to label "better hygiene" as a requirement for training and employment. Christine, who really wanted to be self-supporting, was therefore given a more concrete reason for better grooming. She responded positively almost immediately and began to take better care of herself.

Similarly, Henry had been ill for a number of years during which time his personal hygiene had deteriorated badly. He seemed to regard his control over this issue as crucial, and refused all attempts on the part of his family or his clinicians to get him to take better care of himself. In fact, the issue had become such a power struggle between Henry and his mother that the clinician had suggested and enforced the idea of "shelving" the problem until other issues had been dealt with successfully. Months later, the following discussion occurred shortly after he entered a vocational training program and spontaneously began washing his face.

CLINICIAN: What has made you decide to start washing your face?

HENRY: Well, I had these blackheads on my nose for about 10 years, so. . . .

CLINICIAN: And they're going away?

HENRY: . . . maybe 11 or 12 years. No, they won't go away. It will be a long time before they go away.

CLINICIAN: But what I am hearing is that you are beginning to take a little more interest in your appearance?

HENRY: Yeah.

CLINICIAN: And the message to your mother is that it will happen, but give it time?

HENRY: I don't know if it will happen.

FATHER: Don't make any promises. (*Smiling*)

CLINICIAN: Yeah. (*To parents*) Well, as I said, since we have talked about this for 2 years and I have not had any more success than you have had, I don't know whether it's worth getting into it again. I think we may as well let Henry decide. . . .

MOTHER: Oh, I really am pleased that you are washing your face. I noticed that your face seemed clean, but I thought—it never entered my mind you were washing it. I thought just that you weren't getting it dirty. (*Laughs*)

CLINICIAN: (*To Henry*) Our agreement last time was that if somebody says something to you at work, if your supervisor deals with it, that you would take that as an important message.

HENRY: Yes, I notice him coming around, sniffing me.

CLINICIAN: (*Laughing*) Yeah. Take that as a subtle hint. The time is coming.

HENRY: They don't say anything. They sort of stand there. (*Laughs*)

CLINICIAN: Probably paralyzes the vocal cords. (*All laugh*)

When Henry's vocational counselor did mention the issue of hygiene, Henry immediately began to shower, shave, and change his clothes more regularly. A major problem for Henry and his family was thus resolved without further direct efforts in family sessions.

SUMMARY

The areas of social and vocational rehabilitation are difficult ones to negotiate for the patient with schizophrenia. In the past, patients often remained isolated and dysfunctional, less as a result of the acute symptoms of their illness than as a result of the lack of skills necessary to negotiate the complexities of maintaining a social and vocational life.

Today, with patience and a carefully laid out step-by-step approach, reintegration into both milieus can be achieved for many patients. If the principles of temporarily lowered expectations, the provision of a relatively low-stimulation environment, making only one change at a time, and keeping goals small, can be applied in a flexible manner to the tasks of vocational and social functioning as they are applied in the area of family functioning, some success is possible. Although not easy, families and available community resources can be used to help patients achieve goals commensurate with their capabilities and learn new skills that will enhance their quality of life.

CHAPTER SIX

THE FINAL STAGES OF TREATMENT

Sometimes what I went through seems like a dream. I look back, and I'm amazed that I could have spent so much time in bed doing nothing.—Patient, 2½ years after hospitalization

Although the length of time needed varies dramatically, many patients do achieve the primary goals of psychoeducational treatment: a relatively stable psychological state and a level of social and work functioning commensurate with their basic abilities. However, patients achieve significantly varied levels of adjustment dependent upon the severity of the illness and its aftereffects, the stresses they experience, and the abilities and resources available to them. Some patients do so well that it is difficult to believe that they have had a mental illness. By this point in treatment, they have social and family relationships that are spontaneous and effective, and are able to work or engage in vocational training near the limit of their capacities. Their family members are appropriately involved with them, but not to the exclusion of active social lives of their own. In other words, no major illness-related problems interfere with the lives of the patient or family members as they wish to live them. Most patients, however, do not recover so fully. Entering this stage of treatment, some patients remain behind their peers in accomplishing the usual developmental tasks of young adulthood. Despite months or years of symptom free functioning, they are unable to form or maintain good social relationships or to emancipate from their families of origin. Still other patients at this stage are not particularly well, but are functioning better than they have in the past. They do not cause major turmoil in their families, and some are able to meet the requirements of relatively undemanding employment.

   While patients who do not attain at least a low level of stable functioning should be continued in treatment using the methods described in earlier chapters, there comes a time when the treatment contract should be renegotiated or terminated for all those patients who have shown signs of progress in accomplishing the goals of treatment, and who have maintained gains for an extended period of time. In other words, decisions must be made about the relevance and focus of continued treatment.

When the need to focus directly on the crisis of the illness has diminished, many patients and families become increasingly aware of other problems in their relationships with one another. Many of these issues are not directly related to the illness or the initial treatment contract. Family conflicts, marital problems between the parents of patients, or, if patients are married, marital and sexual issues of patients and their spouses may become more obvious and distressing.

This is not to say that clinicians have a right to assume they can work on these problems or that family members will want to do so. If these issues do not relate to the accomplishment of the goals of the initial contract, the contract must be renegotiated before any of these topics can be addressed. At this point, the clinician, patient, and family are faced with four choices: (1) Treatment sessions can continue to focus on goals related to the original contract, (2) treatment sessions can move to a focus on the more traditional topics of family or marital psychotherapy using more traditional methods, (3) treatment sessions can become less frequent and focus on maintaining the present level of functioning, preventing the development of other crises, and giving an ongoing sense of "lifeline," or (4) treatment can be terminated.

RENEGOTIATING THE CONTRACT

As in the establishment of the original treatment agreement, contract renegotiation must involve input from patient, family members, and clinician. When it is necessary to renegotiate and implement a new contract, however, it is important to avoid sudden major shifts in therapeutic style or strategy, so as not to upset hard won stability. As stated previously, change is usually stressful, including change within the therapeutic environment. In other words, no matter what additional goals are established, the achievement and maintenance of original goals remain an underlying concern.

Occasionally, in discussing contract renegotiation, family members, patient, and clinician may disagree about future treatment goals or even about the need for continuing treatment. In general, when conflict occurs over unattained goals which clinicians believe are crucial to patient survival, it is appropriate and ethical that clinicians do all they can to convince patients and families that continued treatment is in everyone's best interest. This is particularly true when the issue of termination is raised by patients who have had a history of rapid decompensation. In such cases, it is important for both patient and family to maintain a connection with the therapeutic system to allow for rapid intervention should the need arise.

When conflict occurs over treatment recommendations that involve desirable but not essential changes, clinicians should be prepared to accede to the wishes of patients and families. For example, if there is marital conflict between the parents of a stable patient, the parents' must be allowed to decide whether or not they wish to deal with their own problems through therapy. This might even be true when the marital problems are between the patient and his or her spouse. In the following example, a patient, Phil, and his wife had no interest in working on their marital issues and, in fact, were contemplating termination.

CLINICIAN: Last time we discussed a few issues that still concern the two of you and I thought today we might discuss how best to approach them.

PHIL: Yeah, well, Pam and I talked more about it. (*Pause*) You know, we're really thankful for your help. I remember what I was like when we first me—a mess. But I . . . we have come a long way. I'm working, and Pam and I are doing a lot better. I'm even helping out with the kids, and I never used to do that.

PAM: That's right, now he does help.

CLINICIAN: I remember too, and you're right. You folks have come a long way and it's taken a lot of effort on your part. . . .

PAM: And yours.

CLINICIAN: Thanks, but you're the ones who have done the work. Now—

PHIL: Excuse me, but as I've said, we've talked about it and we've decided not to work on the things we talked about last time. In fact, we want to talk more about maybe not coming anymore.

CLINICIAN: I see. We talked about that last time also, and I thought . . . I've got to say again that I'm really uncomfortable with you terminating. I'd prefer—

PHIL: You used a good word, "uncomfortable." Well, we're really uncomfortable coming here—more and more. I mean, I know I had to, but I'm not that way now. Nothing personal, but coming here is a downer. And, I'm doing well.

CLINICIAN: Yes, you are, and I can understand your feelings about coming here. I also know things are a lot better at home. But I still think it's important that we continue to meet. Look, I hate to bring back bad memories, but before your last hospitalization, you also thought things were going better.

PHIL: Yeah, but this time I've been okay for over 2 years.

PAM: He really is doing well, and he deserves a chance to try it his way. I know that last time we talked about the problems we're still having, but—things aren't perfect—but they are a lot better.

CLINICIAN: I know. You know, if you come in we don't have to focus on your relationship. But, your symptoms come on pretty fast, and I believe both of you would be better off being connected, even loosely, with the system. If you had diabetes, and were doing well, you'd still come in for regular checkups.

PHIL: Well . . . that's true. But, this place. . . .

CLINICIAN: I'll tell you what. How about if we negotiated a compromise. The two of you come in, say, every 3 months for a session and medication check. In between, at least for now, I'll call once a month to see how things are. That way you only have to come in four times a year, and as time goes on we can knock that down even more.

PHIL: That sounds a lot better.

In this example, the clinician, who had hoped to work with this couple on their marital issues, found it necessary to modify her expectations based on their wishes. Nevertheless, she did attempt to convince Phil and his wife to stay in treatment, in part because of Phil's past history of rapid decompensation and loss of insight as he became ill. Although she was not able to negotiate a contract of monthly sessions as she originally preferred, she was able to gain their agreement to have phone contact and periodic "checkups." She went along with this compromise because she believed some contact would be better than none, and she did not want to risk alienating the couple. Renegotiation of contracts at this stage often requires that clinicians make compromises.

Continuing to Focus on Original Goals

As we discussed in previous chapters, it is advisable to establish an arbitrary time limit for the initial treatment contract because patients, family members, and clinicians themselves often need some sort of yardstick against which to assess progress towards goals. However, patients and families often do not respond to treatment within these time frames. Some people achieve their goals faster than anticipated, while others move toward their goals at an almost imperceptible pace. When goals and goal attainment are out of sync, renegotiation of the treatment contract can be used to help families and patients to alter their expectations about the time it will take to achieve goals, or to begin to alter the goals themselves.

It is important for clinicians to be able to differentiate between those patients who need more time to attain their goals and those patients for whom the original goals were unrealistic. In the latter case, the process of contract renegotiation should first deal with the inevitable frustration that occurs when goals have not been attained. Second, they should help the patient and family to accept the patient's limitations, and finally, to establish more achievable goals.

In the following example, after the clinician attempts to deal with everyone's frustration about Susan's lack of progress toward the originally contracted goals, he then attempts to negotiate less demanding goals for Susan and her family.

SUSAN: I don't think I'll ever be able to get a job.

CLINICIAN: I know you're frustrated. It's hard to take when things don't go according to plan. I do think I'm responsible for some of your frustration since I helped you to establish these goals.

SUSAN: Yeah, well I don't want a job anyway.

FATHER: We don't blame you, but we've been coming to you for almost 2 years, and nothing has changed. . . .

CLINICIAN: Well, that's not quite true. Susan is feeling better and is helping out a lot more around the house. I *do* agree that in terms of our social and vocational goals, not much has happened, and Susan still doesn't have much initiative.

MOTHER: So, now what?

CLINICIAN: I've been talking a lot with the treatment team about that. We believe that we have to accept the messages that Susan is giving us that she's not ready for vocational training or unstructured social interaction right now.

FATHER: What's left?

CLINICIAN: That's what I'd like to talk about. I think at this time we have to alter our goals slightly. I'm not sure this will always be true, but for now, I think that's the reality. However, I still think Susan can be more active than she is now, and enhance her quality of life.

MOTHER: We'd all like to see that. Isn't that true, Susan?

SUSAN: (*Blandly*) I'm okay, now.

CLINICIAN: I'm glad to hear that, and I don't want to do anything to make you unhappy. What I'd like to suggest is that we establish, as a new goal, helping you to get more active outside the house, but that we not worry right now about your vocational skills.

FATHER: (*Skeptically*) What good would that do?

CLINICIAN: We believe that being more active will help to develop Susan's social skills. It's a start toward being able to handle people better—at work *or* play. In particular, there's a place downtown that has a very structured program for patients. It has an activity focus. They go on day trips, prepare and eat lunches together, things like that.

MOTHER: I'm not sure she can even do that. Do you think she can handle it?

CLINICIAN: I think so—for short periods of time. For right now, I think that type of program may be more appropriate than expecting Susan to do things on her own. What do you think, Susan?

SUSAN: I'm not sure. (*Pause*) I don't need it . . . but I'll think about it.

CLINICIAN: If everyone agrees it's worth considering, we can at least discuss it. Let's talk about it again at our next session.

In this example, the clinician accepted Susan's amotivation without allowing her or her family to negate the progress that had been made. He assumed the responsibility for setting unattainable goals to protect Susan and her parents as much as possible from feeling responsible for another failure. He then made concrete suggestions of more appropriate interim goals and a specific way to begin to achieve it. Most importantly, he did not allow either himself or the family to give up hope. While Susan and her family were not ready to move into the final stage of treatment, there was reason to hope that, given more time, at least some of the original goals might still be attainable.

Focusing on Other Issues

If patient and family elect to continue in treatment with a focus on issues not directly related to the initial contract, the length and terms of the new contract should be related to the type and severity of problems they wish to address. In two-parent families in which the patient is the adult offspring, these new problems may or may not involve the patient. The most common problems for parents at this point in treatment include the possible emancipation of the patient, marital discord, difficulties experienced by another child, and, somewhat less frequently, the desire of one parent to have a more independent life outside the family (e.g., a mother's desire to return to work). In families in which the patient is a married adult, the most common complaints at this time are those of a poor sexual relationship, unhappiness with role assignments or the division of responsibility for household tasks, and disagreements about having and/or rearing children. In general, all of these problems can be handled as they would be in most family or marital therapies, but since there are some special issues created by the fact that a serious mental illness has occurred, each of these themes will be briefly addressed.

Emancipation from the Family

The issue with the greatest potential for causing excessive stimulation or even relapse for patients is too early or too rapid emancipation from their families. Unfortunately, if the onset of the illness occurred during a patient's adolescence, which is common, the emancipation process is often impaired. The developmental tasks of adolescence are stressful ones for normal teenagers, and patients with schizophrenia have added difficulty in establishing themselves as separate, independent adults. if the family's style of relating to the patient happens to be protective or intrusive, a common style when any serious illness (physical or mental) has occurred in a family member, both patient and family probably will have more than the usual amount of difficulty and ambivalence about this issue.

It is likely that the increased differentiation and decreased contact between patients and families that spontaneously occurs as patients get better will decrease the intensity of family life and thus lessen the stress to which patients are exposed. However, separation of patient and family can produce stress in and of itself. It was for this reason that the goal of emancipation was avoided during the early phases of aftercare treatment, and even at this phase of treatment is addressed only with caution. However strongly patients or their families desire the patient's emancipation, it is a difficult step. Furthermore, a unilateral push for patient emancipation by clinicians often makes families feel unjustly criticized, causing them to resist, or even to discontinue therapy. Certainly, planning that arranges such "emancipation" by a premature push into a halfway house or transitional living placement is often unsuccessful. Even after months of gradual preparation, many of these patients and families react to the introduction of the issue of separation with great anxiety. At times, this anxiety is exacerbated by the fact that both patient and family see complete separation or complete enmeshment as the only options. This sort of polarized view is to be avoided for patient survival, for the well-being of the family, and for the survival of the treatment relationship.

It is for these reasons that the simple, structured tasks described in Chapters 4 and 5 are strongly suggested as first steps toward laying the groundwork for the patient's emancipation. These small but increasingly complex tasks allow patients gradually to assume more responsibility before becoming integrated into the world beyond their family. At the same time, repeated, successful task performance allows family members to be reassured about patient ability to function independently before giving up active parenting responsibilities.

As stated repeatedly throughout this manual, the key to the effectiveness of this entire treatment program is the idea of making only one change at a time. Even at this late point in treatment, this message must be stressed repeatedly for two reasons: First, during this phase of treatment, patients often become impatient because they feel better but have become acutely aware that they are far behind their peers in their accomplishments. When they begin to feel good, therefore, they often try to do everything simultaneously. Clinicians must be careful to limit overambitious behaviors in a nonjudgmental way. Second, clinicians, particularly young ones, so highly value emancipation that they tend to push for its attainment whether or not it is realistic to do so. This push is often reinforced by lingering beliefs that families of patients are disturbed and destructive, and therefore patients should be helped to "escape" as soon as possible. While there may be exceptions, it is our experience that most families are not destructive. When they behave in ways that are not helpful, it is most likely that they are anxious, unaware of the patient's needs, or unaware of effective means of coping with difficult behaviors. However, even if a particular family situation happened to be a chaotic or a destructive one, it would still be necessary to prepare the patient for independent living, and to help him move toward independence by taking one step at a time.

Generally speaking, formal emancipation should not become a focus until patients have been working, without experiencing a crisis, for at least 6 months, and then only if this is a goal to which patients or families clearly agree. When it is determined that such a goal is appropriate, it should be approached by first helping the patient to develop the basic skills necessary for independent living before actually facilitating a separation from the parental home. These skills may include the ability to manage money, to care for an apartment, to deal with household crises, and to maintain a schedule. Thus, movement toward emancipation involves assigning tasks in these areas while respecting the inevitable mixed feelings and difficulties that are likely to arise. Dealing with the ambivalence both patients and families have about this goal is central in setting a pace that everyone can tolerate. After all, many of these patients have been dysfunctional for years, and their families are naturally concerned about their ability to manage on their own.

The following example comes from a session immediately after it was decided that independent living would be the next primary goal for Dave, a 24-year-old young man who had been doing well since a psychotic episode 2 years earlier. He had never lived on his own, having been ill for 6 years.

DAVE: I found a great apartment in the ads.

CLINICIAN: Oh?

DAVE: Yeah, I went to see it. It's great, furnished, near the buses, and I can afford it.

CLINICIAN: Sounds good. We might think about it, but I thought we had agreed to put that off for just a little while, while we worked toward—

DAVE: I'm ready now.

CLINICIAN: Okay. Well, before we discuss that, how did the task we assigned last time go?

MOTHER: Not great. At least I couldn't live on what he bought. [The task had been for Dave to go food shopping and buy food for himself, for 1 week. His mother was to go along but not offer advice.] I know I was supposed to keep quiet, but I just couldn't. I mean, he just bought garbage—no vegetables, fruit, or meat. Just chips, ice cream, pop and beer, and candy.

DAVE: Well, that's what I like!

CLINICIAN: Me, too. I sometimes eat the meal just to get the dessert. But, I know I have to eat a semi-balanced diet. . . .

DAVE: No one wants me to live on my own. My mother even said she's afraid.

MOTHER: Well, I am, I guess.

CLINICIAN: To be honest, I don't think the time is right. I think it's great that you found a place on your own initiative. I do want to see you move, but I also want to make sure the move is a success. Right now, I'd like to stick to our agreement, and work on some of those things that will make it go better in the long run. When it's time, I'll be your biggest supporter.

DAVE: It's a nice apartment.

CLINICIAN: I hear that, but I'm sure other nice ones will be available.

In the above example, the clinician attempted to reinforce Dave's enthusiasm, and even to normalize, at least partially, his selection of junk food. At the same time, he set limits on Dave's desire to move out precipitously, maintaining instead a steady pace toward the goal of independent living. He explored Dave's response to the assigned task to assess his skills in managing a budget and his readiness to live on his own. Later in the session, he returned to the issue of the mother's ambivalent feelings.

CLINICIAN: Dave mentioned that you had some feelings about his leaving.

MOTHER: Well, I know it's the best thing for him . . . but . . . I guess I'm afraid. I mean what if he has problems?

CLINICIAN: That's an important question. He will have problems. He will make mistakes, but I think he's almost ready to handle those problems and mistakes. We've discussed it some but I think it's worth talking about a lot more.

MOTHER: How do you think he'll handle it?

CLINICIAN: First, I believe Dave knows his early warning signs. Second—

DAVE: I do.

CLINICIAN: Good. Second, moving out of the house doesn't mean you won't have contact with each other, and it doesn't mean terminating treatment. We'll continue to meet, in fact more frequently around the time of the move.

MOTHER: I know, but . . . I don't know. I hate to say it. It sounds selfish.

CLINICIAN: I think it's important to share what you're feeling now.

MOTHER: Well, Dave is all I have now. He's my company, and we get along well together since he's better. Ever since Don [her husband] died, I haven't had many friends. I guess I'm afraid of being alone. I know that sounds terrible.

CLINICIAN: I don't think so. I think it shows how much closeness there is. That isn't bad, that's good. I can certainly understand your mixed feelings. I don't have the perfect solution, but two things come to mind right now.

MOTHER: Yes?

CLINICIAN: First, with your permission, I would like to work with you more to help you develop your own social life. Second, I think it's going to be very important for both of you that you have regular visits after Dave moves out. You know, dinner a couple of times a week, things like that. Especially since he says he doesn't know how to cook.

MOTHER: I'd still worry about him of course, but that would make it a lot better. Would you do that, Dave?

DAVE: That would be fine with me. (*Smiles*) Chips get boring.

While the issue was far from resolved, a genuine discussion about Dave's leaving home had begun. His mother had begun to share her worries about Dave, and her own fears of loneliness. By adding the goal of expanding the mother's social network to the treatment agenda, the clinician acknowledged the appropriateness of her feelings and her need for ongoing support and contact. As these discussions continue over time, and as various tasks are successfully completed, Dave and his mother will be helped to find ways to be more comfortable with his eventual emancipation.

In many communities, programs are available which provide structured living situations that can be used to allow a gradual movement toward increasingly independent living. Quarter-way, half-way, or transitional living programs offer options to the "all or nothing" choice of staying in the parental home or moving to an apartment to live completely alone. Some of these programs are designed specifically to offer guidance in the development of independent living skills. Although not appropriate for every patient, programs such as these can help patients to accomplish the goal of emancipation. It should be remembered, however, that even if patients enter a residential living program, patients and families may need help in dealing with their feelings about separating from one another. The following example comes from a session held 3 weeks after Shelly had begun living in a transitional living apartment.

FATHER: I don't know why she bothers to stay there. She might as well pack up her things and come home. After all, she's with us every evening.

MOTHER: That's true. Shelly's eaten dinner with the family almost every night, and then she wants to sleep over. We've said "no" so far, but if she dislikes that place so much. . . .

CLINICIAN: Shelly?

SHELLY: I just don't like it there.

CLINICIAN: How come?

SHELLY: I don't know. There's not much to do and the girls I live with aren't that friendly. Besides Mom invites me over to the house almost every day anyway. Why shouldn't I go home? It's my house, too.

CLINICIAN: I understand that, and I think it's important that you feel comfortable there. But, it does sound as if you want to move back in.

SHELLY: Well, I told you I didn't like the apartment.

CLINICIAN: It doesn't sound like you've given it much of a chance.

FATHER: That's true. But, you know she's right about Evelyn [his wife]. She misses Shelly a lot and worries about her all the time. She likes to have her home.

CLINICIAN: And you?

FATHER: I guess I do too. She's never lived away before.

CLINICIAN: I think everyone's reactions are pretty appropriate. I remember the first time I lived away from home and how much I wanted to go back. And I can also imagine how worried I'll be when my kids start leaving.

MOTHER: It's really nerve-racking—not knowing how she's doing.

CLINICIAN: I understand. But, I also know that we all agreed this was the right step and the right time for it. I wonder if we can't work out some way to make everyone feel more comfortable about Shelly being on her own, but at the same time give the move a better chance to succeed?

SHELLY: I don't know.

CLINICIAN: I think if you were able to make some friends there, you'd feel a lot better about the place.

SHELLY: I guess . . . I really don't know anybody there, except the counselor.

CLINICIAN: Maybe she can help you get more involved and more comfortable.

SHELLY: I really don't want to bother her.

CLINICIAN: That's what she's there for. I'd be happy to talk to her for you to get things started and then you can explain your feelings yourself.

SHELLY: Well, okay, but I miss my family.

CLINICIAN: And they miss you. I wonder if we can't work out a compromise. Say you visit home 3 days a week, meet your mom for lunch 1 day, and have phone contact the other 3 days.

MOTHER: I guess we can try that. Knowing she was coming would help.

The rest of the session was spent clarifying the visiting schedule for the next week as well as discussing in more detail each family member's feelings about Shelly's move. By normalizing and empathizing with everyone's reaction to the separation, the clinician was able to maintain Shelly in the transitional-living setting, buying time to allow a positive adjustment to take place.

While many patients and families have difficulty separating from one another, others come to a point when they find it impossible to stay together. Occasionally, families can no longer tolerate the continuing crises involved in living with the patient and are unable to continue to maintain the patient at home. When a family makes such a decision, the clinician must support their stand and facilitate the patient's move to as appropriate a living situation as possible. Clinicians should never attack families or attempt to generate feelings of guilt about their "abandoning" the patient. These decisions are extremely difficult but sometimes in the patient's best interests, and sometimes necessary for the emotional or even physical survival of the rest of the family. Since most clinicians have no idea what it's like to live with a psychotic patient 24 hours a day, they are in no position to pass judgment. The family in the following example had come to such a decision, which they reported in a session 7 months after the patient, Carl, had been discharged from the hospital.

FATHER: Before you begin, I'd like to say something. Joyce [his wife] and I have talked about this a lot and we've decided—I hate to say it—Carl's got to move out. I feel like a rat, but we can't take it anymore. He paces every night. We don't sleep. We're afraid he'll burn the house down with his smoking. And he's still nasty and rude. I hate coming home. Nobody's happy. Joyce and I fight all the time. I'm burned out. We all are. I . . . I feel rotten, angry, and scared, but we've really thought about it and he's got to get out. We love him, but. . . .

CLINICIAN: Okay, I need a second to react. You've never mentioned this before and you caught me by surprise. Joyce, do you agree?

MOTHER: As John said, we've talked about it over and over. I'm scared too, but I'm afraid if he doesn't go, we'll lose our other children. They never stay home any more. And we all fight. It never was like this before. (Cries) I don't know what to do.

CLINICIAN: Carl, how do you feel about this?

CARL: Screw it. I don't care.

CLINICIAN: Well, I guess you know that under different circumstances, this wouldn't be what I'd like to see. But I certainly empathize with you and what you've been going through. I've never had to live in your situation, and to be honest, I don't know what my reaction would be. I realize you've reached your limit, but I'd like to ask a couple of things from you anyway.

FATHER: Sure, we do care, and don't want to hurt Carl, but. . . . (Long pause)

CLINICIAN: I understand. First, I'd like to ask for just a little more time from you. I know it's difficult but it's important. If this is to happen, I'd like to give it as much chance for success as possible, which means I need some time to see what I can arrange.

MOTHER: We've survived this long. We can do it for a while longer, if we know. . . .

FATHER: Right, as long as we can see a light at the end of the tunnel.

CLINICIAN: Good! Second, I'd like to meet more often now, say once a week, and continue to discuss everyone's feelings about this and to arrange a specific plan. As you said, you do care, and I'd like that caring to continue on everyone's part.

FATHER: I think that's a good idea.

CLINICIAN: Also, I'd like the other kids to come in for a few sessions. Obviously, they have feelings about the situation, and they should be a part of whatever we work out.

FATHER: Fine.

CARL: I don't care. I'd be happy to go tomorrow.

In responding to the decision of the family, the clinician did not attempt to convince these parents that they were making a mistake, since she recognized the pain and thought that had gone into their decision. Through future discussions, there would be time to discover possible alternatives, or time to change the plan if they discovered ways of making the home situation more bearable. Since Carl was unable to talk about how he felt, the clinician chose to deal with the reactions of his parents and the need for a practical plan. She also chose to reinforce the caring element of the parents' statements since, if this plan was to have any chance of success, their involvement would be necessary even after Carl left home.

Parental Issues

When it is no longer necessary to focus their primary attention on the patient, some parents recognize that they have issues with one another that they would like to resolve. For instance, if one parent has been more involved with and worried about the patient, the other may have come to feel neglected. Partners, reacting differently to the illness, may have drifted apart, spending increasingly less time together and less energy on their relationship. It's usually hard to do anything about this problem, or even to discuss it, while the patient is severely ill. During these months or years, parents find it difficult to set limits on their availability to the patient and even more difficult to make what seem to be additional demands on each other.

In the following case example, Craig's mother had devoted almost all of her energy to caring for her son since the onset of his illness, several years earlier. Now, since her son had been asymptomatic and working for several months, she had begun to be concerned about some of the problems in her relationship with her husband. She began to express worries that her husband might leave her, since their life together had become so distant. The following dialogue occurred in a session at which Craig was not present, having been asked by his employer to work overtime.

CLINICIAN: You mentioned a fear that your husband is going to leave you?

ANITA: Yes.

CLINICIAN: Why do you feel that way?

ANITA: Well, because so many people have said they don't know how he can stand it after all these years . . . how he could stay at home and take it.

CLINICIAN: We've pretty much always focused on Craig during

our sessions, but let me ask you a question. If you don't want to answer, that's okay. How would you describe your relationship?

ANITA: Mine and Bill's? I would say it's wonderful, *when* we have a chance.

CLINICIAN: Would you say that honestly or is it just because he's sitting here?

BILL: (*Laughs*) Good question.

ANITA: Well, I'll say that our relationship—love-wise, sex-wise, financial-wise—is perfect, but I'll say this, Bill isn't the easiest person to live with. I would have said that before Craig was born. He's a hard person to live with and I know a lot of people who will back my word up.

CLINICIAN: Okay. (*Laughter*) Okay. We don't need witnesses. You've learned the secrets for doing it though?

ANITA: Oh, yes.

CLINICIAN: But you also said, to balance that, I mean because he is a tough guy to live with, there are a lot of positives in the relationship?

ANITA: Oh, yes. They far outweigh the negatives.

CLINICIAN: Where do you get the sense that he's going to walk out? Is that coming from him?

ANITA: No, he always told me he'd tell me when he's ready to leave. He'd tell me first.

CLINICIAN: But, somehow, you really don't believe him. You told me that you think that one day, he's going to go to work and you're going to have dinner on the table, and he won't come home. . . .

BILL: Just look in the bathroom in the morning, and if my toothbrush is there, I'm coming home. (*Laughter*)

A little later:

ANITA: Seriously, I want the cycle [of needing to be available to Craig] to be broken, believe me. I have been so pleased since he's been working.

CLINICIAN: Craig's been your main job for 25 years, right from the word "go." I don't know if you are ready to retire.

ANITA: I am, believe me.

CLINICIAN: Retirement is tough. . . .

ANITA: I have been so glad to get rid of him for 8 hours, and I often daydream how nice it would be if he'd meet the right girl, get on his own. I can't picture myself being so deliriously happy.

CLINICIAN: (*To Bill*) I get the sense that she's not ready.

BILL: Oh, not from home. No, she's ready to retire, but not from Craig.

CLINICIAN: That's what I mean.

ANITA: Oh, I think I am.

BILL: No, she ain't. *No.*

ANITA: Because when he's working, I look forward to Bill coming home and just the two of us having supper alone together with no friction, no tension.

BILL: Well, you know, whether she believes it or whether she doesn't, we're sitting and eating dinner this evening, you know, and she said, "This is really good." And I said, "Yeah, hey, this is better than what you normally make, I like it." She says, "Yeah, and when Craig comes home, I'll make him some." I mean Craig ain't even there. He ain't out of the house 8 hours yet, and already she's worried about him coming in.

ANITA: Well, no. I just said there was enough for him, too.

BILL: Whoa, whoa, whoa . . . it's automatic with you!

ANITA: (*To clinician*) Do you detect just a little jealousy there?

BILL: This is automatic. See this is what you say. Jealousy! I say you are not ready to give up yet. You're *really* not.

ANITA: Oh, I am, I am.

BILL: You say jealousy. You can call it what you want and I can call it what I want. You wouldn't get out of bed to make my supper at 11:00 at night . . . but you would for Craig, huh? I don't know if it's that you want to make him supper or you want to see him. I really don't know.

ANITA: You're no different. You come home tonight and say, "How was he today?" It's always the first question: "How was he today?" or if he's in the house, (*whisper*) "How was he today?"

BILL: No, I say a few other things. "Any mail?" "Anybody call?" "What's for supper?" And then, "How's Craig?"

CLINICIAN: I don't want to get tied up in this because from as far back as you can remember Craig has required your attention. I'm sure with all the physical ailments and the illness and so on, it's required a lot of going to this place, going to that place, being concerned, coming here, hospitalization, medication, the ups and downs, you know, it becomes something that's tough to ignore, tough not to ask how things are going or to be involved, but—

ANITA: Isn't it tough not to see that they get their nourishment, especially with Craig? He has no appetite, he doesn't want to eat. I'm the one that suffers when he's sick. I'm the only one that gets badgered. My husband's out working all day. He can go up to his dad's in the evening. Where can I go? I don't even have family here. I'm not even close with my neighbors.

CLINICIAN: I think that—

BILL: (*Signaling to interrupt and to wife gently*) You can always go with me.

The clinician continued to help Bill and Anita to express their perceptions of their relationship and what they needed from each other. Gradually, these were translated into goals they cold work on as a couple. By the end of the session, they were able to agree on new goals, and to make a commitment to working on them in treatment. They also agreed that Bill would help Anita to find ways to worry less about Craig in order for her to have the energy to give to the marriage.

Some parental couples have marital issues that do not relate directly to the patient. Long-standing sexual difficulties or problems in communication simply may have been put on a back burner for years. In some cases, partners decide not to confront these issues directly, while in others they actively seek therapeutic help. Again, it should be stressed that it is ultimately the couple's decision, not the clinician's! However, if a couple does decide to focus on more general marital conflict, then treatment becomes more traditional in nature. As the focus shifts to the conflicts and strengths of the parental couple, only they need attend the sessions. Before this move is made, however, the clinician must negotiate this shift in emphasis with the entire family. In part, this is in keeping with the open, collaborative relationship with all family members that has been established and maintained throughout the course of treatment. In addition, the clinician must arrange maintenance contacts with the patient and other family members that may continue to occur independent of the marital sessions. In the following example, the clinician negotiates just such a new treatment plan with the family.

CLINICIAN: (*To patient*) You know last time we saw each other, I met with all of you and then I met for awhile with just your parents.

ELLIOTT: [patient] Yeah, they didn't say much about what that was all about.

FATHER: Well it was about mom and me, not about either of you.

CLINICIAN: Right. Well, I thought we could talk a little bit about it since I need everyone's feedback about some tentative plans.

CARIE: [sister] Okay.

ELLIOTT: (*Somewhat tentatively*) Yeah.

CLINICIAN: Good. Last time we agreed as a group to start meeting less often—about every 3 months for right now. Everyone thinks that things are going well for you, Elliott, and that it's a lot more pleasant at home.

ELLIOTT: Right. I'm okay.

CLINICIAN: At the same time, I felt that perhaps your parents were having some difficulties getting along, and I wanted to discuss that with them.

CARIE: I know that's true. It's been a long time since I've seen them be happy together.

CLINICIAN: And they agree with you. Anyway that's what I talked to them about. And they want to work on getting along better.

ELLIOTT: What's the problem?

MOTHER: Well. I'm not sure I can say.

CLINICIAN: Is it all right if I answer that?

MOTHER: Fine.

CLINICIAN: You know, your mother and father have really had some tough going at home, and they have done a really good job. In other words, we've talked a lot about them as parents, and that was open to the whole family. But as a marital couple some of their problems are only between them and shouldn't be discussed with the whole family.

ELLIOTT: I know anyway, so what's the difference?

CLINICIAN: It may be true that you know the issues, but they do have a right to privacy. Anyway, this is what I'd like to suggest. I'd like to meet with your parents pretty regularly to work on their marriage. At the same time, I'd like to keep to last time's agreement and meet with the whole family to check in and see how things are going every 3 months.

CARIE: That's fine with me.

ELLIOTT: I *guess* it's okay.

CLINICIAN: You don't sound so sure.

ELLIOTT: No, it's fine.

CLINICIAN: Okay. But if any questions or doubts come up about this new arrangement, I'd like you to give me a call. (*To Elliott*) I'm still interested and concerned about how things are going with you.

In this example, the clinician began to sort out two separate treatment contracts to work on two separate issues. She made the basic theme of her discussion with Elliott's parents explicit without sharing any of the details they had discussed with her. In fact, she used this opportunity to further reinforce generational boundaries by labeling the parents' marital issues as private, and not appropriate concerns for Elliott and Carie. Finally she reinforced her long standing relationship with Elliott, and reassured him that this relationship would continue.

Conjugal Issues: Sex Roles, Tasks, and Childrearing

Little attention has been paid to the issue of how schizophrenia impacts on the marriages of patients, perhaps because a relatively small percentage of people with this illness marry (Watt & Szulecka, 1979), and those who do tend to be patients with better premorbid functioning (Gittelman-Klein & Klein, 1968; Held & Cromwell, 1968; Turner, Dopkun, & Labreche, 1970). Nevertheless, marriage is complex and stressful, even for healthy individuals. It is not surprising then that patients who are vulnerable to stimulation, and who are experiencing either the positive or negative symptoms of schizophrenia are likely to have particular difficulty negotiating the vicissitudes of married life. Furthermore, spouses who have had to deal with any type of chronic illness in their partner are often plagued by chronic feelings of sadness, anxiety, and fears of loss of control. When the illness is schizophrenia, these common emotional reactions are probably intensified by the unpredictable nature of the behaviors and symptoms associated with the illness, and the need for a relatively long-term rearrangement of role responsibilities within the home. For the patient's spouse, all of this means at least the temporary loss of a companion and a sexual partner. While the degree of impact of the illness on the marriage also depends on the chronicity of the illness and the quality of the patient's functioning between episodes, it is not surprising that many spouses become less tolerant and more resigned over time, and that many of these marriages end in separation or divorce (Johnston & Planasky, 1968).

Although it would be easy to relate all the individual and marital problems of these patients to the presence of a mental illness, it is probable that many of these marriages also have the same problems and strengths of most other marital relationships. This latter phase of treatment is the appropriate time to deal with more typical marital issues: communication difficulties, childrearing disagreements, sexual dysfunctions, role conflicts, and lack of joint and/or independent social networks for each partner. The recurring nature of schizophrenia is, however, a complicating factor in resolving many of these common problems. The occurrence of acute psychotic episodes influences the level at which patients are able to function, and consequently forces continual readjustment in the relationships of patients and spouses. Since couples must live with the ever present threat of another episode, making these relationships work is likely to demand greater skill than that required of "normal" couples. Both partners must learn to play multiple roles dependent not only on the "life-cycle stage" of the marriage, but also upon the intrusion of a recurring illness.

It is important to give couples the opportunity to address marital issues. In the early phases of treatment, patients and spouses will have been helped to deal with the impact of the psychosis itself, and somewhat later to deal with the deficit state that often lingers for months after an episode. At this point in treatment, patients generally should have regained sufficient energy and strength to begin to perform more normally in the marital relationship. Thus, it should be possible to deal with the long-term impact of the illness on the marriage and, independently of that, general marital issues.

During the course of any chronic illness, there is a risk of dysfunctional habits and secondary gains becoming sufficiently reinforcing so as to inhibit the patient's motivation to "get better." This can also block the spouse's ability to see the patient as a whole person or to give up the power inherent in the caretaker role. Considering the severity of this particular illness, patients and their spouses are especially vulnerable to developing a chronic patient–caretaker pattern in their relationship. Despite the fact that patients are "more stable" at this point in treatment, the resumption of more balanced role responsibilities between partners is often unexpectedly difficult. Therefore, intervention into marital issues must often begin by helping couples to move from the relationship structure which allowed a relatively low level of functioning on the part of the patient, to a more balanced relationship with a gradual acceptance of greater responsibilities by the patient as he or she becomes more capable. These tasks must be accomplished in a way that does not allow the patient role to come to dominate either spouse's view of the patient or the marriage. Unfortunately, the discrepancy between the patient's past and present functioning may be significant, especially if the initial psychotic break occurred sometime after the marriage. Thus, clinicians must also help couples to mourn past competencies, before beginning to assess, negotiate, and eventually assume redefined functional and expressive roles.

As in all marital therapy, only more so, it is particularly important not to establish treatment goals based on a conception of an "ideal" marriage. In many cases, the most realistic goals are limited ones, such as the restoration of a "previously marginal symbiotic stability" (Kerr, 1967), or a decrease in the severity and frequency of marital crises. Thus, clinicians must assess a couple's overall strengths and weaknesses, their goals and their potential for achieving them, and whether or not they desire changes in any areas sufficiently to contract for ongoing marital treatment.

In the following example a clinician had helped Norm, the patient, and his wife, Lynn, to deal with the feelings of frustration, confusion, anger, and sadness that have periodically erupted since Norm returned home from the hospital. Norm's first psychotic episode had occurred after the couple had been married for 3 years. At this point they have been married 18 years, having spent much of their marriage coping with the devastating impact of this illness. They had spent the past three years in the treatment program, and Norm's wife, Lynn, was beginning to become impatient.

LYNN: When will it end? I keep waiting. . . .

CLINICIAN: Waiting?

LYNN: I keep hoping that I'll wake up one morning and things will be the way they once were. You know, Norm, his old self. . . . But its hopeless.

CLINICIAN: I'm confused. I thought things *were* going well. What's been happening?

LYNN: It's the same old stuff. He expects me to wait on him . . . to clean up after him, and he doesn't lift a finger to help. I'm his wife, not his maid. I think he likes me doing everything—waiting on him. That's not the way it used to be, and I'm getting tired of being patient.

CLINICIAN: Norm? Do you like the way things are now?

NORM: No, but I work all day, and I'm tired when I get home. Anyway, her job is to take care of the home.

LYNN: That's it! That really steams me! I work too, and I'm tired too. You know you act like you're still sick and can't do anything. Bull!

NORM: You treat me like I'm sick. Nag at me like I'm a little kid! I'm the man of the house.

LYNN: Then act like it!

CLINICIAN: Okay. I know you're both angry right now, but yelling isn't going to solve the problem. What I hear is that you both want something from the other: Lynn, you want Norm to do more around the house, and Norm, you want Lynn to stop nagging and give you more respect.

LYNN: I guess.

NORM: We never solve anything. We can't talk.

CLINICIAN: You can talk here, and you've just made a good start by telling each other what you need. I wouldn't say it's hopeless, these are conflicts lots of couples have, even when one of them hasn't been ill.

In this example the clinician responded to Lynn's complaints of unbalanced roles, moving the emphasis of treatment from the illness itself to marital conflicts that could occur between any two spouses. The session then focused on helping Norm and Lynn come to some agreement about a division of household responsibilities. At the same time, they were helped to begin to focus on developing better communicative skills. They were asked to speak directly to one another, and to state their needs and requests without attacking one another.

Good communication skills are useful in developing and maintaining a healthy marital relationship. Thus, when the crisis has passed, an important component of the marital treatment of these couples involves monitoring their interactions, and particularly assessing and encouraging clarity and specificity. Throughout treatment, both spouses are encouraged to take responsibility for their own statements and to be supportive of one another. In earlier phases of this treatment, patients will have been encouraged to make sense, while spouses will have been encouraged to reinforce the patient's clarity and to limit any bizarre communications. The focus of communication work becomes more sophisticated over the course of time, shifting to help each spouse to be better able to make their needs known to the other.

The discussion of more emotionally charged issues increases the risk of overstressing the patient and stimulating conflict that cannot be resolved given the couple's current psychological resources. To avoid this problem, the task oriented approach can be continued in this phase of treatment, providing structure and support during these emotional discussions. In addition, clinicians must help couples to translate their complaints and concerns into measurable and achievable goals. This concrete focus helps to prevent discussions from becoming overwhelming or out of control. In the following example, taken from a session 16 months after Angela's hospitalization, her husband, Paul, raised an issue that had surfaced a number of times in the past.

PAUL: I've said it a hundred times. I feel like I'm all alone in the battle. Angela's more like my daughter than my wife.

CLINICIAN: I know you've brought this up before and I've put you off because I didn't feel we were ready to deal with it. But things are going well now, and I think it's important to see if things can be better. Could you be more specific about what you would like to see different, Paul?

PAUL: I don't know. It's just everything . . . a feeling I have.

CLINICIAN: I see. Could you give me an example of when you last felt that way so that Angela and I can understand?

PAUL: Well . . . like, if I have a rough day. Like 2 days ago I had a lousy day at work. I came home from work and started telling Angela, looking for sympathy, I guess, and she just didn't want to hear about it. Not nasty, more like she was a kid who you shouldn't tell your problems to.

CLINICIAN: In other words, you turned to your wife for support and she was unable to give it.

PAUL: Yeah, exactly. It's lopsided with us.

CLINICIAN: I agree. Angela, do you remember the time Paul is talking about?

ANGELA: How could I forget? He wouldn't talk to me for the rest of the night. I don't know . . . I want to help, but . . . I don't know.

CLINICIAN: What keeps you from listening or helping?

ANGELA: (*Pause*) I guess I feel guilty. If I were better then he wouldn't have problems. I guess I feel like I'm the cause of his problems. When he's miserable I feel like I caused it and then I get scared that he'll figure it out too and leave. Sounds crazy . . . well, they say I'm crazy.

CLINICIAN: It doesn't sound crazy to me. Do you think that if you felt less responsible you'd be more comfortable being supportive?

ANGELA: I guess.

PAUL: But it had nothing to do with you. It was just a lousy day. I just wanted you to listen.

CLINICIAN: Angela?

ANGELA: I get scared and don't hear that.

CLINICIAN: Okay, if I understand this, Paul, you're asking for support and caring from your wife, and, Angela, you think you could give it if you didn't feel responsible for causing his problems.

PAUL: Yes.

ANGELA: Yes, it sounds so simple when you say it.

The clinician went on to help Angela and Paul to clarify their respective needs, continuously helping them to state their messages to one another in concrete and simple terms. Then, with the clinician's help, Angela and Paul developed a homework task that would continue to provide some support for Paul, while generally increasing marital communication and understanding. Overall, as in most cases during this phase, the emphasis of marital treatment gradually shifted to the development of better tools for conflict resolution, and an intimacy based on increased equality of the roles of husband and wife.

Problems can occur during this phase of treatment if the clinician has become emotionally overinvolved in a couple's system. For instance, because most of these couples present with one spouse obviously ill and the other appearing significantly more healthy, it is easy for inexperienced clinicians who are unaware of their own issues to begin to covertly align with one partner. If this sort of alignment is a transient phenomena, it need not interfere with treatment. However, if it continues over time, it can impede therapeutic progress. Clinicians must avoid such alignments and avoid assuming the role of adversary or champion of either partner. Particularly at this stage of treatment, it is essential that the clinician's allegiance be neither to the patient, nor to the spouse, but to helping the couple to cope more effectively with the illness and their relationship.

Even when clinicians make a consistent effort to maintain a balanced perspective, problems can arise in the treatment relationship. Patients are frequently already sensitized to criticism and often anticipate rejection based on past experiences. Thus, even benign comments made by clinicians may be interpreted as negative. In particular, when clinicians purposely form a temporary alliance with the spouse in an attempt to mobilize the patient, the patient's response may be one of upset, anger, and resistance to treatment. These reactions are complicated by the fact that many of these patients are unusually passive in stating their complaints about therapy. Since they tend not to verbalize their feelings, clinicians are often unaware that they have made an intervention that has stressed the therapeutic relationship. For this reason, it is necessary for clinicians to ask for periodic feedback to insure that no misunderstanding or alienation has occurred. Repetitive clarification of the clinician's commitment, support, and positive intent is often useful. In the following example, the issue arose after the clinician had given a task to Bud in an attempt to counteract his lack of motivation and activity.

> CLINICIAN: Is that okay with the both of you?
> GINNY: [wife] Fine. If Bud does it, I think it will help.
> CLINICIAN: Bud?
> BUD: (*Pause*) Fine.
> CLINICIAN: It doesn't sound like you mean it.
> BUD: No . . . it's fine.
> CLINICIAN: Hm . . . I'm concerned, Bud. I sense something is wrong but I don't know what. I'm worried that perhaps I did or said something you don't like, but I need a clue from you.
> BUD: No . . . well, its just that I know you don't like me.
> CLINICIAN: Huh? I'm sorry you feel that way. It's certainly not true. Did I do or say something today to make you feel that?
> BUD: You make me feel like I'm lazy and stupid. You and her. The way you talk—all these tasks. Like I'm retarded or lazy.
> GINNY: (*Getting angry*) How can you say that? After all I've done. You must be really crazy to think I don't like you. Well, if that's the way. . . .
> CLINICIAN: Whoa, time out. Let's slow down and discuss this before there's a fight. I think I'm the one that really made Bud feel that way. Bud, I'd like to apologize to you . . . and to you, Ginny. I wasn't aware that I was coming across that way. In no way do I feel that you are stupid or lazy. On the contrary, I respect how much effort it's been for you, and for Ginny, to come this far.
> BUD: Yeah? I appreciate that. I'm sorry for saying those things.
> CLINICIAN: Don't be. I'm glad you let me know.
> GINNY: How about me?
> BUD: I'm sorry. I didn't mean what I said to you either. I was just angry about all these tasks.
> GINNY: Okay, I can understand that.

Helping Bud to express his feelings allowed the clinician to become aware of a potential problem in the therapeutic relationship. If Bud's negative feelings had not been discussed, the result may have been increased conflict between the couple since Bud saw Ginny as aligned with the clinician. Finally, the clinician positively reinforced Bud's honest sharing of feelings since this was unusual for him and clearly quite difficult.

The slow pace of treatment, even during this late phase, often creates frustration for clinicians. When frustrated, clinicians tend to move too quickly, and to focus on highly charged or conflictual issues before couples are ready to do so. Unfortunately, this is counter-therapeutic in that it prematurely escalates the intensity of sessions. Most clinicians can accept the advisability of avoiding a dynamically oriented, emotive approach to working with these couples early in treatment. They can see that such a strategy has the potential for precipitating crises, heightening marital distress, and/or increasing symptomatology. In the latter phases of treatment, however, clinicians often tend to feel they should be able to raise and resolve these issues even if patients have not really stabilized and even if couples have not clearly demonstrated a commitment and ability to work in this way. It remains important that clinicians maintain a style and pace that fits with a couple's level of functioning, insight, and ability to tolerate stress. Even years after an acute episode, patients may continue to be highly sensitive to stressful situations. Therapy must continue to offer more than the usual amount of support even when a move has been made to a direct focus on conflictual areas.

To deal with feelings of anger or hopelessness, clinicians can move therapy along by making frequent use of the technique of re-framing events and behaviors positively. For instance, as in the following example, the strengths and coping skills of both partners can be emphasized, since such strengths and skills must be present for them to have dealt with this illness over time.

CLINICIAN: Chip, you seem sort of down tonight.
CHIP: I guess.
CLINICIAN: What's on your mind?
CHIP: Same old stuff, I just can't seem to get anywhere. Now they're talking about layoffs at the mill. I know Peg's upset . . . I just can't do much right.
PEG: Wait a second. I don't blame you for what's happening. Sure I'm upset but it's not your fault. Hundreds are being laid off.
CHIP: Well, I blame myself.

CLINICIAN: You know, it's funny. I was just thinking, we've known each other about 3 years now, and I think I've heard this conversation at least ten times by now.

CHIP: Huh?

CLINICIAN: I can remember when we first talked about applying for this job, and you were sure that they would never hire you. And even before that when you were sure that Peg would leave you because you were worthless.

CHIP: (*Smiling*) I guess I do tend to look at the worst side of things.

CLINICIAN: I'll say. And you know, the funny thing is that things keep working out okay. I'd say that's an important message about what you have to offer, that you've been able to do all this in spite of the trouble you've had.

CHIP: I guess, but. . . .

PEG: No buts, you're a good person with a lot to offer to me and everyone else.

CHIP: Maybe I am too hard on myself. I guess, considering what we've gone through we've done all right.

CLINICIAN: Better than all right. Damn good, I'd say.

After redefining Chip's struggle over the years as having been a successful one, the clinician was able to focus on the potential layoff, helping Chip to view it in its proper perspective as an event unrelated to his worth and capabilities. The couple then could anticipate the possibility of a period of financial stress, and prepare coping mechanisms to use in case things became difficult.

Many couples express a desire to work on sexual problems at this time. Such problems are common and often involve a lack of desire or ability on the part of the patient. It's sometimes difficult to determine whether these issues preceded the illness or are a part of it. Certainly many schizophrenic patients, especially males, report decreased sexual interest and/or functioning as a result of either their illness or their psychotropic medications (Lyketsos, Sakka, & Mailis, 1983). Furthermore, the need for spouses to play a caretaking role tends to deeroticize the marital relationship. Therefore, some attention to the issue of sexuality is usually important during this later phase of treatment, although not always with the goal of increasing sexual interest or performance. Some couples are quite content to put sex temporarily, or even permanently, on a back burner. It is crucial to help a couple to talk about the issue directly enough to come to some agreement concerning both the importance of the sexual issue and what they want to do about it. In general, it is important to remember that if the issue is raised by either spouse before the patient is functioning in a stable manner or during a time of other major changes, it should be labeled as a problem that will be addressed when the crisis has passed.

In the following example, the clinician responds to a comment by the patient's wife, Marilyn, about the changes in their sex life.

CLINICIAN: What do you mean, "not the same"?

MARILYN: Oh Lord, I mean everything's changed. In the past we'd make love three and four times a week, maybe more. Now I'm lucky if we do it once a month. And then only if I nudge.

CLINICIAN: Wayne?

WAYNE: What can I say? It's true. I don't know why but the desire just isn't there. It's embarrassing.

CLINICIAN: Are you uncomfortable talking about it?

WAYNE: Yeah, but it's okay. I know it bothers her and we fight about it.

MARILYN: Only when I don't let you ignore me.

CLINICIAN: What upsets you the most, Marilyn?

MARILYN: It's funny, but I don't miss the sex that much. I mean I like it, but I can survive without it. It's the other stuff. You know, the romance, the cuddling. Things like that.

WAYNE: Really?

CLINICIAN: You sound surprised.

WAYNE: I am. She never said that.

MARILYN: A hundred times. You just never listen.

CLINICIAN: It sounds like he's listening now.

MARILYN: I need to be held, to have some contact. . . .

WAYNE: I avoided you because I was afraid that . . . you know . . . you'd want to have sex. I miss being close, too.

By helping the couple to redefine their needs, the clinician allowed them to temporarily make up for the loss of a sexual relationship by emphasizing a less threatening kind of intimacy. If the couple is able to get some sort of satisfaction in this way, they may desire a more direct focus on their sexual relationship in the future. As is obvious in this dialogue, it is important that the clinician play a very active role in facilitating the couple's communication with each other. Without prodding questions, dialogue about these problems often grinds to a halt before any issue is resolved.

Ultimately, however, there are times when spouses of patients must be helped to make decisions about their commitment to the marriage, especially those times when continuing in the marriage will probably mean a lifelong obligation to a caretaking role. Some spouses willingly accept this role, others do not. If the marriage is to dissolve, the clinician must help the partners to separate with a minimum of stress and chaos, hopefully well after an acute episode when the patient is at his or her best. During this process, it is crucial to avoid a judgmental stance about the behavior of the departing spouse. No one makes the decision to abandon a relationship lightly, no matter how compelling the reasons. Leaving someone who has a serious mental illness can be even more difficult. Most spouses experience a significant amount of ambivalence, guilt, and anxiety at such a time. Some spouses have emotional problems of their own. It is not the clinician's place to implicitly or explicitly suggest to either spouse that there is a right or wrong way to behave under these circumstances, but rather to facilitate whatever decisions either spouse feels must be made.

If the issue of a possible separation is raised, then it is important for clinicians to assess how serious and eminent the separation might be. Both the pros and cons of such a decision must be discussed fully since, at times, the desire to leave may be more related to a temporary sense of frustration or a need for a time out than a genuine wish to terminate the relationship. If this is the case, then treatment can focus on finding ways to increase support for the spouse. However, if the decision to separate seems irreversible, then clinicians should attempt to negotiate a short-term treatment contract that includes the following tasks: establishing a time schedule that helps to ease the abruptness of this change; helping each partner to better understand the reasons for the dissolution of the marriage; helping each spouse to plan for the separation; and establishing ways of coping before the inevitable stress and pain associated with separation and divorce are in full force. In the following example, Sam wants to separate from his wife, Ann, who has been severely dysfunctional for some time.

SAM: I've thought about everything we've talked about. I can't stop thinking about it. And there's just no way. I still want out.

CLINICIAN: What have you thought about?

SAM: It just isn't what I bargained for. I mean, it's been misery for years. You know, we've been seeing you for at least a year, and I was willing to try, and . . . things have even gotten a little better. Ann tries, but I just don't have the same feelings anymore. I kept thinking that when she got better, I wouldn't feel the way I do. But she's better and I still feel bad. I feel like a bastard, but I'm entitled to some happiness, too.

CLINICIAN: Yes, you are. Ann, what is your reaction to all this?

ANN: (*Crying*) I don't know. I hate him! He doesn't care! I am trying! He hates me! I don't know!

CLINICIAN: (*Gently*) I know that you're hurt and upset. This is a painful time for both of you. Sam, I can't tell you what to do. You've talked about this for weeks and it sounds like you've given a lot of thought to this decision.

SAM: Yes.

CLINICIAN: I'm sure that this has been a difficult time for you both and will continue to be hard. I'd like to help you as much as possible to ease the pain, to help you to understand what's happened, and thus help you to make some plans about how to handle this.

SAM: I'd appreciate that.

ANN: Why bother? It's over. I don't need him. He's all I have. What am I going to do without him? Why don't you just go away?

CLINICIAN: I know it seems as though Sam is all you have, but there are a lot of other people who care about you, your family for instance, and the treatment team.

ANN: (*Woodenly*) I guess.

CLINICIAN: I'd like to see you both, together and separately, as we work this out. It will still be hard, but maybe we can make things a little less overwhelming.

The rest of the session was spent with the clinician helping Ann and Sam to share their feelings as well as helping each of them to identify a support network that could be available to them in this time of trouble. For Ann, it was suggested that a session be held with her parents present since they lived in the area and were still actively concerned and involved with her. Later sessions focused on dealing with the pain of separation, as well as the practical aspects of preparing for independent living.

Moving to Maintenance Sessions

When the patient and family have reached a level of stability and comfort with their present life situation, they may prefer to choose the option of maintenance sessions rather than either ongoing therapy or termination. Maintenance sessions should differ considerably from the working sessions of the original contract. Their primary purpose is to give patients and families a chance to "check in," to maintain already established gains, and to prevent future problems. In general, new issues are not raised during the maintenance phase of treatment since sessions occur infrequently. In fact, in the maintenance phase, the time between sessions gradually increases until 3–6 months pass between meetings.

Most patients and families choose to contract for maintenance sessions rather than to terminate. There seems to be a number of reasons for the popularity of this option. First, patients and families usually want to keep a lifeline to the mental health system. They know that good periods in the past, even when things were going extremely well, were often followed by times of crisis and illness, sometimes with little warning. Maintaining a link with the treatment team provides the comfort of knowing that if a problem arises, help will be immediately available. Second, most patients must continue a program of medication. Continuing to hold family sessions, however infrequently, allows the family to have input into the medication program and to be kept abreast of any changes in treatment plans. Third, having "checkup" sessions provides both patient and family a chance to examine the appropriateness of any independent decisions that they may have made.

The decision to move to maintenance sessions is reached by mutual agreement between the clinician, the patient, and the family. If any one of these parties does not feel ready for maintenance, then this decision is best postponed until everyone is comfortable with such a contract. The following example came from a maintenance session 4 years after psychoeducational treatment had begun. After gradually tapering sessions to once a month, then once every 3 months, the family had been moved to sessions at 6-month intervals.

CLINICIAN: Well, it's been 6 months. Why doesn't someone bring me up to date on what's been happening with everyone.

MOTHER: Where to start? Things have been going really well. Jamie [her youngest daughter] got engaged over Christmas, and. . . .

CLINICIAN: Congratulations, Jamie. When's the big day?

JAMIE: (Smiling) Not until next summer. After I graduate.

MOTHER: We're all excited. Also, Pat [the patient] changed jobs. We all talked about it, and I think the choice sounded like a really good one.

CLINICIAN: Pat?

PAT: It's doing pretty much the same thing, filing, but for a different company. It's nearer home and pays better.

FATHER: We thought maybe we should call you, but then we figured that we all agreed it was a good decision, so why bother you? I mean after 4 years we pretty much know the guidelines.

CLINICIAN: I agree. It sounds like a really good decision. I'd like to hear more, both about the job and the wedding plans. Maybe even about what the two of you [parents] are doing.

During this session, the clinician reinforced the ability of the patient and the family to make independent decisions based on the guidelines of the program, using the treatment team only when necessary. She specifically made an effort to include a focus on the positive events in the lives of the patient and the family to reinforce their growing ability to attend to other people's issues and not focus entirely on the patient's problems.

A maintenance contract should allow for the flexibility of increasing the frequency of sessions if a problem arises or if a major change is about to happen for either patient or family. For example, a maintenance contract often goes into effect while a patient is still living in the parental home. If, in the future, consideration is given to the patient moving out, a temporary increase in the frequency of sessions can be arranged to prepare everyone for this move.

A case can be made for continuing maintenance sessions indefinitely since, in living with any chronic illness, lifetime checkups can be an important and vital part of responsible self-care. The clinician's message about the need for ongoing contact is important in and of itself since it emphasizes the chronic nature of the illness, and discourages false hopes and unrealistic expectations as treatment winds down. Rather, it underlines the messages that by following the rules for survival, staying on medication, and keeping in touch with the clinical team, it is possible to lead a functional and productive life.

The following interchange came from a session 9 months following the implementation of a maintenance contract which had begun by scheduling meetings at 3-month intervals. The session began with the patient's mother giving a general report on the patient's progress.

MOTHER: Things have been "status quo." Kenny is still doing fine. Not much has changed.

CLINICIAN: Good.

FATHER: I agree. I'm wondering if every 3 months is even too often. There really isn't anything to report. We don't really seem to need to come here now.

CLINICIAN: Well, I'm not sure. I guess the length of time between sessions is still negotiable. Maybe at the end of the session, we can discuss it further. How goes it with you, Ken?

KEN: Okay. Nothing special.

CLINICIAN: Any problems or symptoms?

KEN: A few.

MOTHER: What?

CLINICIAN: Like what, Ken?

KEN: Voices, every now and then . . . they've never left me all the way.

MOTHER: We wonder whether they were still going on, but you never said anything.
CLINICIAN: Have they gotten worse?
KEN: Not really. They usually don't bother me too much. Except when I take the bus to work.
CLINICIAN: That's when it's the most uncomfortable?
KEN: Yeah. So I took my last paycheck and bought a tape player with headphones. I wear it on the bus and I don't hear anything.
CLINICIAN: Great idea. It sounds like you feel able to control your symptoms.
KEN: Yeah, I can almost always make them stop.
CLINICIAN: Would you know when they were getting out of control?
KEN: I think so. They're different then, the voices get a lot worse and they say upsetting things.
FATHER: Maybe we have more to worry about than I thought.
CLINICIAN: It is not uncommon for people with schizophrenia to occasionally have symptoms, even after things are going well. Remember, this is a chronic illness and we haven't cured it.
FATHER: I guess we try to forget that.
CLINICIAN: I don't blame you. But as Ken is doing so well, it is possible to get on with your life, even with his schizophrenia. However, it is important to check in regularly.
MOTHER: I think we realize that.
CLINICIAN: Now, what about the two of you?

As in this situation, it is natural for patients, family members, and even clinicians to want to forget past troubles and normalize the situation as soon as possible. While this is a healthy response to a chronically difficult situation, it is important that everyone continue to recognize that the patient has a chronic illness that must be monitored and treated. The clinician makes this point, but then moves on to focus on the parents' issues, so as not to make the patient the center of everyone's concerns or overdramatize the minimal symptoms he has reported.

Termination

Despite the chronicity of this illness, some patients and families choose to terminate treatment. As stated previously it is our belief that any sort of absolute termination from treatment is rarely appropriate. Unfortunately, at this time, there is no cure for schizophrenia. No matter how well patients do, they have an ongoing illness that can have spontaneous recurrences or can be exacerbated by stress. A lifeline to help provides both ongoing support and speedy intervention when needed. However, occasionally patients and their families are determined to try going it alone, and thus deserve the chance to do so.

The clinician's response to such requests should be based on the type of termination being considered. If a patient and family make a unilateral decision to stop family sessions, but the patient is willing to continue in a medication management program, an important link with the system remains which might allow family sessions to be reinstituted if the need arises. Although this type of link may not be an ideal one, since the family is no longer likely to be directly involved in providing feedback regarding medication response or in making treatment decisions, such an arrangement does at least allow a continued monitoring of the patient.

The request to terminate all treatments involves a much greater risk for most patients. First, the patient will no longer have the protection of medication. Even patients who have been stable for a long period of time increase their risk of relapse when they discontinue medication (Hogarty, Ulrich, Mussare, & Aristigueta, 1976). Since several months may pass before patients experience the negative results of medication noncompliance, the patient and the family are likely to have become disconnected from the treatment system. Thus, in general, clinician should make a concerted effort to prevent sudden unilateral decisions to terminate, insisting on discussing the reasons over several sessions, and taking an aggressive stand on the importance of some minimal level of connectedness. In the following example, taken from the final minutes of a final session, the clinician continues to look for a way of maintaining contact.

CLINICIAN: I guess I finally have to accept your message. No more sessions.

FATHER: No, sorry. I know you mean well. . . .

CLINICIAN: I'm out of things I can say to try to convince you otherwise. I have to say again though that I think it's a mistake.

FATHER: (Stiffly) We understand.

CLINICIAN: I don't mean to get you angry at me. It's just that I feel concerned and want things to go well.

FATHER: I know you care. And you've been a big help. We thank you.

CLINICIAN: Okay, no more sessions. But . . . would it be all right with you if I called every so often, just to say hello and see how things are going? After 2 years, I am interested in what's happening.

FATHER: I guess that would be fine.

CLINICIAN: Good.

By focusing on the positive nature of the therapeutic relationship over 2 years, the clinician was able to establish an agreement for very minimal contact. Any sort of follow-up contact is better than none. He can use these "check in" calls to provide a link for patient and family during the time of highest risk, gradually decreasing contact if it does not seem necessary or helpful.

If, despite whatever negotiations the clinician attempts, the patient and family remain firm in their decision to terminate, then it is essential to end treatment with a review of the major problems associated with the illness, the patient's particular prodromal signs, and the strategies that have been developed for coping more effectively. Awareness of the significance of the subtle changes in behavior that may precede episodes helps the patient and family to mobilize the necessary resources before decompensation reaches a point that requires hospitalization. To help facilitate this process, it is important for clinicians to stress that, although termination has occurred, they will remain available to patients and their families should the need arise. Termination of active treatment does not have to mean termination of the therapeutic relationship. Building in phone contact for a period of time following the last session helps to reinforce the clinician's messages of caring and availability.

The following example comes from the termination session with Lois and her family after 2 years of treatment. They were determined to try things on their own. Although the clinician would have preferred a more gradual process, in this case, he was somewhat less worried than the clinician in the previous example.

FATHER: We even had a round table discussion, and we're willing to try it on our own. No sessions—no medication.

CLINICIAN: And everyone agrees?

LOIS: Yes.

MOTHER: Yes.

CLINICIAN: We've know each other a long time, so I feel pretty comfortable that you know how to handle things, but let's review it one more time.

MOTHER: Well, we know what to watch for as signs of trouble.

CLINICIAN: Like . . . ?

FATHER: Well, when she starts to isolate herself.

LOIS: And spend too much time in my room.

MOTHER: And when she starts reading the bible a lot, talking about religion.

CLINICIAN: And what do you do then?

MOTHER: Oh, don't worry, we'll call *fast* if that starts up. We don't want to go through all that again.

CLINICIAN: And, Lois, is it okay if they call?
LOIS: Yes . . . although I may not like it then.
FATHER: Like it or not. . . .
LOIS: I know.
CLINICIAN: All in all, I guess I'd still like to hear from you every now and then for awhile. Would you be willing to check in by phone?
LOIS: Sure.

In this example, the clinician attempted to reinforce everyone's awareness of Lois's prodromal signs. Although Lois currently accepted her illness, during past episodes, she had tended to become both belligerent and less insightful. Thus, some preepisode agreement about how to handle these behaviors was crucial. He also attempted to build in some ongoing contact for a time to give added support.

Helping families and patients to become involved with relevant self-help groups in their area is also very useful. These groups can provide ongoing support and information, while giving patients and families with the opportunity to be helpful to others and even to influence the development of mental health policies. The ability to help and care for others, as any professional knows by personal experience, can in itself be therapeutic because it increases self-esteem and a sense of competence.

Thus far, we have outlined a method of treatment for schizophrenic patients and their families. To give the reader a sense of the way in which patients and their families respond to such a psychoeducational program over time, we will describe the treatment course of two patients: (1) a patient who responded well to the program, gradually moving towards an independent work and social life, and (2) a patient who did not respond well and whose treatment experience eventually ended in relapse and the exacerbation of a chronic course. Each account has been disguised to protect the identities and privacy of these patients and their families. While we believe that this method of intervention has been useful to many, it is not yet clear why some patients and families do as well as they do, while others find the program difficult to follow. Perhaps the reader can begin to find some clues in the following stories.

ANATOMY OF A SUCCESS

Paul entered into the psychoeducational family treatment program at the age of 27. At that time, both he and his family appeared to view the program as just one more hopeless attempt to manage a chronically difficult situation. Eight years and a multitude of approaches to dealing with Paul's illness had resulted in no observable improvement.

Paul is the second oldest of five children from an upper-middle-class family. His father is a self-employed insurance salesman and his mother and one sibling work in the father's business. Two of Paul's siblings are married, have families of their own, and live in another state. The two remaining siblings, Paul, and the parents live together in a suburban community. Paul's parents describe his early development as uneventful with no significant physical or emotional trauma. All in all, they describe him as a healthy, well adjusted, happy child.

Paul's first clear signs of schizophrenia occurred at the age of 19, but his parents describe a deteriorating course for at least four years preceding that time. Up until the tenth grade of high school, he was an average to above average student with a relatively large network of friends. While he was growing up, Paul and his father would talk occasionally about Paul taking over the family-owned insurance business after he finished college. In high school, however, Paul began to associate with a set of friends who were not academically oriented, and who were frequently in trouble. He began to experiment with drugs, eventually stealing from neighborhood homes to pay for these activities.

It was during that time that Paul's parents first brought Paul for professional help, although Paul was against it. The first treatment contact was with a psychologist. Paul's mother, Mrs. M, described her feelings at that time: "We were so relieved. We knew something was wrong but didn't know what to do. And when he told us that Paul was just going through an adolescent rebellion phase, we felt that everything would be okay." Nevertheless, after 5 months of treatment with no significant change in his behavior, Paul dropped out. His parents, though unhappy with this decision, let it stand. As Mrs. M stated, "The psychologist told us Paul refused to cooperate, and that he couldn't help unless Paul's attitude changed."

The family's second treatment experience, and first involvement in family therapy, occurred a year later. Paul's problems had continued to worsen and Mr. M insisted Paul get help. The local mental health center assigned a social worker to the case who began family therapy. Mr. M, years later, still vividly remembers the experience. "We were really torn. Paul was angry that I made him get help, but once we started he loved going and we hated it. I can remember Joyce (his wife) and I getting anxious hours before every session. Every time was the same. Paul would go in with his list of complaints and then this girl, young enough to be our daughter, would support everything he said. We couldn't do anything right. It was clear that she viewed us as the cause of Paul's unhappiness. The worst of it was that we believed her." The family, on Mr. M's insistence, finally stopped going to sessions. As Mr. M simply stated, "I just couldn't take it anymore. The meetings were tearing us up."

Paul had his first significant psychotic episode 2 years later. At that time, his symptoms were characterized by paranoid ideation and extreme withdrawal. He was hospitalized on the psychiatric unit of a local general hospital and diagnosed as having a major depressive disorder. Treatment consisted primarily of the use of antidepressant medications and 14 shock treatments. Upon discharge, the family perceived only minimal changes. Paul refused follow-up outpatient treatment, complaining the the psychiatrists were a part of the plot against him. Between that time and Paul's entrance into the program, Paul had three other psychiatric hospitalizations. During his second hospitalization, his diagnosis was changed to that of paranoid schizophrenia. Various antipsychotic drugs were tried in varying combinations and at varying doses. Paul was involved in individual therapy twice, group therapy once, and finally, attended a hospital day program.

Toward the end of this period, Paul left home and was gone for approximately 18 months. During that time, the family had no contact with him and had no ideas where he was. Mrs. M describes that period: "It was a funny mixture. We were constantly worried about what had happened to Paul. And yet, I hate to say it, but it was also the first time in years that there was peace and quiet." The peace ended when Paul's family received a call from the San Diego police, stating that he was being placed on a plane to come home on the condition that they arrange immediate psychiatric help. Mr. M picked him up at the airport, describing him as "totally disheveled and stinking to high heaven. He couldn't answer my questions. What he said made no sense at all—absolutely none. I mean we had heard his delusions before, but this was different. He was incoherent." When Mr. M took Paul home, Paul's talk was rambling and his behavior bizarre. He refused to eat anything red, and would pace continually, except when hiding behind the living room couch. After 2 days at home, Paul's parents took him to the hospital and committed him against his wishes. Paul was again given the diagnosis of paranoid schizophrenia, and the family was referred to our Schizophrenia Research Project. With much anxiety and doubt, the family became involved in the psychoeducational family program a few days after admission. At intake, Mr. M summarized the results of the 8 years of treatments with a succinct, "Nothing has worked."

During the course of the hospitalization, neuroleptic medications were initiated, and the inpatient unit established the following goals (1) beginning to help Paul gain some control over his symptoms, and (2) engaging Paul in treatment sufficiently to insure at least some chance that he would follow through with the referral to outpatient care. Paul responded slowly but positively to chemotherapy. Nevertheless, by the time of his discharge 4 weeks later, he was still quite symptomatic. His speech was characterized by thought blocking and loose associations. His affect was severely blunted. He was still somewhat paranoid, feeling people were after him because of the robberies he had committed 7 years earlier, and he frequently complained of "voices." The voices, however, made only brief, relatively benign comments. Although he was not particularly enthusiastic about any treatment, he agreed to take medication and to continue in treatment with his family.

This agreement had evolved from multiple "connecting" contacts with the psychoeducational clinician who was scheduled to be primarily involved in Paul's outpatient treatment. The contacts began on the inpatient unit after some of Paul's acute symptoms had abated, initially focusing only on the establishment of a relationship with Paul. Specifically, the family clinician visited Paul on the inpatient unit and had a number of brief conversations with Paul about his background, and particularly the experiences he had had during the preceding 18 months. Although incoherent at times, Paul was enthusiastic about talking about his first experiences away from home. Paul described living on the road, picking up odd jobs, and literally surviving hand-to-mouth. Paul's strength in having survived at all under these extremely difficult circumstances was reinforced. Gradually, these conversations became longer and began to focus on the future and the possible benefits of treatment.

Paul, at first was adamantly against treatment and angry with his parents for having committed him. This opposition was overcome as Paul was able to begin to understand the fear and concern his parents experienced during his absence, their ongoing interest during the roughest of times, and their consistent support during his hospitalization. The consistency of the family's caring messages, coupled with their regular visits, helped to make Paul more receptive to the idea of family treatment. Nevertheless, family treatment was framed not as a way to resolve family conflicts, but as one way of helping Paul to achieve his primary goal of becoming functional enough to make money so that he could eventually leave home permanently. Focusing on the treatment team's ability to help patients to manage life more effectively, including their ability to get him training and a job when he was ready, enabled Paul to view treatment as having a special purpose for him.

Simultaneously, time was spent connecting with Paul's family and convincing them that this type of family treatment would be different from the kind they had experienced before. Although they did not see the family clinician until a few days after the admission, contact was made with them by a member of the research team while they were in the emergency room when Paul was being admitted. Help was offered immediately in the form of support as they were going through the commitment process. Soon after Paul was admitted, the family clinician contacted them to do a family assessment and to explain the policies of the inpatient unit and the initial treatment steps for Paul. The appropriateness of the parents' decision to commit him was reinforced and empathy was expressed for their concerns and anxiety. The clinician offered to be their representative to the unit and suggested beginning a series of family meetings with the purpose of helping Paul. No mention of a long-term treatment contract was made at this time since the family was not ready to make this commitment and the exact direction of Paul's treatment was unclear. Although anxious about meeting as a family, the family did agree to come, especially when they were assured that Paul would not participate as long as he was acutely psychotic. Several sessions were scheduled with Mr. and Mrs. M (as well as two sessions that included Paul's two younger siblings). The purposes of these sessions were multiple: to inform them of Paul's progress; to tell them about treatment plans and to seek their input; to give them an opportunity to express their feelings about his illness and its impact on their lives; to join with them in the role of a helping professional; and to begin to form a treatment contract that would involve their participation over the long haul.

The atmosphere of these initial sessions was positive and collaborative. The family was given an opportunity to review Paul's past treatments as well as their reactions to and involvement in these efforts. As the sessions continued and the family began to feel more comfortable with the clinician, the focus shifted toward the future. It was apparent to the treatment staff, and to Paul's family, that he would be unable to function independently upon discharge. The parents, with much ambivalence, decided that it would be best if Paul returned home. As Mr. M stated, "I couldn't tolerate him living in a rat infested hole. At least if he's home, the basics will be provided for." Paul was agreeable to this plan, though not enthusiastic. With that decision reached, the clinician focused on the importance of collaboration between the family and the treatment team during Paul's recuperation. It was stressed that the purpose of treatment was to help Paul, and that his family was a potentially positive agent of change. The desire to help decrease stress for other family members was also emphasized. Those messages coupled with the family's growing feelings of comfort with the team led them to agree to treatment.

After Paul's symptoms partially abated, he expressed willingness to attend sessions with his family during and after the hospitalization. When Paul joined the family sessions, the sessions began to focus on negotiating a treatment contract. Paul immediately established his goal as "getting money and getting out." The clinician, rather than reinforcing or negating these goals, labeled them as appropriate long-term ones, and then began to focus on the intermediary steps that would be necessary to get Paul to that point. The first step he suggested was a focus on restabilization and recuperation within the home, a step Paul accepted somewhat superficially, complaining he was feeling "very tired." At a subsequent family session, the contractual focus became that of preparing the family to live together again, anticipating potential problems, and establishing the minimal rules for household functioning.

One week before his discharge, Paul's family attended the psychoeducational family workshop. Beforehand, they expressed some reluctance about going since there would be other families there. They were somewhat embarrassed about the issue of mental illness in their family. After receiving some reassurance that the other families were dealing with similar issues, and that they would not have to actively participate, the family agreed to attend. Following the workshop, Mrs. M stated, "It was one of the best things we ever did. For the first time, I feel like I have some understanding about what Paul's been through. Even though I hate to say it, there's also a sense of comfort knowing others have gone through the same thing. This is the first time in 8 years that we have a sense of hope, and of not being alone."

The workshop reinforced the collaborative nature of the treatment relationship and also supplied many of the themes that would be followed and reinforced in treatment. During the session following the workshop, there was a noticeable change in the family's attitude. Topics were discussed more freely and the family was no longer hesitant in sharing concerns or issues. Although he did not attend the workshop, Paul also seemed less belligerent. His parents had discussed with him some of the information they had received about schizophrenia. For the first time, he had asked them a question and began to accept the possibility that he had an illness.

This latter point was significant since Paul had been noncompliant with medication in the past, primarily claiming he didn't need it because he wasn't ill. Although now on an injectable long-acting drug, he had alluded several times to the desire to stop his medicine as soon as possible. During this session, he began to make comments which suggested that he was beginning to see that his medications were necessary.

Following the workshop, Paul and his family began meeting once per week with the family clinician. Each session had a similar structure that afforded predictability and allowed Paul to feel in control and the family's anxiety to continue to ebb. The posthospital sessions had the primary goals of helping Paul to gain better control over his symptoms, to feel comfortable at home, and to help the family readjust to Paul's presence and accept his lack of energy. During this time, the clinician labeled Paul's apparent lack of motivation and interests, as well as the presence of some remaining positive symptoms, as natural sequelae to a psychotic episode. Over time, the family was encouraged to decrease their intense monitoring of Paul and to establish an attitude of "benign indifference" by allowing Paul to set his own pace toward recovery. Tasks were used to help maintain some sense of movement, to build in "times outs" for Paul, and to help the family to accept his occasional withdrawal to his room. At the same time, small tasks were given to encourage Paul to spend a small portion of his day with the family so as not to totally allow him to isolate himself.

During the first year of aftercare treatment, Paul's positive symptoms continued to decrease but his amotivation remained. In fact, his negative symptoms were as severe as those of any patient in the program. Although initially tolerant, 10 months after discharge Paul's parents began to express increased frustration with Paul's seeming lack of willingness to do anything. As his brother, Jack, stated, "He's like a bump on the log. I couldn't sleep as much as he does if I tried." At this time, primarily to give the family a sense of movement, Paul was assigned more tasks that encouraged him to assume some responsibility for chores around the house, such as taking out the garbage or doing lawn work. Paul tended to agree to these tasks during the sessions, but often failed to follow through once he returned home.

In reviewing this period of treatment, the team decided it was in a bind. It could continue to assign tasks, but if they were not completed, the result would be an increase in the family's anger and frustration and an increase in tension between Paul and the team. Stopping the push for Paul to assume more responsibility on the other hand, could tacitly reinforce Paul's lethargy. The team, therefore, began to search for any small piece of data that could constitute leverage for getting positive movement from Paul. The nurse clinician shared her perception that the only time Paul showed anything approaching positive affect was when he discussed the activities he did with his family. After considerable discussion, it was decided to attempt to use this piece of positive data to design a chore-oriented task. At the next session, the family clinician suggested that it was too much to expect Paul to do chores on his own at this point since he did not yet have much initiative. Mr. M was then asked if he would be willing to do a chore with Paul, and he agreed. Paul and his father then discussed what might be a reasonable task they could accomplish before the next session. They decided on trimming the bushes in the yard, with Mr. M taking responsibility for inviting Paul to join him at an appropriate time.

At the next session, the entire family agreed that the task had gone well. Paul and his father had trimmed the bushes and both were pleased about their interaction during this time. This tactic then became the theme for increasing Paul's involvement with the family and eventually for increasing his ability to take greater responsibility. Gradually, more difficult and more independent tasks were assigned. Tasks first involved Paul and his father, then Paul and his brother, moving to Paul working 10 minutes by himself before his father joined him, and finally, Paul initiating and completing a task on his own. Over the next 7 months of biweekly sessions, Paul slowly assumed greater responsibility around the house and became more active within the family. Although progress was extremely slow, in fact at times imperceptible, at the end of 18 months of treatment, Paul and his family were comfortable with each other and with their respective roles and responsibilities in living together. Although Paul's attention span and tolerance for stress remained limited, it was decided that Paul was ready to face the next major step of moving to tasks outside the family.

Paul no longer had any friends in his neighborhood and had not been socially involved outside of his family for several years. Vocationally, Paul had worked at a number of odd jobs before becoming ill, but he had no specific skills and had never stayed at a job for longer than 2 months. Thus, in moving to a focus on these areas, there was no substantial existing base on which to build. After a number of conversations with Paul and his family, it was decided that while both areas were important, Paul's desire to learn to be independent as well as his need for money were a higher priority. Therefore, the development of work related skills was chosen to be the primary focus of the next phase of treatment.

Paul was referred to a local vocational rehabilitation agency. During the referral process the family clinician suggested a meeting with the vocational counselors assigned to Paul. At that meeting the clinical team shared information with the counselors regarding schizophrenia in general, and Paul in particular. His strengths and weaknesses, and especially his sensitivity to stress, were discussed. At the end of the meeting a flexible plan was tentatively formulated which included Paul starting a vocational training program two half-days per week in a mechanically oriented training area. Although the procedures of the vocational program usually involved the simultaneous assignment of several supervisor-counselors, it was agreed that one counselor would take primary responsibility for Paul. This simplified plan allowed Paul greater continuity, and also made it easier to establish collaborative meetings between the two professional teams.

Although the plan was arranged, Paul's start in the program was delayed. Just as he was about to begin, Paul's family mentioned that his younger sister was about to leave home to start college. This involved some stress and readjustment for several family members, and in fact, Paul soon developed a number of prodromal symptoms. Based on the principles of one change at a time. Paul's entry into the vocational program was postponed to insure that he was feeling better and that he and his family had adjusted to the new family structure before adding another possible stress. When, 2 months later, all concurred that the situation had restabilized, Paul spent his first half-day in vocational training. His reaction to that day was: "It was okay. Not as bad as I thought, but am I tired!" He went home and slept for 3 days. Predictably, progress during the course of the vocational program was slow, with gradual increases in the amount of time spent at the rehabilitation center and gradual increases in the complexity of the work tasks in response to Paul's own improvements. Again following the principle of one change at a time, at two points Paul's movement to the next stage of the work program was delayed: once, because Mrs. M became physically ill and required hospitalization, and another time, because Paul joined a social group.

Family sessions continued on schedule of once every 3 weeks during the 14 months Paul was in the vocational program. The foci of these sessions were multiple. Paul and his family continued to refine their awareness about the significance of his prodromal signs and how to deal with them. Paul's maintenance of responsibilities at home was reinforced while care was taken to not increase stress within the family. Paul and his family continued to give the staff feedback about the work program so that alterations could be made to enhance its effectiveness.

The final focus (after 6 months in the vocational program) involved enhancing Paul's social life. With the family's encouragement, Paul asked another participant in his vocational program to go to the movies. The two men went and had a good time. Paul found this so reinforcing that he initiated going bowling with the same man the next week. Paul began to express a greater desire to improve his social life and, following a suggestion by the family clinician, he joined a social organization for people with emotional disorders.

Paul got a job at a local supermarket 14 months after starting the vocational program, and 28 months after discharge from the hospital. Four and a half years later, Paul still works at the same store. He is one of their most dependable employees and has been made head cashier. He has remained involved with the social organization and is currently dating two women. His future plans include moving out of his family's home (a topic only now being discussed in family sessions) and returning to school for training as an auto mechanic. He has not been rehospitalized.

ANATOMY OF A RELAPSE

Jessica was 25 years old when she first entered the psychoeducational treatment program. On entering the hospital voluntarily, Jessica complained of severe auditory hallucinations characterized by voices that said derogatory things about her and ordered that she hurt herself. She was paranoid and continually complained that her family particularly her mother, was against her.

During the 5 years that she had been ill with schizophrenia, she had been hospitalized 15 times in six different private and public hospitals. Her treatments included trials on most neuroleptic drugs, eight shock treatments, several types of psychotherapy, a partial hospital program, and a half-way house. The longest she had been out of the hospital during this entire 5-year period was 7 months.

Jessica was the youngest of five children, the only one still living at home with her parents. Her four brothers, successful businessmen, were all married. Two lived out of state and two lived within a few miles of the parental home. Both Mr. and Mrs. F talked proudly about the closeness of their family and the success of their sons. Their devotion to their daughter was clear, as was the heartbreak they experienced as a result of her illness and its unremitting course. Despite Jessica's illness, family gatherings were common, although Jessica rarely participated in them.

Mr. and Mrs. F were first seen the day following Jessica's hospitalization. They willingly came in for the session and comfortably shared their feelings about Jessica's illness and her treatment experiences. Both were critical of the past efforts of professionals to help her since they had never seen appreciable changes in their daughter's behavior. They particularly focused their anger on those professionals who told them that Jessica shouldn't be allowed to return home. Mr. F stated, "What am I supposed to do, let her walk the streets? Whatever she does, she's our daughter and we have to care for her." The one time Jessica had been placed in a transitional living program she stayed 2 days and returned home at 3:00 in the morning. Neither parent supported her return to the program.

During the course of the initial meeting, both parents expressed a willingness to participate in treatment. As Mrs. F said, "We'll do anything you ask if it will help." At the same time, they also made it clear that they were skeptical that anything would alter the situation. Their skepticism was appropriate and labeled as such. Accepting their ambivalence about the program, the clinician nevertheless asked that Mr. and Mrs. F come in for sessions during their daughter's hospitalization so that they could be kept informed of treatment decisions and give their input into the planning for Jessica's aftercare. Mr. F enthusiastically agreed, and shared his greatest frustration with most treatment systems, that of "never knowing what they were up to" with his daughter.

During the course of the next few sessions, the parents' perceptions of Jessica's problems were discussed. They frequently mentioned their fear that they had caused these problems by "poor parenting." Attempts were made to reassure them of their parenting abilities by emphasizing all they had done to help Jessica, and emphasizing the successful outcome of their parenting with their sons. Although they were repeatedly reassured that they did not cause their daughter's illness, the message was also given that there were probably things that they could do that would help in Jessica's recuperation and recovery. Once again, both parents expressed a willingness to try anything that potentially would help.

Simultaneously, individual contacts were made with Jessica on the inpatient unit. Her symptoms had cleared fairly rapidly after admission to the hospital. She expressed enthusiasm about outpatient treatment as a way of beginning to achieve many of her life goals. At that time, she claimed she wanted to be a song writer and live independently of her family as soon as possible. Treatment was presented as a way of helping her to move slowly toward employment and emancipation. Although upset with the need to move slowly, Jessica expressed a willingness both to participate in family sessions and to take her medication if the eventual goal would be that of emancipation.

Since Jessica's hospitalization lasted only 16 days, the first several of which she was acutely psychotic, only one session involving both her and her family could be held before discharge. During that session, a treatment contract was negotiated which included the long-term goals of employment and independent living and the short-term goals of increased responsibility around the house (as was desired by Jessica). All agreed these were reasonable issues to include in the treatment agenda, and sessions were scheduled to begin on a weekly basis after Jessica's discharge.

While Jessica was still an inpatient, Mr. and Mrs. F attended the psychoeducational workshop with four other families. Mr. F was an active participant, taking copious notes, and asking a number of good questions. Mrs. F participated less actively, but did share many of her frustrations in trying to manage Jessica. Both parents had extremely positive reactions to the workshop, especially commenting on the helpfulness of having a chance to meet other family members with similar problems, and getting "straight answers for the first time in years." During the breaks, they engaged in a number of conversations with other families and exchanged telephone numbers with another couple who were also parents of a chronically ill patient. As Mr. F said, "Other people say how sorry they are, but these people really understand."

On discharge, Jessica immediately became determined to function as though she had never been ill. Thus the initial outpatient family sessions emphasized the need to "slow down." In contrast to Paul who was so completely amotivated in the immediate postpsychotic phase of the illness, each week Jessica would arrive at the family session with a new plan for employment or an ad for an available apartment, and excitedly discuss how she knew she could follow through on each new opportunity. The clinician would respond by labeling each idea as a good one, but emphasizing that it was important that Jessica first be prepared for the demands inherent in working and living independently to insure that the plans would succeed. She stressed the need to develop a routine of getting up at a regular hour, following through on routine tasks and relating appropriately to those around her before moving to these more ambitious life tasks. Having seen so many plans fail in the past, Mr. and Mrs. F were supportive of the "go slow" message. Tasks were assigned that involved Jessica doing chores around the house to operationalize these principles. However, when these tasks were reviewed in subsequent sessions, Jessica would call them "boring" or "stupid," or claim to have just forgotten to do them. The clinician would relabel her noncompliance as Jessica's message that she was not yet ready to take the next step towards independent living.

During these times, Jessica's parents also had great difficulty in following through on the clinician's suggestions to set limits on Jessica's unreasonable behaviors. While insisting that Jessica follow through on any of the tasks that would encourage her to assume increased responsibility, Mrs. F would also continually follow her around the house picking up after her. No consistent limits were placed on Jessica's behavior even when it was obnoxious, despite frequent interventions designed to help the family to do so. For instance, Mrs. F complained that Jessica had no concern for others, giving as an example the fact that Jessica flicked her cigarette ashes all over the floor and furniture, yet Mrs. F would clean up without asking Jessica to help. The clinician tried to increase parental control and Jessica's ability to take responsibility by suggesting to Mr. F that he not buy cigarettes for his daughter until she behaved more responsibly. His response was, "How can I deprive her of one of her few pleasures? She has nothing else."

Both Mr. and Mrs. F were aware of their difficulties in setting limits on their daughter's behaviors and in following through with treatment suggestions. Although apologetic, they stated they were doing the best they could, but that they couldn't ignore their daughter's needs. The positive aspects of their caring were acknowledged, while the need to translate some of this caring into limit setting and structure was emphasized. Pressures to decrease their caretaking behaviors and increase their limit-setting continued. The clinician, admitting that these suggested tasks were extremely difficult, emphasized to the parents that they were necessary sacrifices for their daughter's recovery. Although verbal compliance was obtained, Jessica's parents repeatedly failed to follow through with any part of the treatment plan that required either that they set limits, or be less than constantly available to their daughter. Five months into aftercare treatment, a relatively total impasse was reached.

During the regular meetings of the clinical team, this treatment impasse was discussed in detail. The multiple suggestions made by the clinician had resulted only in increased frustration on the part of both the family and the clinician. No progress was being made although there also had been no increase in psychotic symptoms. After discussing several options, it was finally decided to suggest that other members of Jessica's family attend a session in the hopes that they might offer a greater understanding of how to shift the system in some way, or even be willing to lend support to the requests of the treatment team. When this idea was presented to the family, Mr. and Mrs. F and Jessica readily agreed to have their two sons living in the area come, although Mrs. F stated that they were probably too busy. The clinician called and invited Jessica's two older brothers, and at the next session, Jerry and Ed came with their wives. During the next several months, the addition of these family members proved very helpful. Both of her brothers stated that they perceived that the current level of involvement between their parents and Jessica was not particularly helpful and, in fact, might even be detrimental. They did not think Jessica required the level of parental care she was receiving and they worried about the impact of this stress on the health of their parents. While they stated that their parents were still extremely involved in their lives as well, they felt this involvement was a positive one. After considerable discussion, it was decided that, on a rotating basis, each of the two couples would occasionally provide supervision for Jessica to give their parents "time outs." Once a week, Jessica would spend some time at one of their houses. Everyone agreed that this would give the parents a chance to rest while feeling comfortable that Jessica was safe. These respites also had the added advantage of helping Jessica to get out more, since, although she made multiple plans, she rarely left the house, and never without her mother.

Over the next 10 months of treatment Jessica's two brothers, Jerry and Ed, along with their wives, remained involved in family sessions. When her two other brother's returned for holiday visits, they also attended sessions, participating actively. Significant progress occurred, but very slowly. Jessica became more independent and began to assume a little more responsibility for her own personal hygiene, and for chores about the house. Although she still made grandiose plans, Jessica was more amenable to taking a step-by-step approach toward the achievement of her goals. Her brothers willingly continued to try to act as buffers between Jessica and her parents. Although Mrs. F still complained about her daughter's careless behaviors, she was able to distance somewhat and even to insist that her daughter occasionally wash and iron her own clothes. In time, with encouragement from all of their children, Mr. and Mrs. F planned the first vacation that they had ever taken without their children.

Both parents seemed excited and nervous about the trip with Mr. F stating "we won't know what to do," even though it was only to last 4 days. Three weeks before the planned departure, Mrs. F developed a severe back problem that forced the trip to be cancelled. Over the next 2 months, her physical difficulties continued. She repeatedly missed family sessions complaining of ill health, and her husband reported that hospitalization was being considered. During that time, Jessica stopped spending time with her brothers and stopped going out for any reason, stating "My mother needs me." Although the clinical team continued to urge Jessica to get out of the house, even emphasizing her mother's need for quiet time, Jessica did not manage to follow through on these suggestions during this period. She also began to slip in terms of performing her self-care and her household tasks.

During Mrs. F's recuperation period, she again became much more concerned about Jessica. Simultaneously, Jessica began to act out around the house and to complain of being more bothered by her symptoms than she had been in 17 months. Although her medication was increased and therapeutic contact was increased to two times per week, Jessica's complaints continued to worsen. After 3 weeks (18 months into the program), Jessica, following the orders of the voices, took an overdose of her medication, immediately called for help, and voluntarily signed herself into the hospital.

During the course of the hospitalization, the family clinician continued to meet with Jessica's parents and to act as their representative to the inpatient unit. Despite all of her efforts, the parent's skepticism about the potential benefits of the program had understandably returned, with Mr. F stating, "I guess we knew it wouldn't work. Jessica is just too sick." It was pointed out that Jessica had done extremely well during her time out of the hospital, in fact, better than she had done in the 7 years she had been ill. The clinical team expressed a willingness and interest in continuing to work with her and her family once she restabilized and was able to leave the hospital. Mrs. F responded by saying, "It's just postponing the inevitable."

Although the family agreed to continue treatment following Jessica's discharge, it was evident that their commitment had significantly decreased. Various family members called to cancel appointments and other simply failed to show, some for the first time. When these issues were confronted, they would agree to follow treatment suggestions and attend sessions more regularly. However, their attendance continued to be sporadic, and finally the family terminated treatment. Since that time, 3 years ago, Jessica's illness has developed along an increasingly chronic psychotic course. She has had six hospitalizations in the past 2 years and is currently in a state hospital where she has been for many months, indistinguishable from patients who have been there for years.

SUMMARY

This chapter has described the phase of treatment that occurs after the goals of the basic contract have been reached, that is, after patients have been stabilized at what seems to be their level of optimal functioning. When this has occurred, it is possible to offer patients and their families a number of options. They can begin to work on other issues of their choice; they can gradually move toward less frequent sessions which focus on maintaining the gains that have been achieved; or they can move toward termination. Each of these options has been discussed in detail, including possible additional topics that might be addressed and suggested guidelines for when and how to deal with them appropriately.

For those patients who have been ill for many years, it is generally not advisable to consider termination. Some ongoing supportive contact, however minimal, is recommended since these patients are likely to have periodic exacerbations of their symptoms over the years. At times of crisis, an already existing relationship with professionals makes it possible for patients or their families to get help before things get out of hand, thus possibly preventing the occurrence of full blown episodes. If, for whatever reason, termination must be considered for these patients, it is best conducted in a gradual manner to avoid the stress of sudden change. Patients who have not been chronically ill, on the other hand, deserve a chance to terminate and to try to make it on their own should they desire to do so. Again, it is strongly suggested that this be attempted in a gradual fashion and only after life at home and at work has been stable for some time.

CHAPTER SEVEN

IMPLEMENTATION OF A PSYCHOEDUCATIONAL MODEL: TRAINING AND ADMINISTRATIVE ISSUES

When I came to your training session 2 years ago, the psychoeducational approach seemed clear, simple, and easy to apply. Well, I've been trying to do it at my hospital for quite a while, and I'm not sure what's causing me more trouble, dealing with schizophrenia, or dealing with my hospital system.— *Social worker at a state facility*

The psychoeducational model of family intervention discussed in this book is designed to be relatively simple and straightforward. Nevertheless, the approach is not always easy to implement. Not only is schizophrenia a complex illness about which most mental health professionals have firmly established attitudes and practices, but most psychiatric systems do not emphasize any type of sustained contact with families of patients. Furthermore, the frustration inherent in working with patients who are chronically ill requires professionals with skills that many psychiatric systems have not tended to value or even recognize.

In this chapter we will address these issues by discussing how clinicians should be selected, and by making recommendations for a program of training and supervision. Finally, we will examine the systems issues that are raised by attempts to implement a psychoeducational model in hospitals and clinics not accustomed to involving families.

SELECTION OF CLINICIANS

The interventions of a psychoeducational approach can be conducted by psychiatrists, psychologists, social workers, or psychiatric nurses. In fact, in selecting clinicians for this work, their professional degree is less important than relevant past experience, along with certain personality traits and attitudes toward patients and families. More

294

specifically, two types of past professional experience are crucial: experience working with schizophrenic patients and experience working with families.

Without experience in dealing with the realities associated with the course of schizophrenia, clinicians will often have unrealistic expectations and goals. When progress is not consistent and rapid, they tend to respond with frustration. They either become angry, viewing patients as resistant, lazy, and uncooperative, or they become discouraged, questioning their own skills and abilities. Furthermore, clinicians who have been trained to emphasize short-term contracts with the goal of producing rapid change tend not to be satisfied working with this population. While change does occur, the process requires careful timing, patience, and long periods of waiting. In fact, changes that can be viewed as genuine progress with this population often would be considered insignificant in therapy with a less impaired population. For these reasons, trainees should be selected who not only understand what it means to work with a chronically ill population, but who also have a great deal of patience. Naturally, the development of realistic expectations can be addressed in the training process, but it is far easier if training can begin with the assumption that the clinicians involved have a basic acceptance and understanding of the problems inherent in dealing with schizophrenia at more than an intellectual level.

It is also helpful if clinicians have had some experience working with families. It is difficult enough to learn to help families of schizophrenic patients, without simultaneously having to become comfortable and competent in dealing with families in general. If possible, therefore, training programs should try to select clinicians who have an understanding of the interrelatedness of events and behaviors in family systems, as well as an acceptance of the active and central role clinicians must play in family treatment. It particularly helps if clinicians have achieved some level of comfort with being directive. This model of intervention requires active limit setting with patients who are sometimes psychotic and often in serious crisis. It involves getting very upset family members to go along with suggestions that may not make sense to them. The potential for exacerbating already existing stress and chaos is great unless clinicians can take charge by providing direction and specific help to both patients and families.

It is important also to recognize that certain attitudes are likely to interfere with the development of the collaborative working relationship required by this model. In particular, attitudes reflecting a lack of respect for the relevance of families, as well as those reflecting a tendency to blame families cause major problems in the initial process of connecting, and later in the use of this connection for the best interests of the patient. Lack of respect for both the strengths and problems of patients' families is most common in clinicians with backgrounds in a primarily individual model of psychiatric care. These clinicians tend to place so much emphasis on the individual that they see the family only as a resource for information about, or support for, the patient. Professionals with an individual orientation, be it biological or psychodynamic, often find it difficult to believe that families can be relevant, much less an asset, in the treatment of patients. The "real" treatment, they believe, is accomplished with the patient. Clinicians with a strict biological orientation emphasize the effects of medication, while those with a psychodynamic orientation emphasize the corrective effects of the one-to-one treatment relationship and increasing patients' understanding of why they behave as they do.

Clinicians coming from a family therapy background, on the other hand, tend to have more problems with the issue of blame. Despite their claims of accepting a systems perspective, their view is often limited to seeing the impact of families on patients. They tend to see families as disturbed and destructive, either as the cause of the illness, or in need of maintaining the illness for their own survival. For instance, one such family therapist recently responded to a presentation of this model by commenting, "Your model seems to work fine for the families on your tapes because they are not resistant, but what do you do with the families most of us see who don't want treatment and have a *need* to keep the patient 'sick'?" Attitudes such as these promote an accusatory stance that is inevitably communicated to family members, who, not surprisingly, become resistant. It is also not surprising that professionals with these attitudes are not particularly receptive to learning a psychoeducational approach. What good could it do to support families and teach them other ways of responding to the patient if families "need" to respond the way they do to preserve a precarious family system? When clinicians are this skeptical about the usefulness of the basic tenets of this approach, they are less able to deal effectively with the inevitable problems families encounter as they attempt to accept the program and implement the suggestions made in sessions. Furthermore, families are less likely to follow suggestions that tend to be made with a tentative or even hopeless attitude. For these reasons, it is particularly important to select clinicians who believe in the importance of family involvement in treatment, yet who do not have tendencies to blame the family for the patient's problems.

In screening potential clinicians for a psychoeducational program, objective criteria can be used to evaluate the level and type of prior experience. Screening for the right attitudes and belief systems is somewhat more difficult. In general, it helps to ask about the clinician's beliefs about the cause(s) of mental illness, what treatments they have viewed as of value in the past, and what they see as the rights and responsibilities of both professionals and families. Their beliefs and assumptions, as well as the firmness with which they hold to them, can reveal how compatible their views are with those of a psychoeducational approach, and also how flexible and receptive they are to new information.

TRAINING AND SUPERVISING STAFF

The training of clinicians must cover three areas in order for them to successfully implement this type of family intervention. Specifically, they must be provided with: (1) comprehensive information about schizophrenia, including theories of etiology and information about diagnosis, course, and outcome, (2) information about the needs, problems, and perspectives of families with a mentally ill member, and (3) specific therapeutic skills of use in helping patients and families to deal with their special problems of living with chronic illness.

Even when it is possible to recruit clinicians who have experience working with schizophrenic patients, these clinicians rarely have an adequate understanding of the illness or an up-to-date awareness of recent theories, research results, and treatments. In fact, the interventions of clinicians are most likely to be based on intuition, their original, and thus often obsolescent training, or past experiences that may or may not have been successful.

Therefore one of the first tasks of a training program should be to help clinicians master as much information as possible about the illness and to increase their appreciation of how much is *not* known. While incomplete knowledge can create difficulties at all stages of treatment, incorrect information is worse. Clinicians should be given relevant data about the symptoms, course, and prognosis of the illness, along with the mechanisms of action, effects, and side effects of psychotropic medication. Clinicians must come to understand this information well enough to be able to present the material to families in an understandable way and to make it relevant to their experience and management of the patient. Without this knowledge base, clinicians cannot establish their credibility as experts and may thus impede their ability to be effective facilitators of change. The clinician's need for a sound knowledge base is critical since many families, in attempting to understand the patient and to learn how to help, will have obtained some information about the illness from the literature or from other professionals. In other words, clinicians may encounter very well informed consumers. Even those families who are not particularly well informed about theory and research will have accumulated a great deal of firsthand knowledge over the years. If what clinicians tell them does not fit with and go beyond what they have read or experienced, the information, and perhaps the whole psychoeducational program, will be viewed with skepticism. If clinicians cannot provide satisfactory answers to the questions of family members, not only will these family members become less confident about the program, but clinicians themselves will tend to become defensive and thus not able to be as helpful as they could otherwise be.

Finally, without a good understanding of the illness, clinicians themselves tend to have problems accepting the goals and premises of this treatment program and of the therapeutic behaviors that it requires of them. For instance, unless clinicians know something about the usual course of the illness and the usual rates of relapse, the treatment goals will seem unnecessarily limited. Furthermore, without understanding the patient's problems with overstimulation and amotivation, clinicians may tend to push for a rapid reintegration into community life as soon as the overt symptoms of the psychosis abate. Developing an understanding of what is know about schizophrenia helps clinicians to accept the fact that schizophrenia is a chronic illness for which there is no known cure, and accept the fact that all treatments for schizophrenia have their limitations. Thus, unlike some of the less severe problems treated in various types of psychotherapy, clinicians must learn that success cannot be defined as the elimination of all problems and symptoms. They must learn that, as in the course of all chronic illnesses, there are likely to be periodic exacerbations of symptoms and, of course, the continual possibility of relapse. Thus, it is advisable to begin to help clinicians to define success as the reintegration of patients into their communities within the limits of their functional capabilities, and as the decrease of stress for those who care about the patients' wellbeing.

It is not only an awareness of all of these facts, however, that establishes the credibility of clinicians. Family members also are likely to challenge any clinician who does not have some understanding of what *they* have been through. Clinicians must be helped to develop an enhanced sensitivity to what it means to family members to have someone they care about develop schizophrenia, and to what it means to live with this illness. Sensitivity to these issues is important in the development of attitudes that facilitate the process of connecting and maintaining a working alliance with family members. To maintain credibility with these families, clinicians must not only allow a free and open exchange of information and give up attempts to appear omnipotent, but they must also know about and be willing to discuss the pains and problems of coping with a chronic illness. This type of openness with families is a new skill for many clinicians and one that is not easily acquired.

Finally, clinicians must develop the specific skills necessary for working with families with a seriously ill and disruptive member. In particular, clinicians must be helped to develop skills in the areas of connecting with these families, obtaining a treatment contract, imparting information, avoiding and/or overcoming resistance, controlling sessions, assigning tasks, maintaining an appropriate pace and direction, and providing ongoing support. Since most of these skills have been discussed in various chapters of this book, they will only be dealt with briefly within the description of model training programs. However, it must be stressed again that although many of these basic skills should be present in any family oriented clinician, their application to these families tends to differ due to the chronic, complex, and often discouraging nature of schizophrenia and the resultant weariness of both families and professionals.

DESCRIPTION OF A MODEL TRAINING PROGRAM

Although an orientation to this treatment model can be conducted in many ways, the training program described here is based on the concept of a week-long (5-day) seminar that attends to each of the phases of treatment. The time allotted to the training program is, of course, arbitrary. It could easily be longer if time and resources are available. For instance, it might be very useful to spend 2 days on each topic, with more case examples, videotapes, and role-playing. The training could also be conducted in smaller blocks of time over a longer period, dependent on the availability of staff and the needs of the program. Thus, this outline is intended only as a tentative guide. The training goals related to each phase of treatment are noted in Tables 7-1 through 7-5, while the topics and tasks of each segment of training are summarized in Table 7-6. Each session is then discussed in greater detail.

Session I: The Experience of Schizophrenia for the Patient and Family

This portion of training should facilitate the development of positive attitudes and behaviors toward patients and families and, therefore, is essentially "consciousness raising" in nature. Experiences must be provided that enable clinicians to understand a number of issues: (1) the problems typically encountered by these patients and their families in various stages of the illness, (2) the power of families to influence the patient's behavior, and (3) the potential benefits that can be gained from a psychoeducational approach.

TABLE 7-1

Training goals for the connecting phase of treatment

1. Learn the importance of early contact with family members *during* the initial crisis.
2. Learn to focus on the problems and needs of family members, in addition to the problems and needs of the patient.
3. Learn how to relate to patients during hospitalization (or the acute phase of the illness).
4. Learn to gather information in a supportive and nonaccusatory way (learn to focus on strengths as well as problems).
5. Learn to specifically disavow a family etiology belief system.
6. Learn to perform the role of family representative (transmittal of treatment information and plans to families and communication of family concerns to staff).
7. Learn to develop a treatment contract which includes the length of treatment, frequency of sessions, what can be expected, and the establishment of mutual, specific, and attainable goals.
8. Learn to expect and deal with initial resistance to treatment.

Several types of experiences are recommended for increasing the clinician's sensitivity to the problems of patients and their families. Clinicians may be exposed to the growing body of literature that describes these problems. In addition to literature written by and for professionals, there are many recent articles and books by patients and families that give eloquent descriptions of their personal experiences of mental illness. A listing of some of the articles and books that can be used as assigned readings is included in Appendix A.

Videotapes can be an even more powerful learning experience. Particularly useful are tapes of patients and families describing the impact of the illness and of treatment. Having the opportunity to watch patients and families describe how the illness has affected their

TABLE 7-2

Training goals for the survival skills workshop

1. Learn techniques that help to convince families of the importance of the workshop—why they should come.
2. Learn techniques that create a relaxed, open atmosphere within the workshop.
3. Learn information to be communicated, and how to communicate it.
4. Learn facilitating techniques that help families to ask questions of staff.
5. Learn to state themes repetitively, particularly thoses that communicate that the family is not to blame, that this is an illness, and that there is something they can do to make things better.
6. Learn to make connections between didactic material and the specific problems of families (use of relevant examples).
7. Learn possible coping mechanisms for problem behaviors associated with schizophrenia (violence, rituals, suspicion, etc.).
8. Learn to help families to talk with other families.

TABLE 7-3

Training goals for the reentry and application phase of treatment

1. Learn techniques for maintaining ongoing cooperative relationships with family members and patients.
2. Learn to respect and respond to the pace of the patient and the family.
3. Learn to establish treatment priorities and stick to them.
4. Learn to translate problems into small steps, small tasks.
5. Learn techniques of task development, assignment, review, revision.
6. Learn techniques of controlling sessions, taking a stand, establishing rules.
7. Learn team management techniques (coverage, division of responsibility, consistent messages, etc.).
8. Learn to avoid a focus on insight, dynamics, interpretations.
9. Learn to support the patient and family in coping with negative symptoms over time.
10. Learn to assess and cope with resistances to treatment and change (especially medication compliance issues).

lives can give prospective psychoeducational clinicians a beginning appreciation of the fears and problems of patients, as well as the anxiety, pain, and sadness that occurs in family members when a loved one develops schizophrenia. They can also begin to appreciate the tremendous strength that has been needed to cope with these issues, sometimes over a period of many years. These descriptions can also help clinicians to be aware of the negative effects that well-meaning professionals may have had on patients and families over the years.

No other learning experience is ever as powerful as actually talking to patients and families about their particular issues. For this reason, it is invaluable to invite one or more family members and/or patients to actually participate in the orientation of new clinicians. If there is not a family member within a particular treatment system who is

TABLE 7-4

Training goals for the social and vocational rehabilitation phase of treatment

1. Learn to gradually increase pressure for more functional behavior on the part of patients.
2. Learn to establish links with vocational and social programs in the community.
3. Learn techniques for involving patients successfully in vocational and social programs.
4. Learn to apply the principles of the family program to work on training settings.
5. Learn to redefine false starts and failures less negatively.
6. Learn to help patients and families to cope with residual symptoms without sacrificing the ability to function.
7. Learn ways of helping family members to connect or reconnect with support systems external to the family.

TABLE 7-5
Training goals for the final stages of treatment

1. Learn how to renegotiate a contract to deal with other family issues.
2. Learn when and how to establish a maintenance contract.
3. Learn how to establish an appropriate pace toward emancipation or separation between family members.
4. Learn technique of "letting go" gradually as a clinician.
5. Learn to encourage an institutional transference and to maintain an open door.
6. Learn to make patients and families aware of their own strengths and abilities to manage the illness, with the use of professionals only as needed.
7. Learn to connect patients and families with other resources (self-help groups, etc.).

willing to participate, it is sometimes possible to arrange a speaker through one of the self-help groups that have organized in many communities. In some locations, ex-patient organizations even have speaker's bureaus that can offer this service (Lovejoy, 1984). If this experience cannot be provided within the training program itself, clinicians may be able to attend meetings of self-help groups and/or talk to patients and families informally. In general, it is best for the training program to take the initiative in arranging these experiences since the anxiety common in clinicians new to this model may cause them to delay or avoid such encounters with patients and their families.

Finally, experiential exercises may help to stimulate increased empathy and understanding in those clinicians who tend to maintain a careful emotional distance from patients and families. For instance, trainees can be asked to think about someone for whom they have a special attachment, and then to imagine and discuss what it would be like to have that person develop a severe mental illness that lasted for years. They could be encouraged to share the feelings they believe they would have about such an experience, along with the feelings they think they would have about the usual practices and behaviors of the professionals they might encounter. It can be enlightening to ask trainees to consider what it would be like to be a patient or family member under their own care, and what they think their reactions would be to their own therapeutic style and interventions. Forcing this shift in perspective can provide dramatic insights for clinicians about their impact on their clients.

To help clinicians gain a better understanding of family systems issues, especially the interrelatedness of family behaviors and events, some reading of the family therapy literature is useful. Articles must be selected carefully, however, since many implicitly blame families for the difficulties of patients, and thus can encourage or exacerbate a blaming attitude toward families. This literature can also cause less experienced clinicians to want to explore "interesting" dynamics and processes that should be largely bypassed when working within this model, especially in the early stages of treatment. The most helpful readings, therefore, tend to be those with a concrete practical focus emphasizing structural or problem-centered approaches (Alexander & Parsons, 1982; Epstein & Bishop, 1980; Minuchin, 1974; Minuchin & Fishman, 1981; Pinsof, 1983). Although strategic family interventions should not be incorporated into the model, some of the specific techniques of the strategic approach can be helpful. For instance, the skills of "positive connotation" and "circular interviewing" described by Selvini-Palazzoli and her colleagues (1980) are useful for clinicians who are learning to explore family issues in a nonaccusatory manner.

The final task of this training session, that is, creating an awareness of the potential benefits that can result from a psychoeducational approach, can be accomplished in two ways. First, clinicians can be

TABLE 7-6
Topics and tasks of a model training program

	Topic	Teaching method
Session I (day 1)	The experience of schizophrenia for the patient	Lecture, readings of first-hand accounts, videotapes (Chapter 1)
	The experience of schizophrenia for the family	
	Introduction to principles of psychoeducation	
Session II (day 2)	Information about schizophrenia	Literature, mock workshop (Chapter 3)
	Information about coping with schizophrenia	
	Workshop techniques	
Session III (day 3)	Connecting strategies	Lectures, videotapes, role play (Chapter 2)
	Review of patient's history	
	Review of patient's treatment	
	The role of ombudsman	
	Treatment contracts	
Session IV (day 4)	Early Aftercare issues	Lectures, videotapes, literature (Chapter 4)
	The use of tasks in treatment	Lecture, videotapes, role play, literature (Chapter 4)
Session V (day 5, A.M.)	Vocational issues	Literature, videotapes, role play (Chapter 5)
	Social reintegration	
Session VI (day 5, P.M.)	Emancipation, marital and other family issues	Videotapes, role play, literature (Chapter 6)

assigned articles that describe the encouraging results produced by
programs that provide education or skills training to similar patients
and their families (e.g., Anderson *et al.*, 1980; Berkowitz, Kuipers,
Eberlein-Vries, & Leff, 1981; Falloon, Boyd, McGill, Strang, & Moss,
1981; Falloon, Liberman, Lillie, & Vaughn, 1981; Goldstein, 1981;
Goldstein *et al.*, 1978; Leff & Vaughn, 1985; Liberman, Aitchison, &
Falloon, 1979; Snyder & Liberman, 1981).

Second, clinicians can be shown edited videotapes that demonstrate
the progress that occurs in patients and families over the course of
treatment. The opportunity to see actual changes in patients over
time can be a powerful tool in establishing the credibility of the approach.
Clinicians who have been exposed to tapes which have been edited
to include excerpts from several years of treatment, are more likely
to become convinced that the model is effective, and thus are more
likely to be able to communicate its potential benefits to families and
patients.

Session II: Information about Schizophrenia/Coping

The manner in which information about schizophrenia and its
management is transmitted to families is crucial, and requires special
attention and skill on the part of the clinicians. A great deal of information is provided during the survival skills workshop, so clinicians
should be specifically prepared to handle this important event.

While knowledge about schizophrenia is vital to clinicians who
must design, conduct, and/or participate in educational workshops,
knowledge alone is not sufficient to make these workshops successful.
In training, an overemphasis on the information provided, without
consideration of the impact of other aspects of these workshops, would
misrepresent the psychoeducational model. Providing information
alone, or providing information in combination with suggested coping
mechanisms, would probably be insufficient to encourage and maintain
changes in the behaviors of families or patients. In fact, information
alone could intensify feelings of hopelessness by overwhelming family
members with the complexity of schizophrenia. Furthermore, as stated
in Chapter 3, it is our clinical impression that most families leave the
workshop having a beginning grasp of the patient's problems with
stimulation and amotivation rather than an understanding of the role
of neurotransmitters or the complex and sometimes contradictory
information inherent in genetic studies. Even for those who do understand and recall the specifics of the scientific information, it is
questionable whether this is what is useful about the workshop experience.

Generally, families report that what they take away from this
experience is an increased awareness of several general themes: a

family member has an illness that is rooted in biological or cerebral dysfunction; he or she is not to blame for its occurrence; there is hope for the future since new discoveries are being made constantly about the illness and its treatment; the patient cannot control his or her illness and, therefore, is neither lazy nor malicious when symptomatic; while other family members need not center their lives around the patient, they can be helpful by temporarily removing pressure to perform or actively participate in family life; and many other reasonable families are struggling with similar problems. Thus, it is these themes that clinicians must learn to value and emphasize. This is not to say that providing concrete scientific data is not important. All families deserve access to this information. They may not always remember specific facts, but the manner in which information is presented can enable families to judge the competence of staff and to decide whether or not to cooperate with the program.

Because the workshop is important in establishing the relationship between families and staff, the method of presentation can be as important as the information itself. The climate of the workshop can set the stage for making family members a part of the treatment team and for helping families to accept new techniques for managing patients and their lives together. This same climate can then be maintained throughout treatment as information and management techniques are continually shared in a noncritical manner, making it easier for family members to try alternative methods of dealing with one another and the patient. For this reason, clinicians must learn to create an atmosphere that is relaxed and informal, a context within which the staff can begin to demonstrate respect for the opinions and coping abilities of family members.

To create this atmosphere, the clinician must learn the therapeutic skills of maintaining a nonjudgmental stance, using easily understandable concepts and terms, and maintaining a repetitive emphasis on certain key points (i.e., that the patient's illness is a serious one, that it takes time to recover, and that the family is not to blame). The easiest way to teach these skills is for prospective psychoeducational clinicians to actively participate in a workshop. This can be accomplished in at least two ways: A workshop can be given to families as trainees observe; or a workshop can be run *as if* it were being given to family members. In either case, experienced clinicians can serve as role models for trainees. It is not enough, however, to simply allow trainees to observe either real or simulated workshops. Trainees must understand how and why the workshop is organized as it is.

Without knowing the assumptions and premises of the workshop, many trainees attempt to duplicate the information portion without grasping the essential philosophy or the importance of the process. In particular, emphasis should be placed on *why* information is conveyed in the way it is, and how specific structural aspects of the workshop act to promote interaction and the free exchange of information and ideas. More specifically, trainees should be helped to understand why patient descriptions of their own experiences are used, why detailed biological explanations are given, why descriptions of normal coping mechanisms precede suggestions for coping with schizophrenia, and so on (see Chapter 3). Offering the opportunity for beginning clinicians to play a teaching role in subsequent workshops helps to further their understanding of the material while beginning to develop their leadership skills and solidifying their knowledge base.

Session III: Connecting with Families

While all family therapists must learn to form a therapeutic alliance with the families they treat, there are special skills the psychoeducational clinician must develop in this regard. Trainees should be helped to see that the connecting process with the families of schizophrenic patients is complicated by the nature of the illness and its treatment. Specifically, because the illness is a chronic one which is incompletely understood, these families usually will have had years of negative experiences with treatments and professionals of various sorts. They are, therefore, likely to be resistant, angry, and hopeless as well as unusually sensitive to any implied criticism of their behaviors.

For these reasons, clinicians must be trained to respond quickly to families, maximizing the opportunities provided by a crisis to prove to families that they can be useful in some way. To be able to gain a family's trust, clinicians must be trained to communicate care, support, and acceptance by eliciting and responding to the views and concerns of family members. It is important to offer specific training in asking nonjudgmental questions about the patient's illness and the past attempts to cope with it, as well as the family's perceptions of their own current needs and problems. Most importantly, however, clinicians must be trained to handle anger and resistance without taking it personally, while at the same time continuing to reach out to family members. They must be helped to learn to deal appropriately with anger and criticism relating to past treatments, and to handle any anger that is currently being directed at them or other members of the team.

In this model of intervention, clinicians also connect with families by becoming the family's representative to the rest of the treatment system. This part of the connecting role requires special training as well, since it is easy for clinicians to become involved in defending one part of the system against another. For instance, clinicians can easily become angry at the treatment system for not dealing appropriately with families, or for failing to give families the information they require. Conversely, clinicians can become angry or defensive with those families who seem to provoke physicians or nurses or who reject reasonable treatment plans, putting them in an awkward, defensive position with their colleagues. To prepare clinicians to handle the role of family representative, training must emphasize skills in diplomacy and in demonstrating respect for families, other professionals, and other treatments. Training must also stress the need to involve everyone in a step-by-step decision-making process that should include an extended discussion of the tension inherent in the clinician's role as buffer between two systems (the treatment team and the family), neither of which is consistently happy with the other. Since this role in any system is not an easy one, clinicians should be prepared for the problems that they will face.

To be equipped to handle the connecting phase of treatment, trainees must also be taught skills that will enable them to arrive at a treatment contract with families which roughly specifies the goals, content, length, rules, and methods of the psychoeducational family program. The contracting skills specific to the treatment of this population primarily involve the ability to translate the overwhelming problems of this illness into specific, attainable, and mutual goals which can be accomplished in the time allotted. These skills are based upon a genuine understanding of the problems and deficits created by the illness, and a realistic awareness of what can be done about them. Clinicians must be trained to maintain a careful balance between offering families hope and not promising the unattainable. In particular, clinicians must be taught never to promise, or even imply, that it is possible to cure the illness, *only* that it *may* be possible to alter its course and to diminish the frequency or intensity of crises. This latter point is an important one since offering too much hope can create as many difficulties as offering no hope. Clinicians must be helped to understand the patients, families, and professionals who form unrealistic expectations about the patients' abilities can magnify the significance of temporary symptoms or temporary setbacks. This magnification, in and of itself, can increase stress and lead the patient and family into a downward spiral, rather than toward restabilization, and it can decrease appreciation for any actual small gains that have been made.

To develop contracting skills, clinicians should be exposed to videotapes, discussion, and role play. In these experiences, trainees should be taught that contract negotiations usually must be preceded by an open discussion of the family's healthy skepticism about the program and about the patient's chances of living more comfortably with his or her illness. In addition, clinicians must be taught how to explicitly delineate short- and long-term goals. Both patient and family are more likely to be able to maintain a sense of progress if they occasionally can see that some specific goals, however small, have been attained. Clinicians must be helped to use these small positive experiences to help families and patients to believe that eventually the larger goals on the agenda will be addressed.

In general, the art of skillfully formulating an appropriate contract evolves with experience. However, early training in contracting, coupled with an understanding of the illness, can begin to help trainees to help families and patients establish reasonable priorities and sequential goals (e.g., increased ability to function at home before beginning job training). Furthermore, clinicians can be taught to use contracts as general guides to decide when to push for more (i.e., when it is necessary to counteract the patient's and/or family's sense of hopelessness) and when to tone down aspirations (i.e., when they seem unrealistic and doomed to fail).

Finally, training in connecting skills would be incomplete without some attention to helping clinicians to learn how to deal with initial resistances. In this model, a good deal of potential resistance is avoided by the way in which families are approached and the focus of the sessions. For instance, connecting with family members by listening, empathizing, and being of practical help in a time of crisis makes resistance less likely. The fact that the focus of sessions is on sharing both information and pragmatic management techniques, rather than on eliciting highly personal, emotional material, also tends to decrease anxiety and resistance. Nevertheless, initial resistances occur often enough that clinicians should be prepared to deal with them effectively. With sufficient preparation, clinicians can learn to engage even very resistant families.

Training, therefore, should emphasize diminishing initial resistances by learning to demystify treatment by being very explicit about what will be done and how it will be accomplished. Since most people fear the unknown, and most people don't know what to expect of a treatment program, this sort of information is particularly important. Clinicians must also be taught that if families remain skeptical about committing themselves to treatment after such information has been shared, they must walk a fine line between imposing unwanted treatment on families and providing a family with a chance to make a genuinely *informed decision* to accept or reject this particular form of professional help. To handle these situations, clinicians should be taught to offer trial contracts of shorter duration where the primary purpose is simply to prove the goodwill and skill of the treatment team. The experience of the authors would suggest that a positive decision about treatment is more likely if clinicians can learn to convince families to attend the workshop, since it is a powerful forum within which to demonstrate the competence of the clinical team and the possible benefits of the psychoeducational approach. Clinicians can be trained to involve families in the workshop by presenting the positive aspects of the workshop, offering families the opportunity to come with the assurance that there will be no pressure to participate verbally, sharing the positive responses of other families to past workshops, and even promising that if they are not "sold" after attending a workshop, they will not be pursued further.

In addition to the need to learn to handle initial family resistance to becoming involved in the patient's treatment, some attention to handling resistance to change is also essential. Clinicians must learn to work with families who fear change, and who are apprehensive that new behaviors may make things even worse. These fears can be partly allayed by teaching clinicians to work toward the family's goals at the family's pace and by helping clinicians to be more comfortable in dealing with resistance directly. While it is not a major problem when using this model, a wide range of techniques for mastering resistance should be made available to clinicians so that they feel comfortable with families and do not become defensive when it happens to occur (Anderson & Stewart, 1983). Resistance caused by fear and skepticism, for instance, can sometimes be overcome by an emphasis on the time-limited nature of the treatment contract. Thus, clinicians can be taught to say, "You've tried it your way for 7 years and it hasn't gotten better, give us just 1 year. You can always go back to what you are doing now."

Videotapes can be used extensively to demonstrate and teach the techniques of connecting and responding to resistances. However, while simply seeing tapes of families and patients as they progress is of value in changing attitudes, videotapes must be used differently to teach these specific skills. If clinicians not familiar with this model of intervention simply watch a tape of a family session, they tend to feel that not much is happening. They fail to see the significance of the clinician's interventions (or *lack thereof*), or they may feel that this type of treatment is simple. Videotapes, therefore, teach little unless they are accompanied by explanations of *why* clinicians behaved as they did at given points in time. In the course of the teaching sessions, therefore, tapes should be stopped frequently and the trainees asked to comment on what they are seeing and to relate the intervention used to the underlying theory of the model. The training should also stimulate a discussion of feelings about the process of therapy. As time goes on, trainees can be encouraged to design appropriate interventions for the families they are observing on tape before they actually view the ones used by the clinician.

Session IV: Early Aftercare Issues

The training that will enable clinicians to deal effectively with the early outpatient phase of treatment should begin with a comprehensive description of the most common problems encountered in the first year after an acute episode of a psychotic illness. This is important since relatively inexperienced clinicians often focus on the impact of the more dramatic psychotic symptoms of schizophrenia and minimize or underestimate the impact of the negative symptoms that often characterize the first year of recuperation. Understanding that symptoms such as amotivation and disinterest are a significant part of the illness prevents clinicians from viewing patients as willfully malingering or resistant to treatment. An awareness of these problems also helps to increase clinician sensitivity to subtle changes in patients that may indicate an increase in their ability to tolerate greater pressure to function more adequately. To be able to help families during this phase, clinicians must also have a full understanding of the impact of living not only with the patient's bizarre behaviors, but also with his or her bland affect, amotivation, and lethargy. Without an appreciation of the impact of these symptoms, clinicians may tend to be too critical of occasional impatience on the part of family members, or insufficiently supportive of them during this frustrating time.

Other themes that clinicians must learn to handle during this training session include: the natural tendency of family members to overmonitor the patient for fear of another crisis; the patient's desire to discontinue medication prematurely; the desire of patient and families to forget the illness (particularly after a patient's first episode); the patient's general isolation and withdrawal; and, of course, the possibility of the reemergence of symptoms. When clinicians are taught to expect these phenomena, they are less likely to overreact when they occur.

There are a minimum of five core skills that clinicians must learn and develop for use during this phase of treatment. These include skill in controlling sessions, assigning tasks, translating problems into small steps, providing genuine support, and dealing with resistance to change.

Controlling Sessions

Using a family model in working with any sort of severely distrubed patient requires clinicians to be in control of sessions and able to set firm, consistent limits. Without controls, family sessions can become chaotic. Since many clinicians, especially those trained in individual therapy, are unaccustomed to being directive or controlling, the development of these skills requires unusual attention and a repetitive emphasis during training. One way clinicians can be taught to maintain control in sessions is through the use of the treatment contract described earlier. Throughout the course of treatment, the contract can be used to give both clinicians and families a map to follow, defining appropriate topics for sessions in given phases of the illness. For instance, by learning to remind patients and families of the contract, clinicians can more easily limit tangential discussions and untimely topics. They can also use the contract to emphasize the priorities that were established by mutual agreement, in order to postpone goals that are too ambitious (i.e., a move to an apartment or a new job) until success is achieved in accomplishing smaller tasks (i.e., getting up in the morning, doing chores around the house, etc.).

Even when clinicians have learned to carefully structure sessions and use the treatment contract, however, it is possible that patients could become psychotic or threaten violence within sessions. Thus, clinicians also must be taught other methods of limit setting and controlling inappropriate behaviors. If patients or family members cannot accept such limits, clinicians must be taught how to stop an out of control session, and how to reschedule it for a time when everyone is under better control. As time goes on, the need for clinicians to control psychotic behaviors within therapy decreases, but the ability to keep things under control and the ability to set limits remains important. For instance, throughout the course of treatment, clinicians must be able to set limits on plans that are too ambitious, or plans that may threaten the stability of the patient or treatment alliance. When a recently discharged patient seeks permission to hitchhike across the country, clinicians must not only learn to firmly refuse, but to help family members to understand and support this stand. These limits are necessary to enable effective treatment to occur, and clinicians must learn to handle them in an unprovocative manner that does not threaten the collaborative relationship. Again, it is helpful if clinicians learn to continually emphasize that they are using their expertise to accomplish the goals established by the patient and the family. In training, clinician should be taught to use a series of interventions beginning with rational explanations (stressing the step-by-step nature of progress), escalating to direct confrontations of problematic behavior only when necessary.

Learning the skills necessary to control sessions also must extend to learning the skills necessary to control who attends sessions. When a patient or a family calls to cancel an appointment, clinicians must learn to assess the reasons for cancellation, and, if indicated, to stress the importance of the session and insist that the patient and the family attend. Consistent attendance is crucial to prevent crises before they are out of control.

Translating Problems into Small Steps

The slowness of progress and change for the chronic schizophrenic patient is one of the most difficult things for families, and clinicians, to accept. Without a strong focus on this issue in training, inexperienced clinicians will either become inpatient and try to push for more than patients can tolerate, or they will become so afraid of crises or relapse that they will allow patients to stagnate. Learning to maintain a pace that requires patients to perform near the limit of their abilities without going beyond that limit is the art of successfully conducting psychoeducational therapy. As we have mentioned, providing clinicians with a good understanding of the illness helps them to go slowly. Beyond this basic understanding of the illness, however, it is necessary to acquire several other skills in order to tolerate the slowness of change during this time. In particular, clinicians must learn to repeatedly translate overwhelming problems into small steps toward improved functioning, and translate these steps into concrete tasks that help in their achievement. Thus, the ability to design and assign tasks of gradually increasing difficulty is central to the model. Tasks give a sense of activity and progress and help to operationalize the themes and goals of the program. The effective design and assignment of tasks, however, requires sophisticated clinical skills. The training program should help clinicians to master several issues regarding tasks: choice of an appropriate task; the actual assignment of tasks; dealing with the response of the patient and family to task assignment; posttask evaluation; and, finally, task reassignment.

Assigning Relevant Tasks

Since most patients with chronic schizophrenia tend to be initially functioning at a relatively low level, clinicians must learn to assign beginning tasks that require only minimal skill and effort. Neither patients nor families need the sense of failure that accompanies being unable to perform what appears to be a simple assignment. Clinicians, too, often need the experience of seeing patients and families succeed. Programming for success usually means that clinicians must begin by designing small structured tasks that involve such elementary things as encouraging the patient to physically care for him- or herself, to do simple household chores that require relatively little time or effort, or even just to get out of bed at a certain hour. Tasks asked of family members must be small as well since adaptive behaviors learned over the years can be hard to change.

Learning to effectively assign tasks that are sufficiently small is difficult for many clinicians. They are aware that these patients and their families have a serious problem, but they are also aware that they are adults. Most adult schizophrenic patients resent tasks that would seem more appropriate for a 7-year-old. For this reason, clinicians must be taught to give a reasonable rationale for each task they assign. They must learn to make statements such as: "I know this may seem to be a simple task, but it's a part of getting you back into a routine. Tolerating routines is important in getting and keeping a job." It sometimes helps to teach trainees to use analogies related to physical illness or injuries. For instance, after having a broken leg, the first steps must be with the aid of crutches, then a cane, than a slow walk, all before being able to run or move freely. Clinicians also must be taught to relate assigned tasks to the goals desired by patients (i.e., "I know you want to get back to work. Well, staying out of bed for 8 hours is a first step. It's one of the prerequisites of most jobs.").

Clinicians must also be taught that task compliance is greater if patients and family members participate in task design and selection. They must learn, therefore, to ask patients and family members for their opinions about tasks that would be appropriate to their current problems and goals. Clinicians can also be trained to ask potentially resistant patients for their ideas about how they might attempt to *avoid* doing a particularly important task. In this way, resistances can often be anticipated and avoided (Martin & Worthington, 1982). In general, clinicians should be taught that early tasks for patients should usually involve doing something *with* a family member rather than doing something alone. Initiative is low immediately following a psychotic break and thus task compliance is greater when a family member is involved in the process. Finally, clinicians must be taught that tasks will not be taken seriously unless they, as clinicians, consistently follow through in subsequent sessions by asking how the tasks went, rewarding attempts to comply with assignments, and redesigning tasks that did not achieve their desired ends.

It is evident that task selection requires careful thought and a sensitive assessment of patients and families. These skills can best be taught through case presentations, followed by role playing in which trainees attempt to design and implement task-oriented interventions. During the process, trainees should be exposed to multiple examples of patients at different stages of recuperation and treatment, each time being asked to design a series of tasks that would best help to move the patient and family toward their next goal. A thorough discussion of the reasons for choosing a particular task, potential problems with compliance, and likely patient and family reactions to the experience should be a part of each case example used in training.

Attention to the process of task evaluation can also help clinicians to learn to maintain an appropriate pace in treatment. By learning to listen to the feedback that they get from patients and their families about the tasks assigned, clinicians can insure that their expectations and interventions relate to the tolerance level of all concerned. Rather than establishing a program and sticking to it, clinicians must learn to modify their own behaviors based on the response of patients and families to their interventions. However, because change occurs so slowly, clinicians must also learn to simultaneously attend to their own and everyone else's morale, doing so by learning to consistently be aware of any progress that has been made, however minimal it may be.

Providing Support

As implied throughout this book, the provision of ongoing support, in practical ways, is crucial for families. Clinicians, therefore, must come to acknowledge and respect families as the primary caregivers for patients. To be truly supportive, clinicians must know how to firmly refuse to allow things to get out of control, to refuse to side with the patient against the family or vice versa, to be consistently available in crises, and to give practical suggestions that enable the patient and the family to cope with one another on an ongoing basis.

Clinicians must also be helped to understand that rapid reassurance and/or artificial praise is not supportive. Many inexperienced clinicians become so upset by the pain families experience that they rush to provide reassurance. Unfortunately, this tends to leave family members feeling misunderstood or cut off prematurely. Similarly, overemphasizing patient accomplishments only decreases the clinician's credibility and makes patients feel embarrassed. Patients know that performing many of the small tasks that are assigned is not a major achievement in the larger scheme of things. Training clinicians to provide genuine support means training them to be optimistic, but to stay firmly anchored in reality rather than becoming overly enthusiastic.

To do this, clinicians must learn to accept the limitations imposed by the illness. With or without treatment, schizophrenia is a chronic illness and over 80% of this population is likely to have positive symptoms recur at some time in the future. Thus, being supportive means helping family members and patients to achieve as much as possible within these parameters. It is easy for any clinician, but especially an inexperienced one, to lose sight of these issues once the acute symptoms are under control, and especially when the patient begins to exhibit a little more energy. When this occurs, clinicians can inadvertently begin to support unrealistic goals, forgetting the need to go slow and the need to remind family members of the patient's limitations. Therefore, clinicians must be helped to remember that while significant change is possible, expectations must be tempered by an awareness of the realities of schizophrenia and knowledge of the patient's basic skills and abilities.

Dealing with Impasses in Ongoing Treatment

When patients and families become locked in power struggles, despite efforts on everyone's part to avoid them, clinicians must be able to defuse the situation. To do this, they must practice techniques such as relabeling and reframing to make it possible for one side or another to change their attitudes or behavior. For instance, this problem often arises early in treatment around the issue of hygiene, with patients neglecting the care of their bodies while their family members nag them to assume responsibility for some modicum of self-maintenance. Because the impasse that occurs in such situations is one that is upsetting to everyone involved, clinicians must be able to decrease tensions. The effective use of the skill of relabeling (perhaps defining the patients' apathy regarding their personal appearance as part of the illness) often enables family members to back off, which in turn allows patients to become less resistant to basic self-care. Teaching clinicians to reframe a patient's lethargy as part of a need to recuperate from an acute psychotic episode, also gives clinicians a tool to help families to remain patient during difficult times.

Clinicians must also learn to deal with another set of behaviors that can interfere with treatment, those which tend to occur when things are going well or at least when the overt psychosis is under fairly good control. At such times, patients, and sometimes families, are apt to make requests to discontinue medication or even treatment. Clinicians must be taught to reinforce the information provided in the workshop about the course of the illness and the importance of medication and treatment for at least the high-risk period of the first year or two following the episode. They must be prepared to be highly directive and insistent with patients and families about the benefits of maintaining the contract during this time, but if all else fails, they must be prepared to agree to a compromise to avoid losing patients altogether. For instance, clinicians can be taught to suggest holding sessions at greater intervals rather than agreeing to complete termination, or they can be taught to negotiate a contract that allows slowly decreasing medication with the understanding that, if symptoms reappear, the patient would agree to an increased dose.

Overall, during this training session, clinicians must be helped to understand that they can be powerful agents of change. However, unlike the mandate of therapists in more traditional psychotherapies, they must be helped to accept that their mandate is a limited one. They must appreciate that their alliance with both patient and family is formed to deal with the impact of a severe chronic illness, and that this type of alliance limits the problem areas they are entitled to explore. Unless the contract is renegotiated, clinicians must learn to maintain a focus only on guiding the family and patient in their attempts to cope more effectively with the crisis and its aftermath.

Session V: Vocational Issues and Social Reintegration

One of the primary training goals of this session must be helping clinicians to learn when it is appropriate to begin to approach the issues of work, training, or social contacts outside the home. Since work is often highly valued as a sign of normalcy and success, it is often a covert or overt goal of patients, families, and clinicians from the very beginning of treatment. Clinicians must be taught from the outset, however, that approaching this goal too early can lead to an increase in stress, a higher risk of failure, and thus an increase in the potential for patient relapse. Clinicians must be helped, therefore, to appreciate that the areas of vocational and social rehabilitation are difficult ones that they must learn to approach slowly, taking a methodical approach to the attainment of each goal, even in the later stages of treatment. For these reasons, this training session must include experiences that sensitize clinicians to the factors that make a patient ready for work or a vocational training program. To make these judgments, clinicians must develop the ability to assess patient skills, strengths, and weaknesses as well as their potential impact on vocational performance.

This training session must also focus on helping clinicians learn how to formulate tasks that will help patients develop more complex skills, especially those that will increase their ability to cope with the demands of employment. Since the things that upset patients in vocational and social situations tend to be minor stresses or routines that many people would not notice, it is important that trainees be sensitized by exposure to specific examples of patients struggling with these small, but potentially overwhelming issues. The use of videotapes of patients discussing work problems and satisfactions helps to give trainees a sense of the difficulties patients can encounter in vocational environments. Simultaneously, these same tapes can be used to increase the trainee's optimism about the illness since tapes of patients at this stage of treatment clearly communicate the fact that some patients are eventually able to work.

Clinicians must also be trained to assess the best possible route for the patient's return to the work world. Obviously, formal employment and sheltered vocational training require different levels of functioning. Therefore, it is important that clinicians be able to judge which alternative is best for a particular patient, and be aware of available vocational training programs and the levels of functioning they require. Having a representative from a vocational training agency come to the training session to discuss expectations, routines, and programmatic issues helps clinicians understand the specific issues inherent in the system that patients will have to be helped to negotiate.

Clinicians must also be taught to expect and handle the typical mistakes that are made during this phase of treatment. These include starting work before the patient is ready, starting at a level that is too complex or too simple, underestimating the patient's problems with attention, concentration, or motivation, and insufficient preparing of the patient for getting along with supervisors and co-workers or for accepting independent responsibility. The use of discussion and role playing to focus on these problems helps clinicians to be less anxious about making mistakes, to properly prepare ways of avoiding these pitfalls, and to begin to develop therapeutic techniques to deal with these situations successfully.

Learning to deal with issues related to the social reintegration of the patient requires many of the same skills of clinicians as those needed to help patients to return to work. Clinicians must be helped to understand that patient isolation and withdrawal mostly evolve from the illness, and that increased social contact can only be facilitated when patients have recovered sufficiently to tolerate the stimulation and stress inherent in social interaction. The ability to recognize when patients are ready to begin to socialize will increase naturally as clinicians become experienced, but a basic understanding of the ways of evaluating these issues can be developed through discussion and videotape review of specific cases. Once again, clinicians must become familiar with possible community resources that may help in facilitating social interaction for patients. In most communities, there is usually at least one agency that will provide a listing of social agencies and self-help groups. These formal listings are a place to start, and many more resources can be discovered informally as time goes on.

When the social reintegration of the patient is being discussed, simultaneous attention should be paid to the social networks of other family members. In response to the time and energy required to deal with schizophrenia, many family members eventually find themselves socially isolated. Therefore, clinicians must be taught to help family members to connect with a social network without implying they, as family members, are "patients" themselves. Furthermore, they must learn to do this slowly and tactfully since family members are often uncomfortable about attending to their own needs and/or beginning to spend less time with the patient. Teaching clinicians to label the increased social contacts of family members as important for the patient or important for maintaining the family's ability to cope over the long haul, helps in connecting or reconnecting family members with others outside the home.

Session VI: Dealing with Other Issues

The primary focus of this final session of the training series should concentrate on helping clinicians to deal with emancipation difficulties, marital problems, other family concerns, and how and when to renegotiate the treatment contract to deal with these issues. Since the course of treatment has been highly structured and low-key, the move into dealing with these topics is always a difficult one for patients and families. These topics are frequently emotionally charged, ambiguous, and impossible to approach with the same clarity and structure as more concrete issues. Because they require a greater stress tolerance on the part of patients and greater confidence on the part of families, clinicians must be taught to leave these topics until the later stages of treatment. In fact, these issues are purposefully presented at the very end of the training seminar to underline the metacommunication of their appropriate place within the sequence of treatment.

Special attention must be given to the topic of emancipation, since it is frequently mishandled by clinicians. Many young trainees, often still fresh from dealing with their own "emancipation," tend to measure the success of treatment by how quickly they can help the patient to leave home. This rapid approach to the highly complex and emotional process of emancipation often produces disastrous results for both patients and families. Thus, training clinicians to deal with the emancipation process begins by giving the message that the issue can only be approached if patients and their families are ready to deal with it and if patients have demonstrated that they have the skills that will give them at least some chance of success.

In beginning to deal with emancipation everyone must first be given the opportunity to share their thoughts and feelings. While it is not possible, nor even desirable, to avoid emotional reactions to this topic, clinicians should be taught to approach it in a controlled and structured manner. Creating a protected atmosphere will help to avoid some of the escalation of conflict and hurt feelings that can otherwise occur. Clinicians must learn to assign tasks that move toward the goal of emancipation, and to read the responses to these task assignments as signals of the level of everyone's readiness to cope with an eventual separation. They must learn to discourage a focus on emancipation during crisis periods. Finally, clinicians must be made aware that not all patients will ever have the ability to establish themselves in totally independent living situations. They must learn to respect this as a real possibility, assess it realistically, and plan accordingly.

Again, giving clinicians the opportunity to view videotapes that show patients and their families struggling with the patient's emancipation helps prepare them to deal with the difficulties of this portion of treatment. In addition, discussions focusing on the way clinicians emancipated from their families of origin can help to sensitize them to the multitude of feelings associated with becoming independent and leaving home, even without the complication of a major psychiatric illness.

In order to facilitate graduated moves towards emancipation, it is also important for clinicians to become aware of possible, structured, and transitional living arrangements available in their community. These living settings can be used as stepping stones for patients on their way toward more genuine independence, or even as permanent quarters for patients who cannot stay at home, but who cannot function completely independently. Inviting a counselor from one of these agencies to speak at this training session can help trainees to become aware of such facilities, to appreciate the types of problems that arise for patients as they leave home, and even to learn about solutions to specific problems that have worked for some patients in the past.

Trainees must learn to evaluate a wide range of issues for possible inclusion in the contract in the later phases of treatment. Since many of these general issues seem particularly interesting to clinicians, it is important in this phase of training to reemphasize the primary goals of treatment. Unless clinicians are able to maintain a focus on the goals of decreasing stress for family members and the patient, and helping the patient to become more functional, sessions during the later stages of treatment can easily become tangential, fragmented, and diffuse. Thus, it is necessary for clinicians to develop skill in deciding when it is essential to deal with an issue and why. They must learn that if a highly emotional issue is acting as an impediment to the patient's adjustment, it must be dealt with directly and immediately, whereas if that same issue is not interfering with major treatment goals, it can be made an optional part of the treatment agenda or postponed until a time when there is likely to be more energy available to work toward its resolution. When issues must be postponed, clinicians should be empathic and supportive about the frustration of not dealing with important topics, while at the same time, helping families to understand and accept the need for occasional delays.

Finally, clinicians must also learn to accept that a psychoeducational approach allows the patient and family to make their own decisions about when and whether they want to deal with any specific family issue. To learn the skills of involving patients and families in this type of contract renegotiation, clinicians must be helped to genuinely accept the fact that this treatment approach is based on a cooperative relationship, one which almost never involves unilateral decision-making on the part of professionals about treatment. Part of the training process, therefore, must simultaneously help clinicians to recognize the opportunity they have to help effect change, while stressing the need to avoid the abuse of that opportunity by ignoring the rights of patients and families. Although clinical experience and ongoing supervison are essential in helping clinicians to truly internalize these skills and attitudes, early discussions and role playing about these negotiations allow clinicians to become more sensitive about their role and their impact on patients and families.

TEACHING AND SUPERVISION IN AN ONGOING PROGRAM

However comprehensive the initial training program, the constantly changing state of the field is such that some mechanisms should be established to help clinicians keep up to date on the literature about new developments in theory, research, and practice. The same holds true even for experienced staff members. New information about schizophrenia and its treatment is becoming available constantly. In fact, family members themselves often seek out the latest information and ask clinicians about it. Thus, a group norm should be established which encourages each clinician to maintain an awareness of the most up-to-date information. A journal review system can be established with each team clinician responsible for reviewing a key journal and for circulating relevant articles that are discovered. This review system should be broad, covering journals addressing professionals of various subspecialties, as well as journals or magazines written by nonprofessionals or patients and their families. Clinicians also should try to be aware of any presentations in the mass media that may stimulate questions from program participants.

Once beginning clinicians have assumed responsibility for ongoing treatment with patients and families, the refinement and maintenance of specific skills can be facilitated by using four basic techniques: observation of videotapes, cotherapy, live supervision, and peer group consultation. The viewing of videotapes is particularly useful because clinicians, even when they watch their own tapes independently, can gain a different perspective on the major issues of family sessions and how they are managing them. Removed from the tension of the session, it is easier to watch their own interventions with less defensiveness, and to develop more effective alternatives. Reviewing videotaped sessions with a supervisor, or even with other clinicians, provides more opportunities for learning. The detailed discussion of sessions that becomes possible through the use of tapes can stimulate the development of new interventions and creative suggestions from those who are not as directly involved in the treatment.

Cotherapy, while not cost effective in the long run, is very useful in training. By carrying one or two cases in conjunction with someone more experienced with a psychoeducational model, trainees can begin to gain experience without being overwhelmed by having to assume total responsibility for how things go. As trainees feel more comfortable, they can gradually assume primary responsibility within sessions and for the development of interventions and tasks. If cotherapy is to be used as a training tool, however, it is important that each treatment session be preceded and followed by a meeting of the two clinicians involved. This insures that the two clinicians are working consistently towards the same ends, and helps to avoid power struggles or misunderstandings.

Live supervision, that which enables the supervisor to observe a session *while it is occurring* and to call in to make suggestions, is extremely valuable. It not only can assure that a psychoeducational model is actually being followed, but it can also be effective in breaking therapeutic habits left over from other kinds of therapy training. Since most clinicians will have been trained in other models, it is natural that they might occasionally revert to using old, comfortable methods from time to time. Tendencies to focus too heavily on why people behave as they do, or tendencies to stimulate dramatic family interactions can be interrupted immediately by the observing supervisor. Live supervision also can help clinicians to acquire the basic specific technical skills required in putting the principles of the model into practice. The principles of this model of intervention are easy to grasp, but less easy to apply consistently on a day-to-day basis. It is invaluable to have a consultant who, by virtue of being out of the room, maintains a different, less involved perspective. For instance, the consultant can interrupt sessions so that clinicians can quickly learn to take control by taking an active stand. They can also learn to maintain an appropriate focus without alienating any of the participants. Even more importantly, live supervision can help to decrease reactivity on the part of clinicians as they inevitably become emotionally involved in these family systems.

As the clinician's caseload grows, it is neither practical nor necessary for a consultant to observe all family sessions. Furthermore, over time, clinicians become better able to determine when they need consultation. Thus, this type of supervision can become less frequent, perhaps on an "as needed" basis, or it can be discontinued altogether. A peer group of clinicians using this model can be a good practical solution to the problem of ongoing supervision. They key requirement for such a group to work well is the establishment of a climate that is sufficiently supportive to enable clinicians to feel free to expose their practice, and yet sufficiently confrontational to enable them to get honest and direct feedback about their therapeutic errors. The establishment of a basic rule regarding criticism is particularly useful. That is, when clinicians criticize an intervention made by one of their colleagues, they must also make positive suggestions about how the incident could have been handled differently. This helps to increase cooperation and to decrease "one-ups-manship" and the need to become defensive. This type of peer group supervision has the added advantage of establishing a relevant support network of clinicians who are committed to working with difficult but similar patients and problems. Thus, such groups can often become a resource for coping with discouragement and therapist fatigue, in addition to their primary function of focusing on improving each clinician's work with families.

SYSTEMS ISSUES IN IMPLEMENTATION

The primary systems issues encountered when attempting to initiate a psychoeducational program include: (1) getting a mandate to do the program, (2) working cooperatively with various aspects of the system, and (3) dealing with the ramifications of instituting a treatment program that differs from the treatment offered by the larger health system in which it functions.

Getting a mandate to establish a psychoeducational program is not always easy. Some helping systems are reluctant to involve families in the treatment process at all, much less educate them about the illness and its management. The professionals in systems that maintain a strong intrapsychic or biological focus often are not interested in family feedback or participation. Aside from their practical use in contributing information to the assessment of the patient, family members are viewed as unnecessary, irrelevant, or perhaps even harmful to the patient's treatment. Many of these systems see themselves as having a mandate to care for the patient, without any responsibility to consider the well-being of other family members, even if that well-being could make a contribution to the course of the patient's illness. Professionals in some treatment systems fear involving family members because they feel they will not be able to manage families once they become involved. Professionals in other systems fear the potential militancy of families, particularly those who have become members of self-help groups. They do not like the idea of being more accountable for their treatment decisions and do not want to deal with pressures to explain their actions. Finally, professionals in some treatment systems retain the belief that families are somehow responsible for causing and maintaining schizophrenia, and thus discourage the development of any program requiring family involvement.

Hospital administrators are also not always eager to support programs such as these. The fact is that many patients can be kept out of hospitals for extended periods of time with the combined efforts of the family and a competent psychoeducational team. This is not particularly welcome news to hospitals whose own survival is related to keeping inpatient beds occupied. The economics of health care simply don't support outpatient treatment. A treatment facility can collect several hundred dollars a day for hospitalizing a patient, but only a few dollars a visit for an outpatient contact, and none at all for the multitude of phone contacts necessary with and for these patients. It is not surprising, therefore, that many hospitals prefer to emphasize inpatient programs.

Furthermore, programs such as these require that different parts of systems cooperate with each other. Inpatient clinicians must consult with outpatient clinicians and *vice versa*, attending each other's meetings to coordinate the care of patients. Medical and nonmedical personnel must also work together. Each unit and each discipline, however, may have different and even conflicting philosophies and priorities, giving rise to communication problems, tendencies to distrust one another's input, and games of one-ups-manship, as each professional or unit seeks to prove that they have a better understanding of patients and how to treat them. Since the family clinician is established as the family's representative or link to the hospital system and vice versa, this individual can come under considerable strain.

The role of "go between" is always a difficult one. It is particularly problematic when mistakes are made in the process of caring for patients, or when someone on a treatment team makes it difficult to defend decisions that upset patients or family members. Nevertheless, maintaining the role of ombudsman in these situations allows family clinicians to be helpful when families bring their tension and anger into family sessions. It is important that clinicians learn to listen to the complaints of families and patients, and never to exclusively defend the actions of the staff.

Clinicians must also learn that giving family members a chance to express their anger must be followed by acknowledging their right to be angry. Only then can they look for ways to restabilize the situation, right the wrong, and/or repair the therapeutic relationship. In one last example, a resistant and very paranoid young man, Henry, was admitted to a psychiatric hospital only after major efforts on the part of his parents. Shortly thereafter, it was necessary to transfer Henry to a medical hospital for a minor but urgent operation. It was planned that he would be transferred back to the psychiatric unit as soon as his medical condition improved. Due to faulty communication, however, Henry was discharged from the second hospital instead of being sent back to the inpatient psychiatric unit. When his father went to visit, Henry was in the lobby with his bags packed. His father, confused and upset, took him home. Both parents, furious, asked for an emergency session with the family clinician which their son refused to attend.

MOTHER: How could this have happened? I'm enraged. I'm thinking of suing both hospitals.

FATHER: I couldn't believe it! He was standing in the lobby with this smile on his face. There was no one else even there. Where the hell were the doctors? Didn't they know he was sick? Now, we'll never get him to come back.

Both parents continued to express anger and upset for some time. Finally:

CLINICIAN: What can I say? It never should have happened. I certainly don't blame you for being outraged. I know Henry is still pretty sick. I had hoped he would be in the hospital a while longer. But, I'm glad that you called so I could see you right away to discuss what to do now.

FATHER: What *can* we do?

CLINICIAN: Well, you told me before that option number one is out. Henry is refusing to come back to the hospital right now.

FATHER: That's right. And I don't think we can get him to change his mind.

CLINICIAN: Would he be willing to come in to see me—as long as it's not on the unit?

MOTHER: Maybe. I'm not sure.

CLINICIAN: If we can't get him to come back in, I'd like to have frequent contact with him for awhile. I'd like other folks on the team to see him, too. With an all out effort . . . maybe we can work this thing out with him at home.

MOTHER: We'd appreciate that. He was getting better when this happened.

CLINICIAN: How about if I call Henry right now? He knows you're with me. We can see if he'd be willing to come in today or tomorrow.

In this example, the clinician allowed Henry's parents to vent their perfectly understandable anger and upset without intruding, becoming defensive, or making interpretations. Only when they had expressed their feelings did she acknowledge that their anger was reasonable and only then did she attempt to move toward a resolution of the problem. At no time did she defend the actions of either hospital system, since Henry's discharge was clearly undesirable and a serious error on the part of the medical staff. Although the decision to discharge Henry was not made by the family clinician, or the psychiatric staff, she had to take the responsibility for the error, respond to the anger of the family, and pay an emotional price for playing a go-between role in the treatment system. The clinician must learn to live with the negative feelings everyone expresses without also becoming negative.

The tension inherent in the role of family representative may, in fact, be intensified by the provision of information to families and patients. One result of a program such as this is that families, after having been exposed to an educational workshop and/or provided with information over the course of time, may come to be more aware of the current state of the art regarding schizophrenia and its treatment than many of the professionals they encounter. Thus, when professionals make inaccurate statements or errors in judgment, families are more likely to challenge them. If these professionals respond defensively, increased ill feeling may be stimulated in families as well as increased ill will from other professionals toward psychoeducational programs. Again, family representatives must help families and professionals to work together while dealing with their own feelings about being in the middle of such conflicts.

All of these potential systems problems increase the importance of working as a team when using a psychoeducational model. The team approach not only increases the likelihood of continuity of care for patients and families, and the likelihood of mutual support for professionals, but it specifically avoids the competition that can otherwise develop between medical and nonmedical staff. Whatever the etiology of schizophrenia, there is a good deal of evidence that both medication maintenance and psychotherapy contribute to patient functioning and community tenure (Cole et al., 1964; Cole et al., 1966; Hogarty, Goldberg, & Schooler, 1974; Mosher & Keith, 1980). Nevertheless, many combined family and medical approaches to treatment fail. A major reason may be the need of professionals in each of these specialties to prove that their particular intervention is the most important one. When such battles occur, medically oriented staff become less receptive to the possible benefits of psychosocial interventions and tend to retreat to their biological and pharmacological strongholds.

Staff in both specialties can become more involved in their disagreements with one another than in working together toward their common goal of helping patients.

This competition is particularly destructive to those wishing to promote family care since they tend to be less central and/or powerful in a medical hierarchy. Thus, family clinicians who take an adversarial stance with medical staff tend to lose these power struggles and eventually leave hospital settings, giving up on the idea of cooperating with a medical model. Meanwhile, the individual or biological treatment of the patient becomes the sole focus of psychiatric settings, and what limited work is done with families is assigned to an inexperienced person without training, supervision, or support. Consequently, the message family members receive regarding their involvement is an ambivalent one at best, and attention to the needs of family members inevitably decreases.

Some of these systems problems can be avoided by establishing a team approach and scheduling frequent meetings to encourage communication, sensitivity, and respect for the contribution of colleagues to patient care. For such a team to work well, the explicit message of the system must be one that supports and values collaboration directed toward the achievement of the major goals of patient recuperation and reintegration into their communities. Achieving these goals requires the cooperation of the patient, the family, the psychoeducational treatment team, the medical staff, and the larger treatment system. It is no more possible to parcel out ultimate responsibility for treatment success than it is possible to establish ultimate responsibility for treatment failure. Since everyone on a team is sensitive about who receives the credit or the blame, it is important that everyone be prepared to give credit for success to others, and to assume more than their fair share of responsibility for failure. The recipe for success is much like that of a recipe for a successful marriage: each partner must be prepared to give 90%.

In the best of all possible worlds, the psychoeducational team should be allowed to remain involved with patients over time, whether they relapse or not. The chronic and episodic nature of this illness makes it likely that patients will become worse and/or require hospitalization from time to time. An arbitrary division between inpatient and outpatient units breaks the continuity of care so vital to these patients. If outpatient clinicians can maintain an involved stance during hospital admission, it helps ease the inpatient staff's sense that they are left to pick up the pieces after a crisis, helps patients to make the transition between units, and increases the likelihood of patient cooperation with aftercare. Finally, ongoing involvement of the team also allows them to continue their own learning process by facilitating assessments of the impact of any mistakes that may have been made and encouraging the development of ideas about how these mistakes can be avoided in the future.

SUMMARY OF IMPLEMENTATION ISSUES

The encouraging results produced by psychoeducational models of family intervention are leading professionals in many settings to attempt to duplicate these efforts. However, many professionals who attend teaching sessions on this model are primarily interested in exploring the *educational* aspects of the program since they are the most concrete, dramatic, and unique. It is extremely important, however, not to oversimplify the concept of psychoeducational programs or to underestimate the level of skill necessary to conduct them.

While it is not yet known what makes these models at least somewhat more effective than others, it can be assumed that simply giving families information about schizophrenia and telling them to tone down the intensity of their family life is probably not enough to cause change on an ongoing basis. For most patients and their families, schizophrenia is a chronic illness that will require attention for many years. Because disruptions in the relationship with treatment systems are extremely upsetting for patients and families dealing with these chronic, severe problems, programs offering only brief educational interventions without consistent follow-up may not be truly helpful. In fact, they may even add to the problems and frustrations faced by these patients and their families by implying that this is a guide for successful management of patients, without offering to help families to follow it. In order to be genuinely helpful to seriously ill patients, emphasis must also be given to the application of the principles of the educational phase, and to facilitating the use of a family's own coping skills so that they can continue to use this knowledge after active treatment has ended. These tasks are not accomplished in one workshop and not without a good deal of professional energy and an extended commitment to families.

For these reasons, any model of training and supervising clinicians to work with schizophrenic patients using these interventions must build in long-term supports not only for patients and families, but also for staff. Long-term supports will help to prevent clinicians fatigue and burnout. For instance, on our particular project, we chose to employ each family clinician half-time, leaving the rest of their time to teach or work with problems other than schizophrenia. This policy insured that clinicians would have a variety of experiences to help prevent frustration, discouragement, and staff turnover. If a program is located with a large, well-structured institution, staff fatigue can also be mitigated by the use of a multidisciplinary team and the use of the backup system of the larger hospital to handle some of the inevitable emergencies.

A well-functioning team allows one clinician to cover for another, and cushions the impact of having to deal with the many crises that can occur, particularly early in treatment. A larger psychiatric hospital usually has services that can absorb the burden of night calls, contacting clinicians only when absolutely necessary. Policies such as these, however, require administrative support that is not always easy to arrange since a team approach takes more therapeutic time and produces less income. Furthermore, the administration of many institutions does not favor half-time assignments, and many other facilities do not have emergency rooms to take the calls that come in the middle of the night. Therefore, in designing psychoeducational programs and in training clinicians to operate within these models, attention should be given to the context in which the program operates, and the specifics of how it must be modified accordingly.

Although we strongly encourage the use of a team format when implementing this model of treatment, many aspects of the approach can be used by the private practitioner. Certainly, educating patients and families about schizophrenia and its treatment would be a beneficial and important component of any treatment. While it is unlikely that private practitioners will have the resources to provide an all-day multiple family workshop as described here, the same information can be conveyed to the individual family over the course of a number of sessions.

At the same time, it is important for private practitioners to establish a working alliance with the patient and family by connecting with them in a way that emphasizes their power and ability to effect positive change. Using the notion of establishing a realistic treatment contract helps both patients and families to be more clear about what they can expect from the practitioner, and what they can expect in terms of future change. Similarly, private practitioners can use the techniques outlined to support patients and families during the process of stabilization and recuperation, providing structured and concrete methods of management.

The primary difficulties associated with attempting this approach in private practice are related to the lack of support available to clinicians, patients, and families. Patient and family isolation can be modified to some extent by encouraging the use of existing self-help or advocacy groups in the community. For private practitioners, however, solo treatment of patients and families with this illness can become a significant problem. The absence of a treatment team or backup services means that they must assume the entire responsibility of treatment. Since this approach stresses the availability of the treatment team and encourages patients and families to contact them with questions and concerns, private practitioners may get an unusually high number of telephone calls, at least during the initial phases of treatment. The usual clinical response to this is to establish firm boundaries, which can be negatively misinterpreted by the patient or family and reinforce their sense of mistrust or resistance to treatment suggestions. Thus, private practitioners who use this model must be prepared to be available during crises, and to handle them alone. Thus, they will also have a higher risk of "burn out" unless they have access to colleagues that can cover for them and offer them ongoing support. Ultimately, if a program can be developed that offers practitioners the experience of success and the potential to change patients and families, it may be seen as worth the money and energy required.

SUMMARY: A FINAL LOOK

This manual has described a program for schizophrenic patients and their families that begins with the patient's admission to the hospital and continues for several years after discharge. As a psychoeducational program, it stresses the provision of information and the development of problem-solving skills by patients and families in a structured, step-by-step manner. Its goals include decreasing the distress and increasing the coping skills of family members, and increasing the functioning of the patient. The program is based on the assumptions that:

- The provision of support and information to family members will decrease anxiety and maximize the family's use of internal and external resources.
- Medication combined with the protection and support of a temporarily low-stress environment will eventually allow an increase in the patient's ability to tolerate stimulation and give him or her time to overcome some of the problems related to amotivation and hopelessness.

Long-term goals should include the development of a more sophisticated group of mental health consumers, the increased use of extrafamilial support systems, and the facilitation of the patient's maximum level of independence.

The most important question about this model is "Does it work?" The answer seems to be a highly qualified "Yes." The treatment of schizophrenia requires a somewhat limited definition of success. As families are told during the workshop, anyone who claims to have a permanent "cure" for this illness should be regarded with generous quantities of skepticism. *There is no known cure for schizophrenia at this time.* Nevertheless, it is possible to help most patients and their families to avoid many crises, prolonged hospitalizations, and the disruption and "deskilling" that result. It also is possible for some patients and families to learn to live with the illness, and even occasional relapses, without constantly having the symptoms of the illness dramatically disrupt their lives together.

One of the qualities that appears to contribute to the success of psychoeducational programs is that the goals established cooperatively by patient, family, and clinician are grounded in an understanding of the realities of the illness and how it can impact on individual patients. An understanding of the limitations produced by the illness allows for the setting of reasonable goals. This alone is a crucial contribution since it helps to avoid exposing everyone to the repeated, frustrating, negative experiences that occur when patients are asked to respond too quickly or at levels beyond their abilities. Repeated failures decrease the patient's self-confidence and the family's ability to maintain hope. Thus, the requirement of a long-term commitment from patients and families to these programs is viewed as critical in avoiding repeated crises and relapse. The particular psychoeducational program described here asks for a minimum of 1 to 2 year's participation. Even after that, regular "checkup" appointments are scheduled to insure maintenance of gains and prevention of future crises. The need for a long-term contract may cause frustration at the beginning of treatment, but over time, the reassurance inherent in having "lifeline" to help when needed more than outweighs the disadvantages.

Why a Psychoeducational Approach?

This family approach is based on the establishment of cooperation and communication between professionals of various disciplines. In this way, the psychoeducational model attempts to provide a coherent structure to the overall treatment process, and continuity of care for patients and families, while avoiding both pointless power struggles between professionals, and the clinician fatigue that results. In this collaborative approach, clinicians are able to support patients, families, and one another when fatigue and hopelessness set in.

Psychoeducational interventions are suggested as an alternative to traditional family therapies with chronically ill populations since traditional family treatment strategies are often unsuccessful and at times even stimulate noncompliance, crises, and relapse. There are probably several reasons for the failure of more additional family approaches. Perhaps the most significant is the number of potentially negative metacommunications inherent in the practice of traditional family therapy that needlessly erect obstacles and resistances to change, and that exact an unnecessary price from families in terms of pain, guilt, and anxiety. For instance, many family therapists suggest that schizophrenia is best treated through family sessions without medication or other treatments. For families of schizophrenic patients this communication implicitly suggests that we know what schizophrenia is (a family disease), what causes it (families), and what cures it (family therapy). This message can have a number of undesirable effects. It may suggest to families that it is not necessary to cooperate with others on the multidisciplinary team, and it may encourage noncompliance with medication programs. This message not only dramatically increases the patient's risk of relapse but also creates problems with colleagues. To suggest cavalierly that family therapy is *the* method of treatment is evidence of unwarranted arrogance when there is so much evidence that medication programs are a vital part of patient care.

Furthermore, and unfortunately, the recommendation of family therapy often makes families feel that professionals are suggesting that they are to blame for the patient's illness. In fact, while claiming to have a systems focus, some family therapists actually do begin their assessments by attempting to determine how families may have caused the illness, or how they are keeping a poor, struggling, young person sick. If a family happens to behave in an unusual manner, they seldom consider the possibility that these behaviors may be *responses* to years of living with the bizarre behavior of the patient, not preexisting causes. Yet, patients *do* influence their families in addition to being influenced *by* their families.

Thus, the implicit or explicit message that the patient is not "ill" but is rather a symptom of a "family problem" is not a helpful one. This message requires that families, in order to be helped, deny their version of reality. With little respect for the family's perspective, professionals present the view that the patient's inappropriate, bizarre, or severely depressed behavior is a response to family tensions or communications. Even if this were true, the message that such illnesses as schizophrenia or manic depressive disease are solely family problems leaves families feeling confused, helpless, and angry at both the patient and professionals. This communication is reminiscent of what R. D. Laing called "mind bending," a process viewed as destructive between parents and their children, but now apparently regarded as therapeutic when dispensed by professionals. Furthermore, defining the family as the problem too often decreases parental authority by putting parents in a "one-down" position, confused and anxious about their abilities to manage their own children. This is counterproductive to the very goals most family therapists seek to attain, that is, the reinforcement of healthy generational boundaries, clear power structures, and effective communication between family members.

The negative effects of this message are exacerbated by another metacommunication of many family therapy approaches; that increased understanding or better communication will enable the patient to function better. Unfortunately, when illnesses are sufficiently severe to require hospitalization, patients frequently are beyond their own and their family's control. When things have gone this far, increased understanding or better communications in and of themselves may or may not help patients to function. Furthermore, sessions that attempt to increase family understanding and communication without clearly tying this focus to the patient's ability to function tend to alienate families from the professionals who are attempting to help them.

This is not to say that traditional family therapy will never work with chronic patients. Clearly, many of our senior colleagues report success in this regard, although usually without the support of data from controlled clinical trials (Andolfi, Angelo, Menghi, & Nicolò-Corigliano, 1983; Haley, 1980; Selvini-Palazzoli, Bosclo, Cecchin, & Prata, 1978; Whitaker, 1974). We do not doubt the fact that some patients and some families will respond, whether through the sheer force of the therapist's personality and persistence, or because they manage to take what positive things the therapist can offer and ignore the negative. Nevertheless, it would seem that an approach to families that offers education, support, and concrete advice is a more humane and more effective first alternative.

The family approach proposed here specifically attempts to avoid the pitfall of unwittingly increasing the anxiety of family members by implicitly blaming them for the patient's problems. Messages are given to families that specifically undercut the attribution of family causality for the illness. Information is given which allows family members to decrease their anxiety and concern about the patient and use their energy to cope with the difficulties inherent in the illness.

Finally, this model recognizes that the family is *not* the "patient." Families are involved in treatment because a member of their family is severely ill. Therefore, the goals and efforts of the program remain patient focused. When, as can happen, the years of dealing with a chronic illness come to have a depleting effect on the family constellation, families can be offered additional help. Problems such as that of increased isolation, blurred generational boundaries, or grief related to the loss of the patient's functioning are all common. These issues become a focus because they can interfere with the family's ability to effectively cope with the patient and the illness as well as interfering with the quality of life of all family members. Thus, the treatment program recognizes that all families not only can benefit from receiving up-to-date information about the illness, but also can benefit from help in dealing with stresses that have developed in relation to the illness.

This psychoeducational family treatment approach offers certain advantages over individual treatment or the exclusive use of chemotherapy. These approaches tend to underestimate the catastrophic impact of schizophrenia on others in the patient's environment. While chemotherapy is viewed as a necessary component of treatment, it is not sufficient to deal with the multitude of problems that arise as a result of this disorder. Similarly, individual therapy relies on the internal strength, motivation, and insight of the patient to gain cooperation in treatment and to create change. Complete reliance on patient motivation is risky considering the frequent loss of initiative and skill associated with schizophrenia. Thus, the involvement of family members in the patient's treatment should not be viewed as a luxury dependent upon their availability or the interests of specific clinicians. Rather, it should be viewed as a necessity in order to keep patients involved in treatment, to maximize the potential gains they can achieve from it, and to decrease the stress experienced by all. In general, families are extremely influential forces in the lives of patients, and are powerful agents of change. While this program is described as a program for chronic schizophrenic patients and their families, the principles are sound and likely to be applicable to family work with any long-term serious physical or mental illness.

BOOKS, ARTICLES, AND PAMPHLETS FOR RELATIVES AND NEW STAFF

American Psychiatric Association. (1981). *A psychiatric glossary: The meaning of terms frequently used in psychiatry*. Washington, DC: Author.

Appleton, W. S. (1975). Mistreatment of patients' families by psychiatrists. *American Journal of Psychiatry, 131*(61), 655–657.

Arieti, S. (1979). *Understanding and helping the schizophrenic: A guide for family and friends*. New York: Basic Books.

Bachmann, B. J. (1971, April). Reentering the community: A former patient's view. *Hospital and Community Psychiatry*, 35–38.

Bernheim, K. F., & Lewine, R. R. J. (1979). *Schizophrenia: Symptoms, causes, treatments*. New York: W. W. Norton.

Bernheim, K. F., Lewine, R. R. J., & Beale, C. T. (1982). *The caring family: Living with chronic mental illness*. New York: Random House. Includes a glossary of terms, medications, and self-help groups listed by state.

Chamberlain, J. (1979). *On our own: Patient controlled alternative to the mental health system*. New York: McGraw-Hill.

Creer, C., & Wing, J. (1975). Living with a schizophrenic patient. *British Journal of Hospital Medicine, 14*, 73–83.

Creer, C., & Wing, J. K. (1974). *Schizophrenia at home*. London: Institute of Psychiatry.

Hatfield, A. B. (1978). Psychological costs of schizophrenia to the family. *Social Work, 23*(5), 355–359.

Hatfield, A. B. (1979). The family as partner in the treatment of mental illness. *Hospital and Community Psychiatry, 30*(5), 338–340.

Hatfield, A. B. (1982). *Coping with mental illness in the family: The family guide*. Washington, DC: National Alliance for the Mentally Ill.

Holden, D. F., & Lewine, R. R. J. (1982). How families evaluate mental health professionals, resources, and effects of illness. *Schizophrenia Bulletin, 8*(4), 626–633.

Kanter, J. S. (1984). *Coping strategies for relatives of the mentally ill*. Washington, DC: National Alliance for the Mentally Ill.

Kint, M. G. (1977). Problems for families vs. problem families. *Schizophrenia Bulletin, 3*(3), 355–356.

Korpell, H. S. (1984). *How you can help: A guide for families of psychiatric hospital patients*. Washington, DC: American Psychiatric Press.

Kreisman, D. E., & Joy, V. D. (1974). Family response to the mental illness of a relative: A review of the literature. *Schizophrenia Bulletin, 1*(10), 34–57.

Lamb, H. R., & Oliphant, E. (1978). Schizophrenia through the eyes of families. *Hospital and Community Psychiatry, 29*(12), 805–806.

L. Bete Channing Co., Inc. (1979). *About schizophrenia.* South Deerfield, MA: Author. Pamphlet for distribution at workshop.

Lovejoy, M. (1982). Expectations and the recovery process. *Schizophrenia Bulletin, 8*(4), 605–609.

Lovejoy, M. (1984). Recovery from schizophrenia: A personal odyssey. *Hospital and Community Psychiatry, 35*(8), 809–812.

McDonald, N. (1960). The other side: Living with schizophrenia. *Canadian Medical Association Journal, 82,* 218–221.

National Schizophrenia Fellowship (1974). *Living with schizophrenics: By the relatives.* Suney, England: Author. Available from National Schizophrenia Fellowship, 78 Victoria Road, Surbiton, Surrey KT6 4JT, England.

O'Brien, P. (1978). *The disordered mind: What we know about schizophrenia.* Englewood Cliffs, NJ: Prentice-Hall.

Park, C. C., & Shapiro, L. N. (1976). *You are not alone: Understanding and dealing with mental illness.* Boston: Little, Brown.

Patterson, D. Y. (1980). *Living with schizophrenia.* Princeton, NJ: E. R. Squibb & Sons. Pamphlet for distribution.

Peterson, R. (1980). What are the needs of chronic mental patients? *Schizophrenia Bulletin, 8*(4), 610–616.

Rosenhan, D. (1973). On being sane in insane places. *Science, 179,* 250–259.

Schizophrenia Bulletin. Very often issues contain a first-hand account of the illness, written by a patient. These brief accounts can be valuable handouts for relatives attending workshops or for new professionals who wish to increase their understanding of the patient's experience of schizophrenia.

Seeman, M. V., Littman, S. K., Plummer, E., Thornton, J. F., & Jeffries, J. J. (1983). *Living and working with schizophrenia.* Toronto: University of Toronto Press.

Torrey, E. F. (1983). *Surviving schizophrenia: A family manual.* New York: Harper & Row.[1]

Vine, P. (1982). *Families in pain: Children, siblings, spouses and parents of the mentally ill speak out.* New York: Pantheon Books. Contains a glossary of terms, state statutes concerning emergency involuntary hospitalization and civil commitment, sophisticated drug tables (including generic and brand names, dosages, side effects, and other concerns), and lists of resources.

Wasaw, M. (1982). *Coping with schizophrenia: A survival manual for parents, relatives and friends.* Palo Alto: Science & Behavior Books.

Willis, M. J. (1982). The impact of schizophrenia on families: One mother's point of view. *Schizophrenia Bulletin, 8*(4), 617–620.

1. Royalties from this book have been donated to the National Alliance for the Mentally Ill. Also a booklet containing excerpts from the text is available free of charge from E. R. Squibb & Sons, Inc., Princeton, NJ 08540. The booklet is suitable for distribution to relatives at workshops.

Wing, J. K. (Ed.). (1975). *Schizophrenia from within*. Survey, England: National Schizophrenia Fellowship. Available from National Schizophrenia Fellowship, 78 Victoria Road, Surbiton, Surrey KT6 4JT, England.

Wing, J. K. (1978). The social context of schizophrenia. *American Journal of Psychiatry, 135*(11), 1333–1339.

Wing, J. K., & Olsen, R. (1979). *Community care for the mentally disabled*. Oxford, England: Oxford University Press.

LIVING WITH SCHIZOPHRENIA EVALUATION FORM

Group leaders _____
Date _____
Your name (optional) _____

We are interested in your response to today's meeting. Your impressions will be of help to us in planning future sessions. Please answer each question by circling the number which best describes your response.

1. All in all, how helpful was the meeting for you?

1	2	3	4	5
Not at all	A little bit helpful	Somewhat helpful	Moderately helpful	Extremely helpful

2. How well was the meeting organized?

1	2	3	4	5
Not at all	A little bit organized	Somewhat organized	Moderately organized	Extremely organized

3. Was there enough time allotted for questions and discussion?

1	2	3
Not enough time	Enough time	Too much time

4. Did you learn anything about the causes of the illness?

1	2	3	4	5
Nothing	A little bit	A fair amount	A moderate amount	A great deal

5. Did you learn anything about the symptoms of the illness?

1	2	3	4	5
Nothing	A little bit	A fair amount	A moderate amount	A great deal

6. Do you feel you understand the problems produced by this illness any better?

1	2	3	4	5
Not at all	A little bit	A fair amount	A moderate amount	A great deal

7. Did you learn anything about the purpose of medication?

1	2	3	4	5
Nothing	A little bit	A fair amount	A moderate amount	A great deal

8. Do you feel this session will help you to cope better with the illness?

1	2	3	4	5
Not at all	A little bit	A fair amount	A moderate amount	Very much so

9. Do you feel it was helpful to hear other patients and families talk about the illness?

1	2	3	4	4
Not at all	A little bit	A fair amount	A moderate amount	Very much so

10. Do you feel any more hopeful about the illness?

1	2	3	4	5
Not at all	A little bit	A fair amount	A moderate amount	Very much so

11. Do you feel that it was helpful to talk about things in this group?

1	2	3	4	5
Not at all	A little bit	A fair amount	A moderate amount	Very much so

12. What suggestions would you make about future groups? _____

REFERENCES

Alexander, F., & Selesnick, S. T. (1966). *The history of psychiatry.* New York: Harper & Row.

Alexander, J. F., & Parsons, B. V. (1982). *Functional family therapy: Principles and procedures.* Carmel, CA: Brooks/Cole.

American Psychiatric Association (1980). *Diagnostic and statistical manual of mental disorders* (3rd ed.). Washington, DC: Author.

Anderson, C. M. (1977). Family intervention with severely disturbed inpatients. *Archives of General Psychiatry, 34,* 697–702.

Anderson, C. M., Hogarty, G., Bayer, G., & Needleman, R. (1984). Expressed emotion and the social networks of parents of schizophrenic patients. *British Journal of Psychiatry, 144,* 247–255.

Anderson, C. M., Hogarty, G., & Reiss, D. (1980). Family treatment of adult schizophrenic patients: A psycho-educational approach. *Schizophrenia Bulletin, 6*(3), 490–505.

Anderson, C. M., & Janosko, R. (1979). Family therapy with paranoid patients. In J. H. Masserman (Ed.), *Current psychiatric therapies* (Vol. 19; pp. 107–116). New York: Grune & Stratton.

Anderson, C. M., & Meisel, S. (1976). An assessment of family reaction to the stress of psychiatric illness. *Hospital and Community Psychiatry, 27*(12), 868–871.

Anderson, C. M., Meisel, S., & Houpt, J. (1975). Training former patients as task group leaders. *International Journal of Group Psychotherapy, 15,* 32–43.

Anderson, C. M., & Stewart, S. (1983). *Mastering resistance: A practical guide to family therapy.* New York: Guilford Press.

Andolfi, M., Angelo, C., Menghi, P., & Nicolò-Corigliano, A. (1983). *Behind the family mask: Therapeutic change in rigid family systems.* New York: Brunner/Mazel.

Andrews, G., Hall, W., Goldstein, G., Lapsley, H., Bartels, R., & Silove, D. (1985). The economic costs of schizophrenia. *Archives of General Psychiatry, 42,* 537–543.

Angst, J., Baastrup, P., Grof, P., Hippius, H., Poldinger, W., & Weis, P. (1973). The course of monopolar and bipolar psychoses. *Psychiatria, Neurologia, Neurochirurgica, 76,* 489–500.

Anthony, W. A. (1977). Psychological rehabilitation: A concept in need of a method. *American Psychologist, 32*(8), 658–662.

Arieti, S. (1980). Psychotherapy of schizophrenia: New or revised procedures. *American Journal of Psychotherapy, 34*(4), 464–476.

Autry, J. H. (1975). Workshop on orthomolecular treatment of schizophrenia: A report. *Schizophrenia Bulletin, 1*(12), 94–103.

Bateson, G., Jackson, D. D., Haley, J., & Weakland, J. (1956). Toward a theory of schizophrenia. *Behavioral Science, 1,* 251–264.

Beels, C. C. (1975). Family and social management of schizophrenia. *Schizophrenia Bulletin, 1*(13), 97–118.

Beeson, P. B., McDermott, W., & Wyngaarden, J. B. (1979). *Cecil textbook of medicine.* Philadelphia: W. B. Saunders.

341

Begley, S., Carey, J., & Sawhill, R. (1983, February 7). How the brain works. *Newsweek Magazine*, pp. 40–47.

Berkowitz, R., Kuipers, L., Eberlein-Vries, R., & Leff, J. (1981). Lowering expressed emotion in relatives of schizophrenics. In M. J. Goldstein (Ed.), *New developments in interventions with families of schizophrenics*. San Francisco: Jossey-Bass.

Bleuler, E. (1950). *Dementia praecox or the group of schizophrenias* (J. Zinkin, Trans.). New York: International Universities Press. (Original work published 1911)

Bowen, M. (1960). Family concept of schizophrenia. In D. D. Jackson (Ed.), *The etiology of schizophrenia*. New York: Basic Books.

Bowen, M. (1961). The family as the unit of study and treatment. *American Journal of Psychiatry, 31*, 50–60.

Breier, A., & Strauss, J. (1984). The role of social relationships in the recovery from psychotic disorders. *American Journal of Psychiatry, 141*(8), 949–955.

Brinson, L. (1980). Reducing disincentives and fostering the rehabilitation of the mentally ill. In L. G. Perlman (Ed.), *Rehabilitation of the mentally ill in the 1980's* (pp. 25–41). Washington, DC: National Rehabilitation Association.

Broen, W. E., & Storms, L. H. (1966). Lawful disorganization: The process underlying a schizophrenic syndrome. *Psychological Reviews, 73*, 256–279.

Brown, G. W. (1959). Experiences of discharged chronic schizophrenic mental hospital patients in various types of living groups. *Millbank Memorial Fund Quarterly, 37*, 105–131.

Brown, G. W., & Birley, J. L. T. (1968). Crises and life change and the onset of schizophrenia. *Journal of Health and Social Behavior, 9*, 203–214.

Brown, G. W., Birley, J. L. T., & Wing, J. H. (1972). The influence of family life on the course of schizophrenic disorders: A replication. *British Journal of Psychology, 121*, 241–258.

Brown, G. W., Monck, E. M., Carstairs, G. M., & Wing, J. K. (1962). Influence of family life on the course of schizophrenic illness. *British Journal of Preventive and Social Medicine, 16*, 55–68.

Buchsbaum, M. S., DeLisi, L. E., Holcomb, H. H., Cappallet, J., King, A. L., Johnson, J., Hazlett, E., Dowling-Zimmerman, S., Post, R. M., Marihisa, J., Carpenter, W., Cohen, R., Pickar, D., Weinberger, D. R., Margolin, R., & Kessler, R. M. (1984). Anteroposterior gradients in cerebral glucose use in schizophrenia and affective disorders. *Archives of General Psychiatry, 41*, 1159–1166.

Bunney, B. S. (1984). Antipsychotic drug effects on the electrical activity of dopaminergic neurons. *Trends in Neurosciences, 7*, 212–215.

Calev, A., Venables, P. H., & Monk, A. F. (1983). Evidence for distinct verbal memory pathologies in severely and mildly disturbed schizophrenia. *Schizophrenia Bulletin, 9*, 247–264.

Carpenter, W. T., & Heinrichs, D. W. (1983). Early intervention, time-limited, targeted pharmacotherapy of schizophrenia. *Schizophrenia Bulletin, 9*, 533–542.

Carpenter, W. T., McGlashan, T. H., & Strauss, J. S. (1977). The treatment of acute schizophrenics without drugs: An investigation of some current assumptions. *American Journal of Psychiatry, 134*, 14–20.

Cohen, B. P., & Camhi, J. (1967). Schizophrenic performance in a word communication task. *Journal of Abnormal Psychology, 72*, 240–246.

Cole, J. O., & Davis, J. M. (1969). Antipsychotic drugs. In L. Bellak, L. Loeb (Eds.), *The schizophrenic syndrome* (pp. 478–568). New York: Grune & Stratton.

Cole, J. O., Goldberg, S. C., & Davis, J. M. (1966). Drugs in the treatment of psychosis: Controlled studies. In P. Solomon (Ed.), *Psychiatric Drugs* (pp. 153–180). New York: Grune & Stratton.

Cole, J. O., Goldberg, S. C., & Klerman, G. L. (1964). Phenothiazine treatment in acute schizophrenia. *Archives of General Psychiatry, 10*, 246–261.

Corbett, L. (1976). Perceptual dyscontrol: A possible organizing principle for schizophrenia research. *Schizophrenia Bulletin, 2,* 249–251.

Crow, T. J. (1980). Molecular pathology of schizophrenia: More than one disease process? *British Medical Journal, 280,* 66–68.

Crow, T. J. (1984, May 7). *Disturbances in the temporal lobe.* Paper presented at the 137th Annual Meeting of the American Psychiatric Association, Los Angeles.

Davis, J. M. (1976). Recent developments in the drug treatment of schizophrenia. *American Journal of Psychiatry, 133,* 208–214.

Dawson, M. E., & Nuechterlein, K. H. (1984). Psychophysiological dysfunctions in the developmental course of schizophrenic disorders. *Schizophrenia Bulletin, 10,* 204–232.

Day, R. (in press). Social stress and schizophrenia: From the concept of recent life events to the notion of toxic environments. In G. Burrows (Ed.), *The handbook of studies of schizophrenia.* Amsterdam: Elsevier/North Holland Biomedical Press.

Day, R., Zubin, J., & Steinhauer, S. (in press). Psychosocial factors in schizophrenia in light of vulnerability theory. In D. Magnusson & A. Ohman (Eds.), *Psychopathology: An interactional perspective.* New York: Academic Press.

Deasy, L. C., & Quinn, O. W. (1955). The wife of the mental patient and the hospital psychiatrist. *Journal of Social Issues, 11,* 49–60.

Diem, O. (1904). Die einfact demente form der Dementia Praecox. *Archiv für Psychiatrie, 37,* 111.

Doherty, E. G. (1975). Labeling effects in psychiatric hospitalization. *Archives of General Psychiatry, 32,* 562–568.

Donaldson, S. R., Gelenberg, A. J., & Baldessarini, R. J. (1983). The pharmacologic treatment of schizophrenia: A progress report. *Schizophrenia Bulletin, 9,* 504–527.

Epstein, N. B., & Bishop, D. S. (1980). Problem-centered systems therapy of the family. In A. S. Gurman & D. P. Kniskern (Eds.), *Handbook of family therapy* (pp. 444–483). New York: Brunner/Mazel.

Erikson, K. T. (1962). Notes on the sociology of deviance. *Social Problems, 9,* 307–314.

Falloon, I., Boyd, J., & McGill, C. (1984). *Family care of schizophrenia.* New York: Guilford Press.

Falloon, I., Boyd, J. L., McGill, C., Razoni, J., Moss, H. B., & Gilderman, H. M. (1982). Family management in the prevention of exacerbations of schizophrenia. *New England Journal of Medicine, 306,* 1437–1440.

Falloon, I., Boyd, J. L., McGill, C., Strang, J., & Moss, H. (1981). Family management training in the community care of schizophrenia. In M. J. Goldstein (Ed.), *New developments in interventions with families of schizophrenics.* San Francisco: Jossey-Bass.

Falloon, I., Liberman, R., Lillie, F., & Vaughn, C. (1981). Family therapy for relapsing schizophrenics and their families: A pilot study. *Family Process, 20,* 211–222.

Falloon, I., Watt, D. C., & Shepherd, M. (1978). A comparative controlled trial of pimozide and fluphenazine decanoate in the continuation therapy of schizophrenia. *Psychological Medicine, 8,* 59–70.

Farkas, T., Wolfe, H. P., Jaeger, J., Brodie, J. D., Christman, D. R., & Fowler, J. S. (1984). Regional brain glucose metabolism in chronic schizophrenia. *Archives of General Psychiatry, 41,* 293–300.

Fish, F. (1961). A neuropsychological theory of schizophrenia. *Journal of Mental Science, 107,* 828–838.

Frazer, A., & Winokur, A. (1977). *Biological bases of psychiatric disorders.* New York: Spectrum.

Freedman, B. J. (1974). The subjective experience of perceptual and cognitive disturbances in schizophrenia. *Archives of General Psychiatry, 30,* 333–340.

Fromm-Reichmann, F. (1948). Notes on the development of treatment of schizozphrenics by psychoanalytic psychotherapy. *Psychiatry, 11,* 263–273.

Gittelman-Klein, R., & Klein, D. F. (1968). Marital status as a prognostic indicator in schizophrenia. *Journal of Nervous and Mental Disease, 147,* 289–296.

Gjerde, P. F. (1983). Attentional capacity dysfunction and arousal in schizophrenia. *Psychological Bulletin, 93,* 57–72.

Goldberg, S. C., Schooler, N. R., Hogarty, G. E., & Roper, M. (1977). Prediction of relapse in schizophrenic outpatients treated by drug and social therapy. *Archives of General Psychiatry, 34,* 171–184.

Goldstein, M. J. (Ed.). (1981). *New developments in interventions with families of schizophrenics.* San Francisco: Jossey-Bass.

Goldstein, M. J., & Kopeikin, H. (1981). Short and long term effects of combining drug and family therapy. In M. J. Goldstein (Ed.), *New developments in interventions with families of schizophrenics.* San Francisco: Jossey-Bass.

Goldstein, M. J., & Rodnick, E. H. (1975). The family's contribution to the etiology of schizophrenia: Current status. *Schizophrenia Bulletin, 1,* 48–63.

Goldstein, M. J., Rodnick, E. H., Evans, J. R., May, P. R., & Steinberg, M. (1978). Drug and family therapy in the aftercare treatment of acute schizophrenia. *Archives of General Psychiatry, 35*(10), 1169–1177.

Gottesman, I. I., & Shields, J. (1982). *Schizophrenia: The epigenetic puzzle.* London: Cambridge University Press.

Griesinger, W. (1965). *Mental pathology and therapeutics.* New York: Hafner. (Original work published 1867)

Gunderson, J. G., Frank, A. F., Katz, H. M., Vannicelli, M. L., Frosch, J. P., & Knapp, P. H. (1984). Effects of psychotherapy in schizophrenia: II. Comparative outcome of two forms of treatment. *Schizophrenia Bulletin, 10,* 565–584.

Gunderson, J. G., & Mosher, L. (1975). The cost of schizophrenia. *American Journal of Psychiatry, 132,* 901–906.

Haley, J. (1980). *Leaving home: The therapy of disturbed young people.* New York: McGraw-Hill.

Hatfield, A. B. (1978). Psychological costs of schizophrenia to the family. *Social Work, 23,* 355–359.

Hatfield, A. B. (1979). The family as partner in the treatment of mental illness. *Hospital and Community Psychiatry, 30*(5), 338–340.

Hecker, E. (1871). Hebephrenia. *Archiv für Pathologische Anatomie und Physiologie und für Klinische Medizin, 52,* 394–429.

Held, S. M., & Cromwell, R. L. (1968). Premorbid adjustment in schizophrenia. *Journal of Nervous and Mental Disease, 146,* 264–272.

Herz, M. I., & Melville, C. (1980). Relapse in schizophrenia. *American Journal of Psychiatry, 137,* 801–805.

Hirsch, S. R., & Leff, J. P. (1975). *Abnormalities in parents of schizophrenics.* London: Oxford University Press.

Hoch, P. H., & Polantin, P. (1949). Pseudoneurotic forms of schizophrenia. *Psychiatric Quarterly, 23,* 248–276.

Hogarty, G. E. (1977). Treatment and the course of schizophrenia. *Schizophrenia Bulletin, 3,* 587–599.

Hogarty, G. E. (1981). Evaluation of drugs and therapeutic procedures: The contribution of non-pharmacologic techniques. In G. Tognoni, C. Bellantuono, & M. Lader (Eds.), *The epidemiological impact of psychotropic drugs* (pp. 249–264). Amersterdam: Elsevier/North Holland Biomedical Press.

Hogarty, G. E. (1984). Depot neuroleptics: The relevance of psycho-social factors. *Journal of Clinical Psychiatry, 45* (Sec. 2), 36–42.

Hogarty, G. E., Goldberg, S. C., & Schooler, N. R. (1974). Drug and sociotherapy in the aftercare of schizophrenic patients. *Archives of General Psychiatry, 31,* 609–618.

Hogarty, G. E., Goldberg, S. C., Schooler, N. R., & Ulrich, R. F. (1974). Collaborative Study Group. Drug and sociotherapy in the aftercare of schizophrenic patients: II. Two-year relapse rates. *Archives of General Psychiatry, 31,* 603–608.

Hogarty, G. E. Schooler, N. R., Ulrich, R. F., Mussare, F., Herron, E., & Ferro, P. (1979). Fluphenazine and social therapy in the aftercare of schizophrenic patients: Relapse analyses of a two year controlled study of fluphenazine decanoate and fluphenazine hydrochloride. *Archives of General Psychiatry, 36,* 1283–1294.

Hogarty, G. E., & Ulrich, R. F. (1977). Temporal effects of drug and placebo in delaying relapse in schizophrenic outpatients. *Archives of General Psychiatry, 34,* 297–301.

Hogarty, G. E., Ulrich, R. F., Mussare, F., & Aristigueta, N. (1976). Drug discontinuation among long-term successfully maintained schizophrenic outpatients. *Diseases of the Nervous System, 57,* 494–500.

Hubel, D. H. (1979, September). The Brain. *Scientific American, 241*(3), pp. 44–53.

Iversen, L. L. (1978). Biochemical and pharmacologic studies. In J. K. Wing (Ed.), *Schizophrenia: Towards a new synthesis* (pp. 89–116). New York: Grune & Stratton.

Jablensky, A., & Sartorius, N. (1975). Culture and schizophrenia. *Psychological Medicine, 5,* 113–124.

Jacob, T. (1975). Family interaction in disturbed and normal families: A methodological and substantive review. *Psychological Bulletin, 82,* 33–65.

Jeste, D. V., Potkin, S. G., Sinka, S., Feder, S., & Wyatt, R. J. (1979). Tardive dyskinesia: Reversible and persistent. *Archives of General Psychiatry, 36,* 585–590.

Johnson, D. A. W., Pasterski, G., Ludlow, J. M., Street, K., & Taylor, R. D. W. (1983). The discontinuance of maintenance neuroleptic therapy in chronic schizophrenic patients: Drug and social consequences. *Acta Psychiatrica Scandinavia, 67,* 339–352.

Johnston, R., & Planasky, J. (1962). Schizophrenia in men: The impact on their wives. *Psychiatric Quarterly, 42,* 146–155.

Jones, J. E. (1977). Patterns of transactional style deviance in the TAT's of parents of schizophrenics. *Family Process, 16,* 327–337.

Kahlbaum, K. L. (1876). *Catatonic or spastic insanity.* Berlin: Springer.

Kane, J. M., Rifkin, A., Quitkin, F., Noyak, D., & Ramos-Lorenzo, J. (1982). Fluphenazine vs. placebo in patients with remitted, acute first-episode schizophrenia. *Archives of General Psychiatry, 39,* 70-73.

Kane, J. M., Woerner, M., & Weinhold, P. (1982). A prospective study of tardive dyskinesia development: Preliminary results. *Journal of Clinical Psychopharmacology, 2,* 345–349.

Kanter, J. (1981, September 14). *Consulting with the relatives of schizophrenics.* Paper presented at Grand Rounds, St. Elizabeth's Hospital, Washington, DC.

Karen, B. P., & Vanden Bos, G. R. (1972). The consequence of psychotherapy for schizophrenic patients. *Psychotherapy: Theory, Research and Practice, 9,* 111–119.

Karlsson, J. L. (1973). An Icelandic family study of schizophrenia. *British Journal of Psychiatry, 123,* 549–554.

Kasanin, J. (1933). The acute schizoaffective psychoses. *American Journal of Psychiatry, 13,* 97–126.

Kerr, J. W. (1967). Conjoint marital psychotherapy: An interim measure in the treatment of psychosis. *Psychiatry, 30,* 283–293.

Kint, M. G. (1977). Problems for families vs. problem families. *Schizophrenia Bulletin, 3,* 355–356.

Kraepelin, E. (1896). *Psychiatrie, ein lehrbuch für studierende und arzte* (ed. 5). Leipzig: Barth.

Kramer, M. (1978). Population changes and schizophrenia, 1970–1985. In L. C. Wynne, R. L. Cromwell, & S. Matthyse (Eds.), *The nature of schizophrenia: New approaches to research and treatment* (pp. 545–571). New York: Wiley.

Lamb, H. R., & Oliphant, E. (1978). Schizophrenia through the eyes of families. *Hospital and Community Psychiatry, 29,* 805–806.

Lang, P. J., & Buss, A. H. (1965). Psychological deficit in schizophrenia: Interference and activation. *Journal of Abnormal Psychology, 70,* 77–106.

Langfeldt, G. (1939). *The prognosis in schizophrenia and the factors influencing the course of the disease.* Copenhagen: E. Munksgaard.

Leff, J. P. (1980). *The combination of psychiatric pharmacotherapy and sociotherapy.* Pre-publication report.

Leff, J. P., Hirsch, S. R., Gaind, R., Rhode, P. D., & Stevens, B. C. (1973). Life events and maintenance therapy in schizophrenic relapse. *British Journal of Psychiatry, 123,* 657–660.

Leff, J. P., Kuipers, L., Berkowitz, R., Eberlein-Vries, R., & Sturgeon, D. (1982). A controlled trial of social intervention in the families of schizophrenic patients. *British Journal of Psychiatry, 141,* 121–134.

Leff, J. P., & Vaughn, C. (1985). *Expressed emotion in families: Its significance for mental illness.* New York: Guilford Press.

Leff, J. P., & Wing, J. K. (1971). Trial of maintenance therapy in schizophrenia. *British Medical Journal, 3,* 597–604.

Leonhard, K. (1961). The cycloid psychoses. *Journal of Mental Science, 107,* 633–648.

Lewine, R. J. (1981). Sex differences in schizophrenia: Timing or subtypes? *Psychological Bulletin, 90,* 432–444.

Liberman, R., Aitchison, R., & Falloon, I. (1979). *Family therapy in schizophrenia; Syllabus for therapists.* Camarillo, CA: Mental Health Clinic Research Center for the Study of Schizophrenia.

Lidz, T., & Cornelison, A. R. (Eds.). (1965). *Schizophrenia and the family.* New York: International Universities Press.

Lidz, T., Cornelison, A. R., Fleck, S., & Terry D. (1957). The intrafamilial environment of schizophrenic patients: II. Marital schism and skew. *American Journal of Psychiatry, 114,* 241–248.

Linn, M. W., Caffey, E. M., Klett, C. J., Hogarty, G. E., & Lamb, R. (1979). Day treatment and psychotropic drugs in the aftercare of schizophrenic patients. *Archives of General Psychiatry, 36,* 1055–1066.

Linn, M. W., Klett, C. J., & Caffey, E. M. (1980). Foster home characteristics and psychiatric patient outcome. *Archives of General Psychiatry, 37,* 129–132.

Loranger, A. W. (1984). Sex differences in age at onset of schizophrenia. *Archives of General Psychiatry, 41,* 157–161.

Lovejoy, M. (1984). Recovery from schizophrenia: A personal odyssey. *Hospital and Community Psychiatry, 35*(8), 809–812.

Lyketsos, G. C., Sakka, P., & Mailis, A. (1983). The sexual adjustment of chronic schizophrenics: A preliminary study. *British Journal of Psychiatry, 143,* 376–382.

MacCulloch, M. J., & Waddington, J. L. (1979). Catastrophe theory: A model interaction between neurochemical and environmental influences in the control of schizophrenia. *Neuropsychobiology, 5,* 87–93.

MacDonald, N. (1960). The other side: Living with schizophrenia. *Canadian Medical Association Journal, 82,* 218–221.

Martin, G. A., & Worthington, E. L. (1982). Behavioral homework. In M. Hersen, R. M. Eisler, & P. M. Miller (Eds.), *Progress in behavior modification* (Vol. 13). New York: Academic Press.

May, P. R. A. (1968). *Treatment of schizophrenia: A comparative study of five treatment methods.* New York: Science House.

May, P. R. A. (1975). Schizophrenia: Evaluation of treatment methods. In A. M. Freedman, H. I. Kaplan, & B. J. Sadock, (Eds.), *Comprehensive textbook of psychiatry* (Vol. 1). Baltimore: Williams & Wilkins.

McFarlane, W. R. (Ed.). (1983). *Family therapy in schizophrenia*. New York: Guilford Press.

McGhie, H., & Chapman, J. (1961). Disorders of attention and perception in early schizophrenia. *British Journal of Medical Psychology, 34*, 103–116.

McGill, C. W., Falloon, I. R., Boyd, J. L., & Wood-Siverio, C. (1983). Family educational intervention in the treatment of schizophrenia. *Hospital and Community Psychiatry, 34*, 934–938.

McLean, C. S., Greer, K., Scott, J., & Beck, J. C. (1982). Group treatment for parents of the adult mentally ill. *Hospital and Community Psychiatry, 33*, 564–568.

Meltzer, H. Y. (1979). Biochemical studies in schizophrenia. In L. Bellak (Ed.), *Disorders of the schizophrenic syndrome* (pp. 45–135). New York: Basic Books.

Minkoff, K. (1978). A map of chronic mental patients. In J. A. Talbot (Ed.), *The chronic mental patient*. Washington, DC: American Psychiatric Association.

Minuchin, S. (1974). Structural family therapy. In S. Arieti (Ed.), *American handbook of psychiatry* (Vol. 2, pp. 178–192). New York: Basic Books.

Minuchin, S., & Fishman, H. C. (1981). *Family therapy techniques*. Cambridge, MA: Harvard University Press.

Mora, G. (1980). Historical and theoretical trends in psychiatry. In H. I. Kaplan, A. M. Freedman, & B. J. Sadock (Eds.), *Comprehensive textbook of psychiatry* (3rd ed., Vol. 1; pp. 4–98). Baltimore: Williams & Wilkins.

Mosher, L. R., & Keith, S. J. (1980). Psychosocial treatment: Individual, group, family and community support approach. *Schizophrenia Bulletin, 6*, 10–41.

Mosher, L. R., & Menn, A. Z. (1978). Community residential treatment for schizophrenia: Two year follow-up. *Hospital and Community Psychiatry, 29*, 715–723.

Murphy, H. B. M. (1978). Cultural influences on incidence, course, and treatment response. In L. C. Wynne, R. L. Cromwell, & S. Matthyse (Eds.), *The nature of schizophrenia: New approaches to research and treatment* (pp. 586–594). New York: Wiley.

Nasrallah, H. A. (1982). Laterality and hemispheric dysfunction in schizophrenia. In F. A. Henn & H. A. Nasrallah (Eds.), *Schizophrenia as a brain disease* (pp. 273–294). New York: Oxford University Press.

Nuechterlein, K. H., & Dawson, M. E. (1984). Information processing and attentional functioning in the developmental course of schizophrenic disorders. *Schizophrenia Bulletin, 10*, 160–203.

Paul, G. L., Tobias, L. L., & Holly, B. L. (1972). Maintenance psychotropic drugs in the presence of active treatment programs. *Archives of General Psychiatry, 27*, 106–115.

Payne, R. W., Mattussek, P., & George, E. I. (1959). An experimental study of schizophrenic thought disorder. *Journal of Mental Science, 105*, 624–652.

Pinsof, W. (1983). Integrative problem-centered therapy: Toward the synthesis of family and individual psychotherapies. *Journal of Marital and Family Therapy, 9*, 19–36.

Plummer, E., Thornton, M. B., Seeman, M. V., & Littman, S. K. (1981, March). Living with schizophrenia: A group approach with relatives. *Canada's Mental Health*, 17–32.

Rabkin, J. G. (1980). Stressful life events and schizophrenia: A review of the literature. *Psychological Bulletin, 87*, 408–425.

Reveley, A., Reveley, M. A., Clifford, C. A., & Murray, R. M. (1982). Cerebral ventricular size in twins discordant for schizophrenia. *Lancet, 159*, 540–541.

Reynolds, G. P. (1983). Increased concentrations and lateral asymmetry of amygdala dopamine in schizophrenia. *Nature, 305*, 527–528.

Sander, W. (1868). Originare paranoia. *Archiv für Psychiatre, 2*, 10–17.

Schlamp, F. T., & Raymond, C. (1971, April). *A study of mentally ill vocational rehabilitation clients.* Project report, Department of Rehabilitation, State of California.

Schneider, K. (1959). *Clinical psychopathology* (M. W. Hamilton, Trans.). New York: Grune & Stratton.

Schooler, N. R., Levine, J., Severe, J. B., Brauzer, B., DiMascio, A., Klerman, G. L., & Tuason, U. B. (1980). Prevention of relapse in schizophrenia: An evaluation of fluphenazine decanoate. *Archives of General Psychiatry, 37,* 16–24.

Schulman, A., Wetterberg, L., Osaba, H., Schulz, S. C., Van Kammen, D. P., Meurice, E., Nedopil, N., & Splendiani, G. (1984). Hemodialysis in chronic schizophrenics. *Archives of General Psychiatry, 41,* 817-818.

Schulsinger, F., Parnos, J., Petersen, E. T. Schulsinger, H., Teasdale, T. W., Mednick, S. A., Moller, L., & Silverton, L. (1984). Cerebral ventricular size in the offspring of schizophrenic mothers. *Archives of General Psychiatry, 41,* 602–606.

Sechehaye, M. (1951). *Autobiography of a schizophrenic girl.* New York: Grune & Stratton.

Sedvall, G., Oxenstierna, G., Bergstrand, G., Bjerkenstedt, L., & Wik, G. (1984, February). *Evidence of abnormalities of CSF circulation in schizophrenia.* Paper presented at Winter Workshop on Schizophrenia, Davos, Switzerland.

Seeman, M. V. (1982). Gender differences in schizophrenia. *Canadian Journal of Psychiatry, 27,* 107–112.

Selvini-Palazzoli, M., Boscolo, L., Cecchin, G., & Prata, G. (1978). *Paradox and counterparadox.* New York: Aronson.

Selvini-Palazzoli, M., Boscolo, L., Cecchin, G., & Prata, G. (1980). Hypothesizing–circularity–neutrality: Three guidelines for the conductor of the session. *Family Process, 19,* 3–12.

Shakow, D. (1962). Segmental set: A theory of the formal psychological deficit in schizophrenia. *Archives of General Psychiatry, 6,* 1–17.

Silverman, J. (1972). Stimulus intensity modulation and psychological disease. *Psychopharmacologia, 24,* 42–80.

Singer, M. (1978). Attentional processes in verbal behavior. In. L. C. Wynne, R. L. Cromwell, & S. Matthyse (Eds.), The nature of schizophrenia: New approaches to research and treatment (pp. 329–336). New York: Wiley.

Singer, M., & Wynne, L. C. (1963). Differentiation characteristics of the parents of childhood schizophrenics, childhood neurotics, and young adult schizophrenics. *American Journal of Psychiatry, 120,* 234-243.

Singer, M. T., & Wynne, L. C. (1965). Thought disorder and family relations of schizophrenics: IV. Results and implications. *Archives of General Psychiatry, 12,* 201–212.

Snyder, S. H., Banerjee, S. P., Yamamura, H. I., & Greenberg, D. (1974). Drugs, neurotransmitters and schizophrenia. *Science, 184,* 1243–1253.

Snyder, K., & Liberman, R. (1981). Family assessment and intervention with schizophrenics at risk for relapse. In M. J. Goldstein (Ed.), *New developments in interventions with families of schizophrenics.* San Francisco: Jossey-Bass.

Spitzer, R. L., Endicott, J., & Robins, E. (1978). *Research diagnostic criteria (RDC) for a selected group of functional disorders* (3rd ed.). New York: New York State Psychiatric Institute.

Spohn, H. E., Lacoursiere, R. B., Thompson, K., & Coyne, L. (1977). Phenothiazine effects on psychological and psychophysiological dysfunction in chronic schizophrenics. *Archives of General Psychiatry, 34,* 633–644.

Springer, J., & Kramer, H. (1928). *Malleus maleficarium.* London: Rodker.

Stevens, J. R. (1973). An anatomy of schizophrenia? *Archives of General Psychiatry, 29,* 177–189.

Stevens, J. R. (1982). The neuropathology of schizophrenia. *Psychological Medicine, 12,* 695–700.

Stierlin, H., Wynne, L. C., & Wirsching, M. (Eds.). (1983). *Psychosocial intervention in schizophrenia: An international view.* New York: Springer-Verlag.

Strauss, E. W. (1966). *Phenomenological Psychology.* London: Tavistock.

Sturgeon, D., Turpin, G., Kuipers, L., Berkowitz, R., & Leff, J. (1984). Psychophysiological responses of schizophrenic patients to high and low expressed emotion relatives: A follow-up study. *British Journal of Psychiatry, 145,* 62–69.

Taube, C. (1974). Readmissions to inpatient services of the state and county hospitals, 1972. Statistical Note 110. Biometry Branch, National Institute of Mental Health.

Tecce, J. J., & Cole, J. O. (1976). The distraction–arousal hypothesis, CNV, and schizophrenia. In D. I. Mostofsky (Ed.), *Behavior control and modification of physiological activity.* Englewood Cliffs, NJ: Prentice-Hall.

Thornton, J. F., Plummer, E., Seeman, M. J., & Littmann, K. (1981). Schizophrenia: Group support for relatives. *Canadian Journal of Psychiatry, 26,* 341–344.

Tienari, P. (1984, October). *The Finnish adoptive family study of schizophrenics.* Paper presented at the VIIIth International Symposium on the Psychotherapy of Schizophrenia, Yale University, New Haven, CT.

Torrey, E. F. (1973). Is schizophrenia universal? An open question. *Schizophrenia Bulletin, 7,* 53–59.

Turner, R. J., Dopkun, L. S., & Labreche, G. P. (1970). Marital status and schizophrenia: A study of incidence and outcome. *Journal of Abnormal Psychology, 76,* 110–116.

Van Putten, T., & May, P. R. A. (1976). Milieu therapy of the schizophrenias. In L. J. West & P. E. Flinn (Eds.), *Treatment of schizophrenia* (pp. 217–243). New York: Grune & Stratton.

Vaughn, C. E., & Leff, J. P. (1976). The influence of family and social factors on the course of psychiatric illness. *British Journal of Psychiatry, 129,* 125–137.

Vaughn, C. E., Snyder, K. S., Jones, S., Freeman, W. B., & Falloon, I. R. H. (1984). Family factors in schizophrenic relapse: Replication in California of British research on expressed emotion. *Archives of General Psychiatry, 41,* 1169–1177.

Venables, P. H. (1964). Input dysfunction in schizophrenia. In B. A. Maher (Ed.), *Progress in experimental personality research* (Vol. 1; pp. 1–47). New York: Academic Press.

Venables, P. H. (1976). Cognitive disorder. In J. K. Wing (Ed.), *Schizophrenia: Towards a new synthesis* (pp. 117–137). New York: Academic Press.

Vine, P. (1982a). *Burying the stigma.* Paper presented to the Family Alliance for the Mentally Ill, New York City.

Vine, P. (1982b). *Families in pain.* New York: Pantheon Books.

Wachtel, P. (1967). Conceptions of broad and narrow attention. *Psychological Bulletin, 6,* 417–429.

Warner, R. (1983). Recovering from schizophrenia in the third world. *Psychiatry, 46,* 197–212.

Watt, D. C., & Szulecka, T. K. (1979). The effects of sex, marriage and age at first admission on the hospitalization of schizophrenics during two years following discharge. *Psychological Medicine, 9,* 529–539.

Waxler, N. (1974). Culture and mental illness: A social labeling perspective. *Journal of Nervous and Mental Disease, 159,* 379–395.

Weinberger, D. R. (1984, May 7). *Neuropathological localization in schizophrenia.* Paper presented at the 137th Annual Meeting of the American Psychiatric Association, Los Angeles.

Weinberger, D. R., Wagner, R. L., & Wyatt, R. J. (1983). Neuropathological studies of schizophrenia: A selected review. *Schizophrenia Bulletin, 9,* 193–212.

Whitaker, C. (1974). Psychotherapy of the absurd with a special emphasis on the psychotherapy of aggression. *Family Process, 14,* 1–16.

Wing, J. K. (Ed.). (1978). *Schizophrenia: Towards a new synthesis.* New York: Grune & Stratton.

Wing, J. K., & Brown, G. W. (1970). *Institutionalism and schizophrenia.* London: Cambridge University Press.

Wynne, L. C., & Singer, M. T. (1958). Thought disorder and family relations of schizophrenics: I. Research strategy. *Archives of General Psychiatry, 9,* 191–198.

Yolles, S. F., & Kramer, M. (1969). Vital statistics. In L. Bellack & L. Loeb (Eds.), *The schizophrenic syndrome* (pp. 66–113). New York: Grune & Stratton.

Young, M. A., & Meltzer, H. Y. (1980). The relationship of demographic clinical and outcome variables to neuroleptic treatment requirements. *Schizophrenia Bulletin, 6,* 88–101.

Zelitch, S. R. (1980). Helping the family cope: Workshops for families of schizophrenics. *Health and Social Work, 5*(4), 47–52.

Zubin, J., Magaziner, J., & Steinhauer, S. (1983). The metamorphosis of schizophrenia: From chronicity to vulnerability. *Psychological Medicine, 13,* 551–571.

Zubin, J., & Spring, B. (1977). Vulnerability: A new view of schizophrenia. *Journal of Abnormal Psychology, 86,* 103–126.

AUTHOR INDEX

A

Aitchison, R., 304, 346n.
Alexander, F., 80, 341n.
Alexander, J. F., 303, 341n.
American Psychiatric Association, 80, 85, 341n.
Anderson, C. M., 2, 13, 73, 74, 125, 304, 309, 341n.
Andolfi, M., 332, 341n.
Andrews, G., 85, 341n.
Angelo, C., 332, 341n.
Angst, J., 80, 341n.
Anthony, W. A., 194, 341n.
Arieti, S., 130, 341n.
Aristigueta, N., 8, 276, 345n.
Autry, J. H., 102, 341n.

B

Baastrup, P., 341n.
Baldessarini, R. J., 99, 343n.
Banerjee, S. P., 96, 349n.
Bartels, R., 341n.
Bateson, G., 15, 341n.
Bayer, G., 125, 341n.
Beck, J. C., 74, 347n.
Beels, C. C., 65, 341n.
Beeson, P. B., 84, 341n.
Begley, S., 94, 342n.
Bergstrand, G., 21, 348n.
Berkowitz, R., 19, 23, 304, 342n., 346n., 349n.
Birley, J. L. T., 2, 9, 114, 342n.
Bishop, D. S., 303, 343n.
Bjerkenstedt, L., 21, 348n.
Bleuler, E., 81, 342n.
Bosclo, L., 332, 348n.
Bowen, M., 15, 342n.

Boyd, J. L., 74, 304, 343n., 347n.
Brauzer, B., 348n.
Breier, A., 196, 342n.
Brinson, 221, 342n.
Broen, W. E., 17, 342n.
Brown, G. W., 2, 9, 13, 16, 115, 125, 342n., 350n.
Buchsbaum, M. S., 20, 342n.
Bunney, B. S., 97, 342n.
Buss, A. H., 17, 346n.

C

Caffey, E. M., 11, 12, 346n.
Calev, A., 18, 342n.
Camhi, J., 18, 342n.
Carey, J., 94, 342n.
Carpenter, W. T., 10, 156, 342n.
Carstairs, G. M., 16, 342n.
Cecchin, G., 332, 348n.
Chapman, J., 86–89, 347n.
Clifford, C. A., 21, 348n.
Cohen, B. P., 18, 342n.
Cole, J. O., 18, 96, 325, 343n., 349n.
Corbett, L., 19, 343n.
Cornelison, A., 15, 346n.
Coyne, L., 20, 349n.
Cromwell, R. L., 262, 344n.
Crow, T. J., 21, 81, 343n.

D

Davis, J. M., 96, 99, 325, 342n., 343n.
Dawson, M. E., 18–20, 343n., 347n.
Day, R., 7, 343n.
Deasy, L. C., 73, 343n.
Diem, O., 81, 343n.
DiMascio, A., 348n.

351

SUBJECT INDEX

A

Acetylcholine, 98
Acute psychotic episode, 58
Adaptation, families, 110–112 (*see also* Coping)
Akathisia, 98, 102
Alcohol consumption, 103, 219–221
Ambivalence, and emancipation, 251–255
Amygdala, schizophrenia, 21
Anger
  in families, 110
  reframing technique, 268
Antipsychotic drugs (*see also* Drug treatment)
  action of, 96, 97
  information to families, 96, 97
  side effects, 97
  and compliance, 160
Anxiety, in family, 109
Arousal, schizophrenia, 18–20, 93
Attention, schizophrenia, 18–20, 86, 92, 93
Attitude
  of family, toward patient, 148
  of patients, toward illness, 163, 164, 191, 192
  of therapists, and success, 296
Auditory hallucinations, 91
Autobiographical reports, 85, 86

B

Benign indifference, 148
Biological theories, schizophrenia, 6
Bipolar disorder, 80
Birth trauma, 104
Bleuler's influence, 6, 81
Brain and schizophrenia, 93–96

C

Caffeine consumption, 102
Capacity theory, 18
Catastrophe theory, 7
Catatonia, 80
Cerebral blood flow, 20, 21
Cerebral ventricles, 20, 21
Childrearing, 261–272
Chlorpromazine, 96
Cholecystokinen, 21
Chronic patients, 193, 275–277, 330
Cigarette smoking, 103
Circular interviewing, 303
Clinician–family relationship
  establishing of, 29, 30
  solidification of, 39, 40
Clinicians
  attitudes of, importance, 295–297
  connecting with patients, 52–57
  control of sessions, 310, 311
  as family representative, 49–52, 307, 325
  frustrations of, 268, 269
  providing support, 314, 315
  selection of, 294–297
  task assignment, learning, 312–314
  training and supervision, 297–322
  and treatment impasses, 315, 316
Cognitive restructuring, 78
Commitment, case history, 34, 35
Communication, family, 121–124, 179, 180
Communication skills
  and marriage, 264, 265
  practice in, family, 200–203
Compliance (*see* Drug compliance)
Conflict resolution skills, 240, 241
Conjugal issues, 261–272 (*see also* Marital conflict)

side effects, 13
Psychotherapy, 12, 13, 102, 333
Psychotic episodes
  drug maintenance treatment, 100
  and relapse, 8, 9
Psychotropic drugs (*see* Drug treatment)

Q

Quarter-way programs, 254

R

Receptors, neurotransmission, 94, 95
Reentry period, 132–193
  crisis sessions, 136–138
  goals and methods, 133–139
  phone contacts, 134–136
  training goals, clinicians, *301*
  treatment session, content, 155–193
  treatment session, structure, 139–155
Reframing techniques, 191, 268, 315
Reinforcement, positive behavior, 200, 201, 206
Relabeling techniques, 191, 315
Relapse risk
  case report, 287–292
  drug discontinuation, 7–10
  family environment, 16, *17*
  family therapy protection, 23–25
  sex differences, 9
  timing of, 133
  vocational rehabilitation, stress, 221
Renal dialysis, 102
Residential living, 254
Resistance
  coping with, 189–193
  to employment, 224–226
  handling of, training, 308, 309
  medication compliance, 164, 166, 167

and split sessions, 153
and task assignment, 313
Responsibility, resumption of, 168–173
Risk, schizophrenia, 104, 105 (*see also* Relapse risk)
Role-playing
  job interview, 227, 228
  supervisor-employee, 241
Routines, and work, 226–229
Rules, establishing of, 116–120, 180, 181

S

Sadness, in families, 110
Schizo-affective disorder, 81
Schizophrenia
  attitude toward, patients, 163, 164
  chronicity of, and treatment, 275–277, 330
  clinician's understanding, importance, 297, 298
  cost of, 85
  definition, 5, 83
  drug therapy, 7–11 (*see also* Drug treatment)
  epidemiology, 83–85
  family environment influence, 15–17
  genetics, 103–106
  history, 80–83
    and treatment, 2–5
  as illness, 83, 330
  informational approach, 71–73, 77–79
  marriage impact, 261–272
  natural environment influence, 13–17
  personal experience of, 85–89
  psychobiology, 92–96
  psychosocial therapy, 11–13
  public experience, 89–91
  relapse risk, drugs, 8, 9 (*see also* Relapse risk)
  and Survival Skills Workshop, 71–131
  theories of, 5–7